D1433866

DATE DUE

Emergency Psychiatry

Emergency Psychiatry

Arjun Chanmugam, MD, MBA
Associate Professor, Department of Emergency Medicine,
The Johns Hopkins University School of Medicine,
Baltimore, MD, USA

Patrick Triplett, MD
Assistant Professor and Clinical Director, Department of Psychiatry,
The Johns Hopkins University School of Medicine,
Baltimore, MD, USA

Gabor Kelen, MD
Professor and Chair, Department of Emergency Medicine,
The Johns Hopkins University School of Medicine,
Baltimore, MD, USA

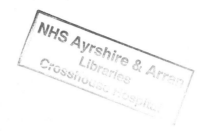
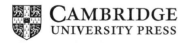

CAMBRIDGE
UNIVERSITY PRESS

CAMBRIDGE UNIVERSITY PRESS
Cambridge, New York, Melbourne, Madrid, Cape Town,
Singapore, São Paulo, Delhi, Mexico City

Cambridge University Press
The Edinburgh Building, Cambridge CB2 8RU, UK

Published in the United States of America
by Cambridge University Press, New York

www.cambridge.org
Information on this title: www.cambridge.org/9780521879262

First published 2013

Printed and bound in the United Kingdom by the MPG Books Group

A catalogue record for this publication is available from the British Library

Library of Congress Cataloguing in Publication data

Emergency psychiatry / [edited by] Arjun Chanmugam, Patrick Triplett,
Gabor Kelen.
    p.   ;   cm.
Includes bibliographical references and index.
ISBN 978-0-521-87926-2 (Hardback)
I. Chanmugam, Arjun S. II. Triplett, Patrick. III. Kelen, Gabor D.
[DNLM: 1. Emergency Services, Psychiatric–methods. 2. Mental
Disorders–diagnosis. 3. Mental Disorders–therapy. WM 401]
    616.89′025–dc23

                                                              2012029376

ISBN 978-0-521-87926-2 Hardback

I dedicate this book to Karen, my wonderful inspiration; to Sydney, William, and Nathan, who all remind me of what is important; and to Teruni and Tamara and my parents, whose support helped make this work possible. May this book serve well those who seek to reduce suffering.

Arjun Chanmugam

For Audrey, Hallie, and Alex, and with thanks to James and Florence for their support and kindness. Thanks too to my colleagues at Johns Hopkins for their wisdom, guidance and unwavering commitment to our shared missions.

Patrick Triplett

To my late parents, Andrew and Susan Kelen, who instilled in me a love for discovery.

Gabor Kelen

Contents

Contributors

Eric L. Anderson, MD
Assistant Professor
Department of Psychiatry
The Johns Hopkins University School
of Medicine
Baltimore, MD, USA

Dennis Barton, MD
Physician Executive, Dearborn
Advisors, LLC
The Johns Hopkins University School
of Medicine
Baltimore, MD, USA

Annette L. Beautrais, PhD
Department of Emergency Medicine
Yale University School of Medicine
New Haven, CT, USA

O. Joseph Bienvenu, MD, PhD
Associate Professor
Department of Psychiatry and Behavioral
Sciences
The Johns Hopkins University School
of Medicine
Baltimore, MD, USA

Ashley D. Bone, MD
Department of Psychiatry and Behavioral
Sciences
The Johns Hopkins Bayview Medical Center
Baltimore, MD, USA

Curtis Bone, MD
Department of Psychiatry and Behavioral
Sciences
The Johns Hopkins Bayview Medical
Center
Baltimore, MD, USA

Sharon Bord, MD
Emergency Department
The Johns Hopkins Bayview Medical Center
Baltimore, MD, USA

Arjun Chanmugam, MD, MBA
Associate Professor, Department of
Emergency Medicine
The Johns Hopkins University School of
Medicine
Baltimore, MD, USA

Michael Clark, MD
Associate Professor and Vice Chair for
Clinical Affairs
Department of Psychiatry
The Johns Hopkins University School of
Medicine
Baltimore, MD, USA

J. Raymond DePaulo, MD
Henry Phipps Professor and Director
Department of Psychiatry and Behavioral
Sciences
The Johns Hopkins University School of
Medicine
Baltimore, MD, USA

Emily Frosch, MD
Assistant Professor
Division of Child & Adolescent Psychiatry
Department of Psychiatry & Behavioral
Sciences
The Johns Hopkins University School of
Medicine
Baltimore, MD, USA

Angela S. Guarda, MD
Associate Professor of Psychiatry and
Behavioral Sciences
The Johns Hopkins University School of
Medicine
Baltimore, MD, USA

James Harrison, BA
University of Pennsylvania School of
Medicine
Philadelphia, PA, USA

Frederick Houts, MD
Instructor
University of Washington School of
Medicine
Washington, DC, USA

Lisa S. Hovermale, MD
Instructor, Department of Psychiatry
and Behavioral Sciences
The Johns Hopkins University School
of Medicine
Baltimore, MD, USA

Geetha Jayaram, MD
Associate Professor
Department of Psychiatry
The Johns Hopkins University School of
Medicine
Baltimore, MD, USA

Patrick Kelly, MD
Instructor
Division of Child & Adolescent Psychiatry
Department of Psychiatry and Behavioral
Sciences
The Johns Hopkins University School of
Medicine
Baltimore, MD, USA

**Gregory Luke Larkin, MD, MS, MSPH,
FACEP**
Department of Emergency Medicine
Yale University School of Medicine
New Haven, CT, USA

Valerie R. Lint, DO, MS
Department of Emergency Medicine
University of Toledo College of Medicine
Toledo, OH, USA
Department of Emergency Medicine
St. Luke's Hospital
Maumee, OH, USA

Cynthia Major-Lewis, MD
Director of Psychiatric Emergency Services
The Johns Hopkins University School of
Medicine
Baltimore, MD, USA

Catherine A. Marco, MD
Department of Emergency Medicine
University of Toledo College of Medicine
Toledo, OH, USA

Darren Mareiniss, MD, JD
The Johns Hopkins University School of
Medicine
Baltimore, MD, USA

Dave Milzman, MD, FACEP
Professor of Emergency Medicine
Senior Clinical Advisor for Research
SMP Medical Director for Community
Outreach
Georgetown University School of Medicine
Research Director Georgetown
University of Washington Hospital Center
Emergency Medicine Residency Program
Attending Physician, Washington
Hospital Center
Washington, DC, USA

Melinda J. Ortmann, PharmD, BCPS
Clinical Pharmacy Specialist
Emergency Medicine
Department of Pharmacy
The Johns Hopkins Hospital
Baltimore, MD, USA

Theodosia Paclawskyj, PhD, BCBA
Assistant Professor, Department of
Psychiatry and Behavioral Sciences
The Johns Hopkins University School of
Medicine
Department of Behavioral Psychology
Kennedy Krieger Institute
Baltimore, MD, USA

Graham W. Redgrave, MD
Assistant Professor of Psychiatry and
Behavioral Sciences
The Johns Hopkins University School of
Medicine
Baltimore, MD, USA

Paul P. Rega, MD, FACEP
Assistant Professor, Department of Public
Health and Preventive Medicine
Department of Emergency Medicine
University of Toledo College of
Medicine
Toledo, OH, USA

Mustapha Saheed, MD
Assistant Clinical Director, Department of
Emergency Medicine
The Johns Hopkins School of Medicine
Baltimore, MD, USA

Eric Samstad, MD
The Johns Hopkins Medical Institutions
Bayview Medical Center
Baltimore, MD, USA

Karen Schwartz, MD
Associate Professor
Department of Psychiatry
The Johns Hopkins University School of
Medicine
Baltimore, MD, USA

Dyanne Simpson, DO
The Johns Hopkins Bayview Medical
Center
Baltimore, MD, USA

Hahn Soe-Lin, MD
Case Western Department of Surgery
Cleveland, OH, USA

Roshni I. Thakore, MD
The Johns Hopkins University School of
Medicine
Baltimore, MD, USA

Glenn Treisman, MD
Professor
Department of Psychiatry
The Johns Hopkins University School of
Medicine
Baltimore, MD, USA

Patrick Triplett, MD
Assistant Professor and Clinical Director
Department of Psychiatry
The Johns Hopkins University School of
Medicine
Baltimore, MD, USA

Crystal Watkins, MD
Assistant Professor
Department of Psychiatry and Behavioral
Sciences
The Johns Hopkins University School of
Medicine
Baltimore, MD, USA

Holly C. Wilcox, PhD
Assistant Professor
Department of Psychiatry and Behavioral
Sciences
Division of Child and Adolescent
Psychiatry
The Johns Hopkins University School of
Medicine
Baltimore, MD, USA

Preface

Emergency Psychiatry is designed for health care providers who may manage patients with acute psychiatric problems or wish to better understand the fundamentals of urgent psychiatric conditions. This concise but practical reference focuses on the management of patients who are thought to be suffering from an acute psychiatric ailment or crisis. The authors are experts in their field, and the editorial team each has considerable clinical experience in emergency psychiatric evaluation and care, including the inherent difficulties associated with many of the conditions and the superimposition of social contexts.

Our goal was to provide a review of the key issues in psychiatry in a comprehensive but succinct format. Although many of the issues discussed in this book are complex and deserving of a more detailed discussion, our primary concern was to provide a review that will help guide practical acute management. Psychiatric conditions are, by their very nature, challenging to manage, but with a good understanding of the pathology and the appropriate resources, patients can be effectively cared for in the acute setting. The editors understand that in some cases, adequate resources for psychiatric patients may be wanting or scarce; it was in fact that very realization which compelled us to create a reference to assist the acute care provider in stabilizing and managing the patient with an acute presentation of psychiatric illness.

Emergency psychiatry is a nascent subspecialty of both psychiatry and emergency medicine. However, many fields of medicine are called on to recognize and manage patients with acute psychiatric conditions and to appreciate the impact these conditions have on other clinical and social conditions. We hope that this book may help to better serve patients and providers and in the process to promote increased recognition of the importance of emergency psychiatry.

Acknowledgement

We would like to thank Melinda Ortmann, PharmD, who was a constant source of information and a key advisor for this book.

Assessment and general approach

Patrick Triplett and J. Raymond DePaulo

Introduction

Clinicians in overburdened emergency departments (EDs) and other acute care environments provide a broad array of services. In addition to handling emergent medical or surgical conditions such as trauma, heart attack, or stroke, ED providers are often the front line of care for patients with psychiatric disorders. Demand for a full spectrum of care provided in EDs continues to grow. The Institute of Medicine report *Hospital-Based Emergency Care: At the Breaking Point*[1] describes the ways in which demand for care in EDs far outpaces supply in the United States. The volume of patients with psychiatric complaints in EDs has continued to grow as part of this trend.[2-7] Increasingly, ED providers are called on to assess and manage patients in psychiatric crisis, often for days at a time.

A number of factors have contributed to this greater use of EDs by patients who are in need of psychiatric assessment and care. These factors include shortages of psychiatrists and other mental health professionals, limited and often fragmented systems of outpatient psychiatric care options, lack of other sources of support for persons with chronic mental illness, and steadily diminishing inpatient psychiatric beds, both acute and long-term. Not surprisingly, patients and families seeking help for psychiatric conditions for which the community provides no other services look to the ED as the provider of last resort. With fewer inpatient and outpatient resources available, patients wait longer in the emergency setting, contributing to crowding, and in some situations adversely affecting staff and patient safety.

Given these circumstances, virtually all ED clinicians will likely provide some psychiatric assessment and care, in spite of often limited psychiatric resources for referral or inpatient care. Regardless of staffing models or location of emergency facilities, there are fundamentals of emergent psychiatric assessment that need to be applied to patients with psychiatric disorders. The most important consideration is the safety of all. This will be a recurring theme throughout this and subsequent chapters. A systematic approach to safety, assessment, stabilization, and disposition is the most effective means to create a secure and effective treatment environment for acute psychiatric conditions.

Practical safety considerations

There are numerous safety, legal, and logistical issues that arise when caring for patients with emergent psychiatric complaints. Prior to a discussion of the fundamentals of patient

Emergency Psychiatry, ed. Arjun Chanmugam, Patrick Triplett, and Gabor Kelen. Published by Cambridge University Press. © Cambridge University Press 2013.

assessment and management, it is important to review some of the issues that form the backdrop against which emergency psychiatry occurs. Instituting a culture of safety and having practice expectations clearly defined in advance will cut down on confusion and enhance patient care and safety.

Triage. ED nurses and physicians routinely perform assessments of acuity of a patient's condition based on a very brief examination. This can be a particularly challenging task in patients with psychiatric complaints. There should be institutional and ED-based policies and protocols addressing the process of ED triage and management of patients with psychiatric and other behavioral presentations. These may vary depending on the availability and organization of psychiatric services. Triage practices should incorporate assessments for severity, risk, and potential need for time-sensitive intervention, and issues pertinent to communication between emergency and psychiatric providers, especially if they are available for rapid consultation. Absence of a policy or established protocols invites a variable approach to patients which can be a serious risk in the ED environment.

Space. Most EDs do not have a space specifically designed to handle patients with psychiatric complaints. In many settings, a space has been carved out of the main ED to prevent "clogging" of medical/surgical beds by longer-stay and occasionally behaviorally disordered patients. Ideally, the area would have maximum visibility for staff and privacy for patients. A thoughtful design would also incorporate safety features including detachable sprinkler heads and lack of other obvious anchoring sites, grounded outlets, and safe restroom facilities for patient/self-care.*

Even in facilities where there is a designated area for patients with psychiatric complaints, crowding of patients can be severe. Without an effective means of communicating concerns between dedicated psychiatric providers and other emergency medicine providers, the risk of adverse events increases. Concerns about a patient's safety and need for observation must also be conveyed directly and plainly to subsequent providers at hand-offs. Similarly, if acuity in the psychiatric designated area (where they exist) is high, or if crowding threatens to surpass what can safely be handled, providers in both areas must be able to convey concerns in order to avoid catastrophe.

Safety meetings. Routine, multidisciplinary meetings to discuss issues related to the care of patients with psychiatric emergencies in the ED can have tremendous impact on safety and the quality of care delivered. The Comprehensive Unit-based Safety Program (CUSP)** has proven to be a successful model in creating and implementing needed change in other medical settings.[8–10] This approach can be adapted to emergency psychiatry. Members of such a group focused on psychiatric care provided in the ED would optimally include ED physicians and nurses, security personnel, legal or other executive leadership, clerical staff, social workers, and others whose work involves patient care.

---

* The National Association of Psychiatric Health Systems (NAPHS) has a list of guidelines for inpatient psychiatric units and many of these guidelines have applicability to designated space for psychiatry in an ED (http://www.naphs.org/Design Guide 4_3 FINAL.pdf). Further discussion of physical space and categorization of types of psychiatric emergency services can be found in the APA Task Force on Psychiatric Emergency Services' *Report and Recommendations Regarding Psychiatric Emergency and Crisis Services: A Review and Model Program Descriptions.*

** The CUSP format is an approach to improving patient safety which involves examining systems of care, introducing evidence-based (when possible), high-impact interventions to improve care, measuring rates and outcomes, addressing cultural issues in the setting and learning from errors.[10]

Communication among providers. In psychiatric emergencies and in the ED generally, communication among providers is fundamental, but is often taken for granted, and when not done well can be a source of confusion and error. Hand-offs at change of shift or patient transfer are particularly fraught with risk and have been recommended as a target for improvement.[11] Clear documentation of medical reasoning and effective verbal communication at hand-offs can help avert disaster. This applies to transfers to inpatient wards, communication with outside facilities when arranging transfers, and interactions with paramedical professionals (e.g. emergency medical technicians (EMTs), clinical aides) involved in patient care. Communication of threats or acts of violence by patients (or even family or friends of patients) is also important and is discussed in the section 'Behavioral alerts and aftercare plans' (below), and in Chapter 10.

Given the number of elements involved in the care of patients with psychiatric symptoms, an operational checklist[12,13] may be a way to keep track of the various forms, documentation, and other elements of communication that a presentation can generate. For example, a patient may present with a somatic chief complaint and later require a psychiatric assessment. In that instance, it is useful for mental health providers to know the status of the workup and plan for medical issues.

Emergency assessment and involuntary commitment. In some settings, police bring patients in their custody to designated facilities or select hospitals for psychiatric assessment. In other places, these patients are taken to the nearest ED. Laws vary by state regarding the process by which people with dangerous behaviors thought to be based on a psychiatric disorder are brought to emergency medical attention. Knowledge of applicable laws is essential. A hospital's legal team is usually willing to provide periodic updates or refresher courses for ED staff on the legalities of a state's emergency involuntary assessment and commitment laws. Reviewing the sometimes arcane details of these laws can help avoid bad outcomes and allow staff to have a greater sense that their decisions, which may run counter to the wishes of the patient, are clinically driven and legally valid. Attention to the details of forms and paperwork is critical. Patients in clear need of involuntary psychiatric care may sometimes be released at a commitment hearing, not because of doubts about clinical judgment, but because of incomplete or poorly completed paperwork.

Reluctant patients. As with all patients seen in an ED, the patient's autonomy must be respected and care provided only to the extent accepted by the patient. For the patient brought by family or friends for psychiatric issues, or for the patient who comes in for a somatic complaint but who appears to require psychiatric assessment, concerns for the safety of the person and others may outweigh patient autonomy. Both situations require judgment on the part of the physician as well as nurses and support staff and may necessitate urgent psychiatric consultation, or even contact with available legal counsel. Here again, ongoing communication of the patient's status between providers is critical (especially when different disciplines are involved). Uninformed staff may mistakenly release a dangerously impaired person in need of further care. Conversely, a lack of adequate communication could result in holding a person against his/her wishes, even through use of force, leading to potential harm to the person.

Patient searches. Formal search policies, reviewed by the hospital's legal team, should be in place. Searches, and confiscation of belts, potential (or actual) weapons, and drugs of any kind, remain important interventions and these should be adequately explained to all patients prior to conducting searches. While some patients may take offense, ED staff have a responsibility to provide (and patients have a right to be seen in) a safe environment in which care is delivered. Some hospitals, often in response to adverse events, insist that all patients who present with psychiatric complaints be stripped and put in a gown. While this may have a practical benefit in removing many (though not all) means of harming themselves or others, it presents a number of problems. The first is a misguided impression that these patients are unquestionably safer in a hospital gown. Standard hospital gowns can easily be anchored for hanging, used for strangulation of others, or even torn up and ingested. Many people find these garments humiliating as they are usually open in the back and offer scant bodily coverage. Forcing patients to wear gowns can often increase the distress of an already stressed patient, compounding the difficulty of discussing intimate issues. For patients with histories of sexual trauma, the violation of personal space and forced stripping can exacerbate mood and anxiety symptoms and even lead to violence. Whatever the policy, forced stripping should not be routine.

Firearms and patients in custody. Prisoners or persons otherwise in custody frequently end up in the ED. They may have an armed police officer or guard at the bedside and may be physically restrained. For hospitals providing care in these circumstances, there should be a policy about the presence of firearms during psychiatric assessment of such patients. The unpredictable behavior that may accompany many psychiatric conditions should be adequate reason to ensure that firearms are highly secure.

Privacy. The Health Insurance Portability and Accountability Act (HIPAA) had a number of aims, including greater security for patients' personal information, but the Act has also inadvertently led some providers to fear disclosing any health-related information, even in emergencies when the information can be critically important. Adding to that is the tradition of keeping psychiatric records sequestered due to the risk of disclosure of intimate, potentially embarrassing information, all compounded by the stigma of mental illness. These are sound reasons for discretion in releasing psychiatric records, but there are times when clinical considerations may be more compelling. Many patients in psychiatric crisis are willing to sign a release form to allow communication between providers and other contacts, though some are not. Determining when a psychiatric emergency is dire enough (and the information critical enough) to go against a patient's wishes for privacy requires experienced clinical judgment, often buttressed by counsel (legal and medical) from others. Exceptions to absolute confidentiality in the ED for patients with psychiatric issues include situations where there is a duty to protect the patient, a duty to warn a patient's intended victims, or a duty to inform legal guardians or surrogates.[14,15]

Privacy is a prized commodity, especially in a busy ED.[16] When possible, the physical space should allow the patient to discuss psychiatric complaints without fear of being overheard by other patients or non-treating staff. In some settings, creating such an environment is no small task, and may involve use of family meeting areas, sound masking devices, and creative use of existing space. The desire for privacy must be balanced with the need for patient safety and ready access to security and other staff if needed.

Collateral informants. In psychiatric emergencies, the people who know the patient best, including physicians, can provide critical information and perspective that a patient may be unable or unwilling to provide. Nevertheless, there may be times to be skeptical about the motives of informants. Providers should seek to verify information whenever possible, and confirming informants' observations is an important strategy. Police and EMTs who bring in patients may also be useful informants, for example, by providing information on where the patient was found and what he or she was doing prior to arrival and during transport.

Fellows, residents, medical students, and visitors. Though common sense goes a long way, it is useful to establish ground rules and expectations prior to allowing a rotation for newcomers in the ED.[17] The level of supervision for the trainee interacting with patients and families should be clear in advance. A primer on confidentiality and basic safety in the area should be provided and should be tailored to the setting. Trainees should not interview patients alone in seclusion rooms. Interviews with potentially agitated patients should be conducted close to security guards and only by experienced and trained team members. In some instances, a gender-appropriate chaperone should be present. Trainees should know how to seat themselves and the patient to allow for the quick egress of the patient and the trainee if needed. Trainees should be told to keep a low threshold for terminating an interview, if the patient appears to be getting agitated or the trainee is otherwise becoming uncomfortable. In many settings, an introductory class is conducted for trainees and new employees (and refresher courses for current employees), with hands-on training to demonstrate take-downs (this should be performed by trained staff only), use of seclusion and restraints, and escape from various holds as well as a detailed description or tour of the setting, including security features, routes of egress, and the operation of emergency alarms. This training should include an explanation of the roles of security personnel, physicians, nurses, and other staff, as well as the alerts used in the facility for agitated and/or violent patients.

Patient visitors in the ED can be a thorny issue. In some EDs, friends, family, or even patient advocates may be allowed to stay with patients undergoing assessment in the ED. Visitors may provide a calming influence for someone in psychiatric crisis. There are times, however, when visitors may actually be a more destabilizing presence for the patient or others in the ED or may simply contribute to crowding in an already congested area. In some settings, limitations on space and concerns about safety can make visitors a significant risk for all involved. A thoughtful policy that reflects the practice at the facility is important and this should be conveyed to inquiring potential visitors.

Assessment

Patients presenting with psychiatric issues may arrive at the front door of the ED self-referred, brought or accompanied by concerned family and friends, or in police custody. The complaints may be straightforward or subtle, and in many cases the complaints may obscure the underlying issue. Patients presenting with somatic complaints may have active psychiatric issues[18] and may even be harboring suicidal thoughts.[19] Many patients who go on to complete suicide have recently seen a physician, though often not for an ostensibly psychiatric chief complaint.[20]

Medical screening. One of the most important tenets of emergency care is that all patients, regardless of presentation, are carefully screened to determine if a medical condition is contributing to their symptoms and behaviors. Only after the extent of medical illnesses are known should an urgent yet careful psychiatric assessment take place, if warranted. The need for obtaining vital signs at triage with patients presenting with psychiatric symptoms is frequently raised. There are a number of medical conditions that can masquerade as psychiatric presentations (see Chapter 5) and vital signs may be the only early clue. A delirium due to some infectious process, for example, may present as agitation and combativeness. Sometimes patients are too agitated for vital signs to be safely read at triage. Once stabilized though, a comprehensive set of vital signs should be obtained.

Laboratory studies and imaging. Routine use of ancillary services, such as electrocardiograms (ECGs), chest x-rays, head CTs, and laboratory panels, including a toxicology screen, for all patients with psychiatric complaints is of questionable utility.[21–29] There is no one-size-fits-all approach to ancillary testing and there are no established or reliable standards for every patient and setting. Not all patients need a full, detailed workup.

Appropriate ancillary investigations are determined by the patient's presentation, an understanding that psychiatric diagnoses in the emergency setting are diagnoses of exclusion, time and resource constraints, and the need to guide stabilization or reversal of acute medical conditions that cause or mimic psychiatric symptoms. Basic metabolic panels and complete blood counts are generally indicated and can be of great utility in ruling in or out organic diagnoses. However, head CTs are not routinely appropriate even in those with an abnormal mental status. CT imaging of the head should be considered in a patient with unexplained new mental status change.

Not all patients need urine drug screens and blood alcohol levels, though these studies may prove instructive. Urine drug screens can be useful in confirming details of patient drug use, prescription or illicit,[17,30] but may not contribute enough to emergency decision-making to warrant routine screens for all patients.[31] General emergency medicine practice is to determine patient sobriety based on physical examination and clinical judgment. With alcohol, there is great variability in effect and tolerance among individuals, thus, basing judgment on levels alone may not always be appropriate. Assessment can be further complicated by the use of benzodiazepines to treat withdrawal symptoms. A full psychiatric assessment of an acutely intoxicated patient, however, is of little utility. Some assessments, such as a focused assessment of safety, are nonetheless an element in the management of intoxicated patients in the ED, who may be (or may become) belligerent, suicidal, or otherwise disruptive to the ED milieu.

Some ancillary studies are impractical and are unnecessary in the emergency setting. At many facilities, thyroid studies, vitamin levels (e.g. B12, folate, thiamine), and therapeutic monitoring levels (e.g. quantitative tricyclic antidepressant levels) are not performed daily or are sent to outside facilities to be performed. In instances of suspected overdose on tricyclics, an ECG will provide more rapid and useful information than a quantitative tricyclic level which may take days to be processed.

ECGs can be useful in emergency psychiatry, as many psychotropic medications used are known to prolong the QTc interval, potentially leading to a fatal arrhythmia. Thus, a screening ECG may be useful if psychotropics are being used or are contemplated. Severely agitated patients may require neuroleptic or other medications emergently, in order to keep themselves and others safe, before a baseline ECG can be obtained. Once the patient is calmer, an ECG should be obtained. Whenever possible, knowledge of a patient's pre-existing risk should determine the aggressiveness with which the ECG is pursued and may lead a provider to choose a different class of medication as an alternative. In many cases pre-existing risk may be difficult to ascertain before medications are given.

Physical examinations. The patient's presentation, elements of the history, and medical conditions being considered will likely determine the focus(es) of the physical exam. Routine disrobing in the ED of every patient with a psychiatric complaint for the duration of their ED visit should be avoided when possible.[32] Patients who are presenting for primarily psychiatric reasons may not be expecting a physical examination. Patients should be told in advance that a physical exam or other contact is forthcoming. The gender identification, trauma history, and/or sexual orientation of the patient might also need to be considered and chaperoning with gender-appropriate staff (and documentation of same) provided for the patient's comfort and dignity.

Psychiatric assessment. Essentially, psychiatric assessment begins at triage with the chief complaint and includes the mode and details of presentation. The following questions are helpful to quickly understand the immediate needs of the patient.

- How did the patient present to the acute care setting? Who else was with the patient at the time of presentation? Was the patient found alone, or brought in by friends or family? Was the patient brought in by emergency medical services? Is the patient in police custody?
- What concerning statements did the patient make? What did others report about the patient?
- How did the patient appear? Was the patient discovered or found somewhere other than where he/she was expected?
- Is he/she here voluntarily? Is he/she in legal custody? Is he/she competent and does he/she have impaired capacity to make some/all decisions?
- Is he/she cooperative?
- What is the reliability of any information obtained?

There are a number of excellent resources that may be consulted regarding the assessment of patients with psychiatric complaints or signs.[33–37] Time constraints in the ED do not usually allow for in-depth assessment of all psychiatric conditions that a patient may have ever experienced, but a focused examination may provide an accurate assessment of a patient's acuity along with important cues for determining the best treatment setting for continued care.

A psychiatric history and mental status exam follow the triage assessment/chief complaint described above. The Johns Hopkins Phipps Clinic psychiatry service has used a standardized approach (see Appendix) for history-taking which covers many psychiatric conditions. The general template can be adapted to the ED setting. The order in which the entire history is obtained is usually not crucial and may be determined to some degree by the chief complaint. The important issue is that fundamentals are covered. Basic history can be supplemented with more detailed history and an examination tailored to the presentation (for example, if an eating disorder or sexual disorder is present). There may not be adequate time to collect in-depth responses to all of these areas of inquiry, but even a skeletal outline with these components may be useful in formulating the likely causes for the patient's presentation and suggest the most appropriate treatment interventions. Listed below are the general topics and a set of questions frequently asked under each topic. In most ED encounters, it is unlikely that all these questions can be asked, but it is useful to have an understanding of what information is needed in a comprehensive psychiatric assessment, in order to apply important elements to a particular patient in the ED.

Family history

In the Phipps history, family history comes soon after chief complaint, though it can certainly be obtained later in the interview.[†] Patients may be unwilling or unable to provide much information and outside informants may be helpful. In the emergency setting, the family history should include a focused history of psychiatric disorders (including substance abuse) in the family, suicides, and any salient family medical issues, including neurologic (e.g. Parkinson's, Alzheimer's, Huntington's) or other somatic disorders that may have psychiatric manifestations. More extensive family history, such as family members' response (or lack of response) to certain psychotropics or more qualitative or quantitative description of family members' psychiatric syndromes might be more usefully explored in a non-emergent setting.

Personal history

Personal history usually includes details of development (including gestation, if appropriate), childhood health and behavior (including abnormalities such as discipline problems, animal cruelty, expulsions, violence, fire-setting, etc.), educational attainment and/or difficulties including any learning disorders or special education (including reasons for leaving school early), work history (profession(s), longest held job, reasons for terminations), military service, relationship history[‡], current social relationships, living arrangements, sexual history, history of abuse, neglect or trauma, legal history, religious or other social history. Further details on any overlap with past psychiatric history or the patient's current presentation may be expanded upon in "past psychiatric history" or "history of present illness."

Substance use history

This should include at a minimum the factors that might lead to adverse outcomes, especially alcohol and benzodiazepine use/dependence. Details here should include any history of delirium tremens, ICU or medical floor admissions for complicated withdrawal, history of hallucinations, seizures, tremors or other signs of physical dependence, and some estimate of amounts and rates of consumption, including last use. For illicit substances and misused prescription medications, route(s) of consumption, along with details of amounts (including monetary cost), rates, and how the drugs are obtained, can be useful information, as can information on repercussions (physical, legal, interpersonal, financial) of drug use. Outside informants may be helpful. Experience with abstinence, inpatient or outpatient detoxification, longest period of sobriety, past rehabilitation programs, and any involvement

---

[†] The Phipps history is based in part on Adolph Meyer's approach to assessment, which entailed a systematic and comprehensive assessment of the patient[33,59] and considered a patient's presentation a culmination of all the biological and environmental influences that have acted upon the patient, not merely their current complaints. The history is described chronologically, beginning with family or genetic factors, then moves on to birth, development, childhood behaviors, and so on, finally reaching the assessment of the patient's current mental state. In most settings, the details of the patient's presentation and recent history are recorded just after the patient ID and chief complaint, the other elements of the history and exam then follow. Again, the order is less important than confirming that the critical elements of the history and examination (as can reasonably be obtained given the circumstances) are acquired and recorded, allowing for an appropriate formulation, risk assessment and plan.

[‡] A description of relationships can be instructive. For example, patients with certain personality disorders may describe a pattern of intense, unstable relationships with family, friends, and romantic partners.

with 12-step programs such as Alcoholics Anonymous or Narcotics Anonymous (if yes, does the patient have a sponsor?) may provide useful information on past successes or pitfalls that will guide treatment decisions. Use or misuse of other substances, such as LSD, MDMA, synthetic marijuana, "bath salts," inhalants, tobacco, caffeine or others would also be listed here.

Past medical and surgical history

This should include a list of currently active diagnoses, past diagnoses and procedures (and dates), allergies, current care providers, and current medications. Any contact information for current providers may also be useful.

Review of systems

This should include a review of all physical systems, as with medical emergency evaluations. The degree of detail in any or all areas may be determined by the patient's past medical history, level of physical or emotional distress, results of lab studies and physical examination, and ability or willingness to answer questions. Knowledge of somatic confounders for psychiatric diagnoses is important.[38] Review of current psychiatric complaints will be addressed primarily in mental status examination and history of present illness.

Pre-morbid personality

This is a description of the person's personality traits, as described by the patient and by outside informants. A description by the patient alone may be of limited utility. Descriptors of stable or unstable temperament, impulsivity, degree of concern for the welfare of others, and how the person handles stress can be important insights that may affect management and care decisions in the ED.

Past psychiatric history

This should include: first psychiatric contact, if any; previous hospitalizations or crises, including ED visits for psychiatric complaints; past trials of psychiatric medications and other treatment modalities (e.g. electroconvulsive therapy (ECT), transcranial magnetic stimulation (TMS), psychotherapy); current psychiatric provider and/or other mental health providers, such as therapists, and duration(s) of care; and any past history of self-injurious behavior, including self-mutilation and suicide attempts. Descriptions of any past prolonged depressive, manic, or hypomanic episodes and any periods of psychosis or other psychiatric syndromes and their treatments, if any, should be included here.

History of present illness

This should include all of the salient factors leading to the patient's current presentation, including descriptors of timing, intensity, duration, psychosocial factors (e.g. job loss, romantic or other relationship issues, financial stressors, non-adherence to treatment), vegetative symptoms (e.g. sleep, appetite, energy), mood or anxiety symptoms (including irritability, panic episodes, anhedonia, diminished self-attitude or vital sense, passive death wish, suicidal or homicidal thoughts and/or plans, observed psychomotor retardation or agitation, pathologic guilt, racing thoughts), or cognitive symptoms (memory problems, problems with concentration or attention). Ongoing areas of concern such as eating disorder behaviors, obsessive-compulsive thoughts and behaviors, psychosis, bereavement, or other psychosocial issues influencing the presentation, substance use, problematic sexual behaviors or others should be described here in sufficient detail. Some assessment of the level of impairment in overall function (such as failures to maintain their role at work, with family, or even care for themselves) including timing, duration, and intensity is important in gauging the severity of a patient's complaints. Outside informants are useful here.

The mental status exam

This should include what the clinician observes and how the patient describes his/her inner state and experience currently. This part of the exam should begin with basic observation of alertness: awake, somnolent, significantly changed or depressed level of consciousness, or completely non-responsive? For patients who are awake, level of alertness should be noted: alert, distractible, fully inattentive. How cooperative is the patient: guarded, defensive, uncooperative? What is the patient's appearance: well-groomed, disheveled, etc. Are there other factors in the patient's physical appearance such as deformities or other abnormalities? Are there any abnormalities in movement, such as tremor or other seemingly involuntary movements?

What is the quality of their speech? Assessment of speech includes a description of rate, rhythm, volume, and tone. Is the speech hard to follow? An example of speech content can be very useful. Psychiatrists will often describe the quality of associations in a patient's speech (how well does an expressed thought link to the preceding one?) and the presence or absence of evidence of disordered thought (for example, formal thought disorder, defined as the patient's subjective complaint of how distorted his/her thinking is from baseline, or some description of speech that suggests underlying disordered thinking, as may be seen in patients with schizophrenia).[35]

How does the patient describe their mood? Mood is the patient's subjective description of his/her inner, emotional experience ("I feel happy/sad/neutral"). How would the clinician describe the patient's affect, and does it match the patient's description of their mood? Affect is the observer's description of the patient's outward appearance ("The patient's affect is euthymic/downcast/euphoric"). Clinicians may also comment on the range of observed emotion a patient demonstrates or appears capable of demonstrating ("The patient's range of affect is normal/labile/constricted"). An important component is to note if the affect is congruent with the stated mood.

Does the patient express any suicidal thoughts? If so, is there a plan? What are the details of that plan? What is the patient's intent to carry out the plan? What are the odds of rescue if the person were to pursue the plan? Does the patient have access to the means to commit suicide (such as access to a firearm)? Are there thoughts or plans to hurt others? If so, what are the details? (Also see Chapter 3.) Does the patient report hallucinations? Are these hallucinations auditory, visual, olfactory, gustatory, tactile? Does the patient describe or appear to be hallucinating currently? Are any delusions (i.e., fixed, false, idiosyncratic beliefs) present? Does the patient describe obsessions, compulsions, phobias, anxieties, or panic symptoms? How impairing are they?

Finally, an assessment of cognition should be performed, including an assessment of insight and judgment. The Mini-Mental State Examination[39] or another screening tool of cognition can provide a useful and quick assessment of global cognitive capacity (though it may not allow a fine-tuned diagnosis of specific deficits).

Formulation. *The Perspectives of Psychiatry*[33] provides a useful framework in the emergency setting for formulating the salient features of patient presentations. The patient's background, complaints, and details of their current condition can be put into four categories of psychiatric interest: (1) the disease perspective, or what the patient *has* (e.g. delirium, depression, bipolar disorder, schizophrenia), (2) the behavior perspective, or what the patient *does* (substance abuse or dependence, sexual disorders, eating disorders; disordered behavior for which there is a biologic and psychological "drive" or motivation), (3) the dimensional perspective, or who the patient *is* (personality traits or disorders and intellectual capacity), and (4) life story issues, or what the patient *encounters* (environmental factors).[33]

The goal of the formulation is to summarize the significant factors involved in the presentation, including possible diagnoses when the true etiology is not, or cannot be, known. It is from this formulation that the clinician can succinctly highlight the patient's most pressing problems and determine appropriate interventions.

Risk assessment and plan. The risk assessment can be the most critical part of ED documentation for patients assessed for psychiatric complaints. As with all other fields of medicine, it is important to document pertinent information and the resulting clinical reasoning. The goal of the risk assessment in emergency psychiatry is to create a record of the thinking behind treatment decisions (most often this concerns the decision to admit or discharge a patient).

Common elements of the risk assessment include the risk of harm to self or others. Though these issues are addressed in detail elsewhere in the text, the suicidal patient in particular is a challenge for providers. The core components of assessing the suicidal patient, beyond considerations of psychiatric illness, personality disorder, substance use issues, and "life story" events, include inquiry into how detailed any existing plan may be, the potential lethality of the plan, the likelihood of rescue, and an assessment of the patient's intent. Access to lethal means (e.g. a firearm) should be assessed, and the feasibility of securing or otherwise rendering such modes of self-harm inaccessible to the patient should be evaluated. These critical questions may seem obvious, but are often overlooked. Positive and negative answers to each element should be documented in the record. Background information on the patient should be factored into the risk assessment of adults (see Chapter 3) as well, including, but not limited to: any history of previous suicide attempts, history of impulsivity, personality disorders or traits, family history or suicide in close contacts, active or past psychiatric disorders, substance use, male gender, older age, feelings of hopelessness, active stressors, and chronic pain. Risk profiles for children and adolescents may differ and are reviewed in other chapters. Though a number of suicide rating scales exist, these generally lack sensitivity and specificity and should not be used alone to access suicidality in the ED setting. They may serve as a supplement to a psychiatric assessment and clinical judgment, but should not replace them.

Finally, when possible, try to find common ground with the patient. Patients in psychiatric distress often have an agenda in mind. In some cases, that agenda may be concordant with the treating team's goals, but in other cases, the patient's agenda may be impossible to accommodate. The patient may present with a list of problems, only a few of which might be reasonably addressed in a health care setting. It is often useful to focus on one or two of what you *both* agree are important and amenable to solution. This is a single-shot version of problem-solving therapy,[40] which is a manualized, focused psychotherapeutic approach to help patients define problems, adopt useful plans to address them, and with successful completion, engender in the patient a sense of accomplishment or mastery. Other patients may deny having any problems at all, despite being brought by others for concerning behaviors. One of the most valuable skills in emergency psychiatry is determining the true areas of concern and the most effective and least restrictive intervention to address the problem(s), while confirming the safety of the patient and others.

Stabilization

Management of the most common acute psychiatric states (including use of seclusion and restraints) is handled in greater detail in a number of the following chapters. In addition to any pharmacologic or psychotherapeutic interventions that may occur, many of the safety issues reviewed in this chapter may play their role in stabilization, even if indirectly, and are no less important. We have also added a number of clinical pointers below that apply to clinical management of patients with psychiatric complaints in the ED.

The prolonged ED stay. Because of the problems with access to inpatient psychiatric beds nationwide, patients are often staying longer in EDs awaiting an inpatient bed and contributing to ED crowding.[41,42] These prolonged stays require more than a single, initial assessment. With prolonged stays, serial reassessment of a patient's psychiatric status is important, as the patient's condition may change with time. It is important to document periodically (for example, during each shift) the updated assessment and include the reasons why a patient is still in the ED. Documentation of reassessments should be clearly included in the medical record as well as the anticipated disposition and patient updates.

Though a multi-day stay with treatment in an ED may lead to stabilization and improvement in a patient's condition, a complete reformulation should usually be discussed with previous providers. Wholesale dismissal of a prior provider's observations can be a mistake. There are times when a patient's first appearance is not a true representation of the risk they will present at subsequent assessments, as seen, for example, with drug-induced states. The ED may then serve as a short-stay psychiatric service; the stressors or intoxicants that led to the patient's presentation may resolve while they are in the ED, allowing for a safe discharge plan. Documentation should convey how the clinical situation has changed during their stay and changes in the disposition plan should be carefully explained.

Disposition

Medical clearance. The idea of "medical clearance" has long been a problematic one and has been the source of some controversy, especially as it applies to patients with psychiatric complaints in the ED.[43,44] An obvious question is: "cleared" for what? Often, the practical response is that the patient is either being assessed for stability for transfer to an inpatient psychiatric unit or discharge with a plan for outpatient follow-up, if needed. Care providers on inpatient psychiatric units have a different set of skills than staff on inpatient medical units and some psychiatric units lack ready access to needed medical or surgical resources. Patients who have serious medical problems in addition to an acute psychiatric issue can be challenging when determining a disposition. The total burden of disease has to be carefully evaluated by the emergency providers when seeking an appropriate disposition. Inpatient psychiatric units are often not well-equipped to manage complex medical diseases, while medical units are not the best environment to manage acute psychiatric conditions. Further complicating these considerations is the association of some psychiatric disorders (and their treatments) with medical conditions and poor medical outcomes.[45-48] The medical screening exam should detail the medical needs of the patient, with treatment recommendations. If the patient needs admission to an inpatient psychiatric unit, a thoughtful medical formulation of chronic and/or sub-acute issues and communication of treatment recommendations can go a long way in assuaging the concerns of psychiatric providers.

"**Frequent fliers.**" Many ED staff can name at least a few patients who seem to present to triage almost every night. Some EDs keep lists.[49] For many of these patients, there may be a known psychiatric component (including drug or alcohol misuse) to their recurrent visits, but in a number of cases there is an undiagnosed or undertreated psychiatric illness. These patients can be a source of frustration and contention for even the most committed health care providers. The challenge in caring for such patients is to assess accurately their needs and to help these patients engage in meaningful interventions. In resource-poor areas, there may not be ready access to capitation programs or ED-diversion resources (e.g. non-hospital "crisis" beds, home visits, education, or other modalities[50]), which can in some instances provide a life-saving intervention. In these instances, creative use of existing resources, including shelters, outpatient physicians, social workers, and families may be the only options.

Behavioral alerts and aftercare plans. Awareness of the risk of violence in the health care setting is on the rise.[51] Providers on the front line must be aware of a patient's history of violence and/or unpredictable behavior in time to plan and keep themselves, the patient, and others safe. Failure to provide a safe work environment, with appropriate safeguards to prevent violent attacks, has led to Occupational Safety and Health Administration (OSHA) fines for hospitals.[52] While many acts of violence cannot be predicted, for patients with histories of harming (or threatening to harm) staff, themselves, or others, protocols and alert systems may help prevent future violence. Ideally, alerts would be triggered at triage (or before, if possible), leading to a coordinated and rehearsed response by all staff, beginning with the triage nurse and clerical staff responsible for patient registration. The details of the planned responses should be applicable to any potential danger, but if possible, planned responses should be tailored to the patient's problematic behavior. For example, a patient with a history of violence directed against providers would be carefully supervised at all times by appropriate levels of security personnel on subsequent visits.

Many departments of psychiatry have developed their own formal or informal behavioral aftercare plans that may be found in discharge summaries or other documents that may or may not be accessible to emergency care providers. These care plans may address problems that run the spectrum of severity from violence and stalking to non-adherence to medication plans or follow-up. While ED providers may not need unfettered access to all psychiatric records, there are times when a patient's potentially dangerous behaviors should be known, in order to prevent the patient, staff, or others from coming to harm. The CUSP format mentioned above can be an effective format for creating an understanding between the disciplines on how such information can and will be shared. Importantly, the behavioral aftercare plan should not be a "do not care" plan, outlining only the care that will not be provided or "banning" the patient from care. The goal is to tailor a plan of care to the patient's problematic behavior(s), allowing providers to safely address the patient's acute medical or psychiatric presentation.

Conclusion

The chapters that follow will cover many of the topics raised here in greater depth as well as others not yet discussed. While the trends of increased use of EDs for patients with active psychiatric issues will likely continue, there are other changes on the horizon that will impact the ways in which care is provided. The broad adoption of electronic medical records in health care settings may allow instant access to needed records, providing a boon to the practice of emergency psychiatry, but it also raises concerns about confidentiality,[53,54] the hazards of "cut and paste" notes,[55] and other potential risks.

The movement toward integrated, collaborative care, and the medical home model[56–58] will influence the ways in which psychiatric care is delivered, including use of emergency care, creating a number of opportunities to improve care as well as pitfalls to be avoided. While the effects of these changes cannot be predicted, the importance of sound fundamentals in the practice of emergency psychiatry and the provision of safe care will continue.

Summary tips

Emergency psychiatry is being delivered in diverse clinical settings, with staffing and resources ranging from sparse to fully staffed and carefully designed psychiatric emergency services with a host of ancillary supports. Below is a shorthand list of tips to be considered, in varying degrees, in every ED.

When possible, get vital signs early.
- Severely agitated patients may refuse, but their agitation may be due to an underlying medical problem.
- Vitals may be useful in detecting medical problems in psychiatric patients.[24]

Do a "chart biopsy" before a psychiatric assessment, if records are available.
- Allows for confirmation of existing information and formulation of necessary questions for the patient and informants.
- Focus can then be on the most salient parts of history and presentation.

See the patient before worrying about disposition.
- Seems simple, but delegating to others or trying to make disposition decisions before seeing the patient can frequently complicate the decision-making process.

Talk to collateral informants.
- Obtaining information, especially from others who know something of the patient, is crucial. Maintaining an objective point of view when speaking with informants helps with diagnostic accuracy. Trust but verify.

When in doubt, send a urinalysis and drug screen.
- *In Urina Veritas* (in urine is truth).
  - Most useful for detection of illicit drugs or misused prescriptions.
  - Some screens will also detect commonly used medications and may be useful in determining prescriptions used in overdoses or adherence to prescribed medication regimen (knowledge of sensitivity and specificity of the screens is useful for the latter).
  - In some older or otherwise susceptible patients, a urinary tract infection may be involved, or even causative.

For women of child-bearing age, check for pregnancy.
- There are psychiatric syndromes associated with pregnancy.
- Some psychiatric facilities do not have easy access to obstetric care.
- Concerns about potential teratogenic effects of medications need to be discussed with patients.

For most patients, send a blood alcohol level.

- Patients may appear sober, but have high blood alcohol levels. Countless patient exams have had to be repeated because the patient was secretly intoxicated.
- The idea of "clinical sobriety" is of little utility for psychiatric assessment.
- The patient's story, mental state, and decision-making are frequently quite different when the patient is sober.

Formulate.

- What factor(s) best explain(s) the symptoms the patient is reporting or demonstrating?
    - Disease (medical and psychiatric).
    - Behavior (substance abuse, sexual disorder, eating disorder).
    - Dimensional traits (temperament, personality disorders, IQ).
    - Life story (environment and social issues).

When in doubt, confer with appropriate consultants.

- Do a risk assessment.
    - Most clinicians do this instinctively.
    - Requires knowledge of epidemiologic and other risks for suicide, violence, or other mishaps due to inability to care for self.
    - Many physicians fail to document their medical reasoning.
    - Explain why the patient is or is not safe for discharge and what factors influence this decision.
    - Include collateral information (other informants besides the patient).

Plan.

- Can this be handled as an outpatient or is inpatient care required?
- When in doubt, confer.

Monitoring patient for safety while in the ED

- Who does it?
- How often?
- Is there a standard in the ED?
- What is the appropriate nurse:patient ratio for the area?
- Is the patient in a safe environment?
- Have sitters and security staff received appropriate training?

Update the patient (and family, friends, when applicable) on estimated length of stays and potential dispositions.

- Patient satisfaction has become a focus in many EDs.
- Informing patients can improve compliance with treatment, safety, and reduce angst.
- Checking in with the patient and family periodically can go a long way in helping reduce the distress associated with an emergency visit.

Establish a routine for rapid assessment and management of severely agitated patients.

- A multidisciplinary approach involving front line staff (physicians, nurses, security, others) is most effective and safest.

Establish a multidisciplinary safety committee or incorporate psychiatry into ED safety committee.

- Ideally this would include physicians, nurses, nurse practitioners, security, clerical staff, legal, administration, other paramedical staff, patient safety experts if available, even residents in training.
- Unfortunately, these committees are often formed only after a bad outcome as part of a root cause analysis. Regular meetings with an agenda can profoundly improve "culture" (including relationships between ED and psychiatric providers), efficiency, and safety.

Be familiar with referral resources.

- Social work, psychiatry, and the local health department may be useful in compiling lists of inpatient and outpatient psychiatric care, emergency phone and other contacts, and substance abuse resources.
- Lists should be updated routinely, as referral resources may change.

Addendum: Full Phipps Psychiatric History.

Psychiatric assessment note

Note: Before starting interview state the limits of confidentiality: i.e. confidential except: self harm, harm to others, history or current sexual/ child abuse, medical emergency, court order/ subpoena.

Date of Evaluation: Time:

Informants and Patient Contacts	Reliability of Informant(s):
Identifying Data and Chief Complaint	Emergency Petition? ☐Yes ☐No

Family psychiatric history

Father
Age, (alive/dead, details of latter if applicable) Health, Education, Occupation, Personality, Relationship with patient, any past psychiatric conditions, treatment

Mother
Age, (alive/dead, details of latter if applicable) Health, Education, Occupation, Personality, Relationship with patient, any past psychiatric conditions, treatment

Siblings (Specify Biologic Relatedness)
Age, (alive/dead, details of latter if applicable) Health, Education Occupation, Personality, Relationship with patient, any past psychiatric conditions, treatment

Extended Family Medical and Psychiatric History
Include Neurological or Psychiatric Illness or Hospitalizations, Substance Use Disorders, Attempted or Completed Suicides

Personal history

Gestation & Birth
Early Development and Milestones Childhood Health

Social position
Home atmosphere

Childhood/adolescence Behavior Symptoms
Fires, Fighting (other children, teachers), Truancy, Animal cruelty, Enuresis, School Refusal

Education
Age at Entry, Highest Level or Grade Completed, Age at Graduation, Academic Performance, Special Education Requirements, Learning Disorder diagnoses

Occupations
Age at Starting Work, Jobs Held, Longest Job, Last Worked, Military Service, current source(s) of income

Menstrual History
Age at Menarche/ Menopause, Regularity of Menses, LMP

Sexual History
Age at First Sexual Activity, Number of Partners, Sexual Preference, Contraception and Safe Sexual Practices, Sexual Abuse (reported?), paraphilias, issues of gender identity

Marital History/ Other Significant Relationships
Duration of Acquaintance, Length of Unions, Age, Health, Education, Occupation, Personality of Spouse(s) and Quality of Relationships

Children
In Chronologic Order Age, Health, Education, Occupation, Personality, and Relationship

Living Situation
Current and any significant past issues

Religious Affiliation

Legal History
Arrests, Convictions, Total Jail Time, Time Served, Solitary Confinement, Current Parole or Probation

Substance use history

Drug	Route	Age at First Use	Current Use And Duration	Maximum Use	Last Use	Longest Abstinence Date/ Length/ Context	Withdrawal Symptoms
Tobacco:			Pack years				
Ethanol	p.o.						
Marijuana							

(cont.)

Drug	Route	Age at First Use	Current Use And Duration	Maximum Use	Last Use	Longest Abstinence Date/ Length/ Context	Withdrawal Symptoms
Cocaine	Intranasal Smoke . IV						
Heroin	Intranasal Smoke IV						
Others Amphetamines, BZD, LSD, MDMA, PCP, Solvents, Caffeine							

Past Medical History (includes surgical history, any history of brain injury):
Allergies:

Current Medications (Include OTCs/herbals):

Outpatient physicians and contact information:

Review of Systems

Constitutional	Fever/sweats/chills Weight loss/gain Fatigue
HEENT, Neck	Dysphagia Vision changes Hearing loss
Pulmonary	Dyspnea Cough Phlegm/blood
Cardiovascular	Chest pain Edema Claudication
GI	Nausea Vomiting Constipation Diarrhea Hematochezia Melena
GU	Dysuria Hematuria Discharge Pain Bleeding
Musculoskeletal Dermatologic	Myalgias Rashes Joint pain/swelling
Neurologic	Headache Numbness/tingling Dizziness Lightheadedness Weakness Seizures
Endocrine	Thyroid disease Diabetes
Heme/Lymph/Immune	Easy bruising/bleeding

Premorbid Personality

Patient Description of personality traits: (e.g. easy-going, worrier, introverted, extraverted, live-in-the moment, consequence-avoidant, stable, unstable, intense or muted emotional responses to events):

Outside informant description of personality traits (and name, relationship of informant):

Past Psychiatric History

Include chronology of psychiatric problems from first onset (including childhood), the associated symptoms including vegetative symptoms, thoughts of suicide or attempts, types of treatments received including medication trials, and their outcomes, any hospitalizations or ED presentations, past neuropsychological testing, including IQ testing, details of current treatment if applicable

History of present illness

Mental Status Exam

Appearance **General** **Behavior**	Level of arousal: Alert Drowsy Somnolent Comatose Cooperative? Grooming: good/fair/poor Disheveled: yes/no Clothing: Own/hospital Eye contact: good/fair/poor Psychomotor agitation or retardation: Abnormal Involuntary Movements:
Speech form and content, **Language** **Associations** **Form of Thought**	Speech Rate: fast/slow/normal Rhythm: normal or absent Volume: very soft/soft/normal/loud/very loud Tone/ Prosody: Pressured: No/Yes Can be interrupted: No/Yes Dysarthric: Yes (slurring yes/no)/No Formal thought disorder: Yes/No Associations: (e.g. loose, intact) Sample of Speech:
Mood, Affect **Self-Attitude** **Vital Sense** **SI/HI/PDW**	Stated Mood: Objectively Appears: Vital Sense (Physical well being): Good/Poor Self Attitude: Good/Poor Hopefulness for the future: Passive Death Wish: Suicidal ideation, intent, plan Details of any thoughts/Intent/Plan to harm self: Thoughts/Intent/Plan to harm others:

(cont.)

Abnormal Perceptions and Illusions	Hallucinations (visual/auditory/olfactory/tactile/gustatory)
Delusions	
Anxiety	Obsessions: Compulsions Phobias Panic attacks/ Free-floating anxiety
COGNITION Intelligence Abstraction General Information	Abstraction: (ex. explanation of parables) Estimated IQ: (ex. Can the patient name the current president? Name prior presidents in order?):
Judgment Insight	
Scales, MMSE	Total score: /30 missed items:

Physical examination

Vital Signs	Wt BMI:		T	HR	RR	BP
HEENT and Neck						
Pulmonary / Back						
Cardiac/ Vascular						
Abdomen	Abdominal circumference:					
GU/GYN						
Skin/Extremities						
Neuro	Cranial Nerves:					
	Motor:					
	Sensation:					
	Cerebellar: Gait:					
	Reflexes:					

Data/Labs:
CXR:
ECG:
RBC folate:
B12:
TSH:
RPR:
Pregnancy (urine/serum) hCG:
Utox:
Serum volatile screen:
UA:

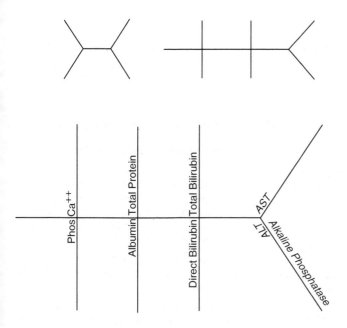

Other:
Formulation

_____

_____

_____

_____

_____

_____

_____

_____

_____

_____

_____

Diagnostic Impression

Axis I	
Axis II	
Axis III	
Axis IV	Acute: Enduring:
Axis V	Current: Past Year:

Risk Assessment:

Consider Family History of Suicide, Past Attempts by Patient, Lethality, Current Mental State, Past Violent Acts Towards Others, Current Thoughts to Harm Others, Unpredictability

Initial Plan

Admission Type, Observation Status, and Initial Treatments Including Medications

References

1. Institute of Medicine, Committee on the Future of Emergency Care in the U.S. Health System. *Hospital Based Emergency Care at the Breaking Point.* Washington, DC: National Academy Press, 2007.

2. ACEP (American College of Emergency Physicians). Study Confirms Emergency Department "Boarding" Major Cause of Crowding. [Online]. Available: http://www.acep.org/webportal/Newsroom/PressReleases/AnnalsOfEmergencyMedicinePressReleases/Arvchive2003/StudyConfirmsEmergency Department BoardingMajorCauseofCrowding.htm Accessed June 7, 2005. Cited in Institute of Medicine, Committee on the Future of Emergency Care in the U.S. Health System. *Hospital Based Emergency Care at the Breaking Point.* Washington, DC: National Academy Press, 2003.

3. Appleby J. *Mentally Ill Face Extra-long ER Waits.* USATODAY.com 2008; Sect. Health & Behavior.

4. Slade EP, Dixon LB, Semmel S. Trends in the duration of emergency department visits, 2001–2006. *Psychiatr Serv.* 2010;**61**(9):878–884.

5. Larkin GL, Claassen CA, Emond JA, Pelletier AJ, Camargo CA. Trends in U.S. emergency department visits for mental health conditions, 1992 to 2001. *Psychiatr Serv.* 2005;**56**(6):671–677.

6. Owens PL, Mutter R, Stocks C. *Mental Health and Substance Abuse-Related Emergency Department Visits among Adults,* 2007. http://www.hcup-us.ahrq.gov/reports/statbriefs/sb92.pdf.

7. Hazlett SB, McCarthy ML, Londner MS, Onyike CU. Epidemiology of adult psychiatric visits to US emergency departments. *Acad Emerg Med.* 2004;**11**(2):193–195.

8. Pronovost PJ, Weast B, Bishop K, et al. Senior executive adopt-a-work unit: a model for safety improvement. *Joint Commission Journal on Quality and Safety.* 2004;**30**(2):59–68.

9. Pronovost P, Goeschel C. Improving ICU care: it takes a team. *Healthc Exec.* 2005;**20**(2):14–20.

10. Pronovost PJ, Berenholtz SM, Goeschel CA, et al. Creating high reliability in health care organizations. *Health Serv Res.* 2006;**41**(4 Pt 2):1599–1617.

11. Kohn LT, Corrigan J, Donaldson MS. *To Err is Human: Building a Safer Health System.* Washington, DC: National Academy Press, 2000.

12. Pronovost PJ, Vohr E. *Safe Patients, Smart Hospitals: How One Doctor's Checklist can Help Us Change Health Care from the Inside Out.* New York, NY: Hudson Street Press, 2010.

13. Gawande A. *The Checklist Manifesto: How to Get Things Right.* 1st ed. New York, NY: Metropolitan Books, 2010.

14. Moskop JC, Marco CA, Larkin GL, Geiderman JM, Derse AR. From hippocrates to HIPAA: Privacy and confidentiality in emergency medicine – part I: Conceptual, moral, and legal foundations. *Ann Emerg Med.* 2005;**45**(1):53–59.

15. Moskop JC, Marco CA, Larkin GL, Geiderman JM, Derse AR. From hippocrates to HIPAA: Privacy and confidentiality in emergency medicine – part II: Challenges in the emergency department. *Ann Emerg Med.* 2005;**45**(1):60–67.

16. Olsen JC, Sabin BR. Emergency department patient perceptions of privacy

and confidentiality. *J Emerg Med*. 2003;**25**(3):329–333.

17. Melchiode GA, Puryear DA, Babick M. The emergency room as a clerkship site. *Am J Psychiatry*. 1983;**140**(7):894–897.

18. Downey LV, Zun LS, Burke T. Undiagnosed mental illness in the emergency department. *J Emerg Med*. 2012;**43**(5):876–882.

19. Claassen CA, Larkin GL. Occult suicidality in an emergency department population. *Br J Psychiatry*. 2005;**186**:352–353.

20. Luoma JB, Martin CE, Pearson JL. Contact with mental health and primary care providers before suicide: a review of the evidence. *Am J Psychiatry*. 2002;**159**(6):909–916.

21. Schiller MJ, Shumway M, Batki SL. Utility of routine drug screening in a psychiatric emergency setting. *Psychiatr Serv*. 2000;**51**(4):474–478.

22. Zun LS, Hernandez R, Thompson R, Downey L. Comparison of EPs' and psychiatrists' laboratory assessment of psychiatric patients. *Am J Emerg Med*. 2004;**22**(3):175–180.

23. Riba M, Hale M. Medical clearance: Fact or fiction in the hospital emergency room. *Psychosomatics*. 1990;**31**(4):400–404.

24. Olshaker JS, Browne B, Jerrard DA, Prendergast H, Stair TO. Medical clearance and screening of psychiatric patients in the emergency department. *Acad Emerg Med*. 1997;**4**(2):124–128.

25. Korn CS, Currier GW, Henderson SO. "Medical clearance" of psychiatric patients without medical complaints in the emergency department. *J Emerg Med*. 2000;**18**(2):173–176.

26. Henneman PL, Mendoza R, Lewis RJ. Prospective evaluation of emergency department medical clearance. *Ann Emerg Med*. 1994;**24**(4):672–677.

27. Broderick KB, Lerner EB, McCourt JD, Fraser E, Salerno K. Emergency physician practices and requirements regarding the medical screening examination of psychiatric patients. *Acad Emerg Med*. 2002;**9**(1):88–92.

28. Anfinson TJ, Kathol RG. Screening laboratory evaluation in psychiatric patients: a review. *Gen Hosp Psychiatry*. 1992;**14**(4):248–257.

29. Janiak BD, Atteberry S. Medical clearance of the psychiatric patient in the emergency department. *J Emerg Med*. 2012;**43**(5):866–870.

30. Woo BKP, Chen W. Substance misuse among older patients in psychiatric emergency service. *Gen Hosp Psychiatry*. 2010;**32**(1):99–101.

31. Schiller MJ, Shumway M, Batki SL. Utility of routine drug screening in a psychiatric emergency setting. *Psychiatr Serv*. 2000;**51**(4):474–478.

32. Stefan S. *Emergency Department Treatment of the Psychiatric Patient*. New York, NY: Oxford University Press, 2006:215.

33. McHugh PR, Slavney PR. *The Perspectives of Psychiatry*. 2nd ed. Baltimore, MD: Johns Hopkins University Press, 1998.

34. Goodwin DW, Guze SB. *Psychiatric Diagnosis*. 5th ed. New York, NY: Oxford University Press, 1996.

35. Sims ACP. *Symptoms in the Mind: An Introduction to Descriptive Psychopathology*. 2nd ed. London: Saunders, 1995.

36. Mayer-Gross W, Roth M, Slater E. *Clinical Psychiatry*. 3rd ed. Baltimore, MD: Williams and Wilkins, 1969:42–46.

37. The American Psychiatric Association published a consensus guideline for psychiatric assessment of adults in 2006 (accessible at http://www.guideline.gov/content.aspx?id=9317).

38. Lishman WA. *Organic Psychiatry: The Psychological Consequences of Cerebral Disorder*. 3rd ed. Oxford; Malden, MA: Blackwell Science, 1998.

39. Folstein MF, Folstein SE, McHugh PR. "Mini-mental state". A practical method for grading the cognitive state of patients for the clinician. *J Psychiatr Res*. 1975;**12**(3):189–198.

40. D'Zurilla TJ, Nezu AM. *Problem-Solving Therapy: A Social Competence Approach to Clinical Intervention (Springer Series on*

Behavior Therapy and Behavioral Medicine). 2nd ed. New York, NY: Springer Publishing Company, 1999.

41. Moskop JC, Sklar DP, Geiderman JM, Schears RM, Bookman KJ. Emergency department crowding, part 2 – barriers to reform and strategies to overcome them. *Ann Emerg Med.* 2009;**53**(5):612–617.

42. Moskop JC, Sklar DP, Geiderman JM, Schears RM, Bookman KJ. Emergency department crowding, part 1 – concept, causes, and moral consequences. *Ann Emerg Med.* 2009;**53**(5):605–611.

43. Reeves RR, Perry CL, Burke RS. What does "medical clearance" for psychiatry really mean? *J Psychosoc Nurs Ment Health Serv.* 2010;**48**(8):2–4.

44. Tintinalli JE, Peacock FW 4th, Wright MA. Emergency medical evaluation of psychiatric patients. *Ann Emerg Med.* 1994;**23**(4):859–862.

45. Frankenburg FR, Zanarini MC. The association between borderline personality disorder and chronic medical illnesses, poor health-related lifestyle choices, and costly forms of health care utilization. *J Clin Psychiatry.* 2004;**65**(12):1660–1665.

46. de Leon J, Diaz FJ. Planning for the optimal design of studies to personalize antipsychotic prescriptions in the post-CATIE era: the clinical and pharmacoepidemiological data suggest that pursuing the pharmacogenetics of metabolic syndrome complications (hypertension, diabetes mellitus and hyperlipidemia) may be a reasonable strategy. *Schizophr Res.* 2007;**96**(1–3):185–197.

47. Daumit GL, Pronovost PJ, Anthony CB, Guallar E, Steinwachs DM, Ford DE. Adverse events during medical and surgical hospitalizations for persons with schizophrenia. *Arch Gen Psychiatry.* 2006;**63**(3):267–272.

48. Brown S, Kim M, Mitchell C, Inskip H. Twenty-five year mortality of a community cohort with schizophrenia. *Br J Psychiatry.* 2010;**196**(2):116–121.

49. Geiderman JM. Keeping lists and naming names: Habitual patient files for suspected nontherapeutic drug-seeking patients. *Ann Emerg Med.* 2003;**41**(6):873–881.

50. Michelen W, Martinez J, Lee A, Wheeler DP. Reducing frequent flyer emergency department visits. *J Health Care Poor Underserved.* 2006;**17**(1 Suppl):59–69.

51. Kelen GD, Catlett CL. Violence in the health care setting. *JAMA.* 2010;**304**(22):2530–2531.

52. Anonymous. Hospital's History of Violence Leads to OSHA Fine. http://ohsonline.com/articles/2010/07/20/hospitals-history-of-violence-leads-to-osha-fine.aspx. Accessed March 1, 2011.

53. Raths D. Stay out of my EMR. Privacy issues are dominating the airwaves as the industry begins to deal with the EMR data-mining minefield. *Healthc Inform.* 2008;**25**(5):43–44.

54. Gaylin DS, Moiduddin A, Mohamoud S, Lundeen K, Kelly JA. Public attitudes about health information technology, and its relationship to health care quality, costs, and privacy. *Health Serv Res.* 2011;**46**(3):920–938.

55. Hirschtick RE. A piece of my mind. Copy-and-paste. *JAMA.* 2006;**295**(20):2335–2336.

56. Katon W, Unützer J. Consultation psychiatry in the medical home and accountable care organizations: achieving the triple aim. *Gen Hosp Psychiatry.* 2011;**33**(4):305–310.

57. Engel AG, Malta LS, Davies CA, Baker MM. Clinical effectiveness of using an integrated model to treat depressive symptoms in veterans affairs primary care clinics and its impact on health care utilization. *Prim Care Companion CNS Disord.* 2011;**13**(4):PCC.10m01096.

58. Sorel E, Everett A. Psychiatry and primary care integration: challenges and opportunities. *Int Rev Psychiatry.* 2011;**23**(1):28–30.

59. Shorter E. *A History of Psychiatry: From the Era of the Asylum to the Age of Prozac.* New York, NY: John Wiley & Sons, Inc., 1997.

Management of agitation and violence

Mustapha Saheed

According to the National Institute of Occupational Safety and Health, approximately 1.7 million people are assaulted in the workplace annually, with a significant percentage occurring in the health care environment.[1] Professionals like police and firefighters are associated with higher rates of fatal violent events. Although health care violence is usually non-fatal, it is more frequent and pervasive. Violence is four times more common in health care settings than in other private industries. The most common settings for these assaults include hospitals (particularly emergency departments (EDs), intensive care units, geriatric and psychiatric floors), nursing homes, and social service agencies. A survey of over 250,000 private industries found that 45% of non-fatal occupational injuries occurred as a result of a health care violence.[2,3] Even more concerning is that these rates appear to be on the rise.[1–3]

Nurses are the most frequently assaulted health care workers.[4–8] Campbell et al., in a survey of health care workers, found over 30% of nurses reported an incident of physical assault.[4] Other research also suggests nurses experience a high incidence of workplace violence.[9] Internationally, similar rates of health care-related violence have been reported.[10–16] The ED is often the site of violence and is clearly a very high-risk area of the hospital.[17–22] A survey of over 3000 registered nurses from the Emergency Nursing Association revealed 25% had experienced physical assault more than 20 times over the preceding three-year period.[6]

Physicians and similar health care practitioners are not immune and also report alarming rates of violence.[20–25] In one survey of over 500 doctors, more than half of the respondents reported episodes of aggressive behavior from patients.[24] Behnam et al., in a national survey of emergency physicians and residents, revealed 21% of physicians reported a physical assault in the previous 12 months.[18] Moreover, the impact of the violence on health care workers is troubling. Kowalenko et al. report that 81.9% of the surveyed emergency medicine physicians were occasionally fearful of their workplace.[20] Forty two percent sought various forms of protection including a gun (18%), knife (20%), mace (7%), and security escorts (31%).

Education regarding health care violence continues to be a significant need, with many physicians and nurses requesting further education in the management of violent or agitated patients.[5,12,26,27] A survey of accredited emergency medicine training programs found only 16% had some training or workshop for the management of violent patients.[18] Similarly, nurses, and other health care professionals, report a paucity of training opportunities.[5,18,20] In response, many major health care societies including AMA, APA, and

Emergency Psychiatry, ed. Arjun Chanmugam, Patrick Triplett, and Gabor Kelen. Published by Cambridge University Press. © Cambridge University Press 2013.

ACEP have policy statements and advocacy goals relating to the reduction of workplace violence. Most recently, the American Association of Emergency Psychiatry (AAEP) has published guidelines on managing agitation through its Project BETA: Best Practices in the Evaluation and Treatment of Agitation. The publication of these high quality guidelines is an important step in improving the consistency and safety in the management of agitated patients.[28] The algorithms from Project BETA are included in this chapter (see Figures 2.1–2.3).

Concern about escalating patient violence is warranted. An eight-month evaluation into the types of weapons confiscated from two large urban EDs revealed over 3706 metallic weapons including 4 guns, 2162 knives, and 633 box cutters/razors.[29] Although controversial, many health care workers report improved perception of safety in departments with metal detectors.[29–35] Additionally, surveys of patients suggest minimal negative perception and strong sense of improved safety with metal detectors.[29–35] However, the evidence supporting the efficacy of metal detectors in preventing crime or as a deterrent is scant, and at least one institution admitted that installation of metal detectors did not decrease weapons discovered in the treatment area.[36] Furthermore, most assaults involving health care workers are non-fatal and do not involve a weapon.[1–3] As such, the utility of metal detectors is likely minimal in preventing most incidents of health care-related workplace violence.

Perhaps the first step in reducing the rates of hospital violence is recognizing the potentially violent or agitated patient. Rapid identification of patients at risk for violence allows for the institution of preventative measures that reduce the risk of injury and minimize escalation.[28,37–41] Early studies initially suggested that health care workers, psychiatrists and psychologists in particular, could not readily identify or predict patients at risk for violence.[42] Reassuringly, as research in the area has improved our understanding of the violent patient, so has the ability to identify patients at risk of committing violent acts.[42–44]

An understanding of risk factors for violent behavior is part of a broader risk assessment. Substance abuse appears to be a risk factor that is highly correlated with violence.[35,45–48] Other risk factors include male sex, age between 15 and 40 years, access to weapons, homelessness, and major psychiatric disorder.[49] A history of prior violence is particularly correlated with a likelihood of future violence. Rao et al. found rates of violence to be 20 times higher in patients with a prior history of violence.[46]

Patients with a history of psychiatric illness have long been associated with violence. In fact, some attribute the increased trend in ED violence to a rise in the proportion of ED patients presenting for psychiatric emergencies.[17,46,50] However, this potential association is controversial. Amore et al. found that patients with positive symptoms (hallucinations, delusions, thought disorders) – as measured by the Brief Psychiatric Rating Scale – were much more likely to be violent during an inpatient psychiatric admission.[51] In contrast, Elbogen et al., in a review of over 34,000 subjects completing surveys for the National Epidemiologic Survey on alcoholism and related conditions, found that psychiatric illness did not independently predict future violence.[47] Another study, by Fazel et al., revealed similar findings: the increased violence associated with schizophrenia was mostly a result of concomitant substance abuse and dependence.[48] Anderson et al. suggest that only a small subset of patients with psychiatric illness and specific symptoms are at high risk for violence.[42] It is likely that individuals who have some active impairment or intoxication are more likely to be at risk for violence than those who simply have a primary psychiatric disease label.[52]

Caution should be exercised when relying solely on risk factor analysis for a risk assessment. For example, racial demographics have been documented to be associated

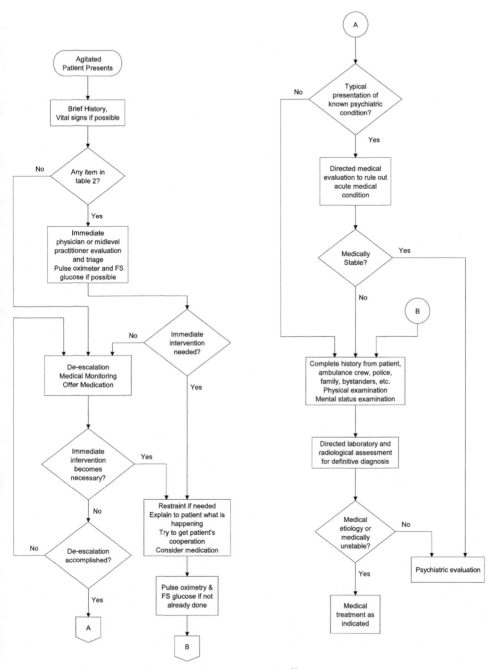

Figure 2.1. Medical evaluation and triage of the agitated patient[38]

with rates of violence.[53,54] In particular, African Americans have increased rates of self-reported violence, arrest, and incarceration.[42,55,56] While this suggests an increased rate of violence, Sampson et al. showed that most of the racial association with violence disappears when social economic status is controlled.[54] Moreover, there is an appropriate ethical

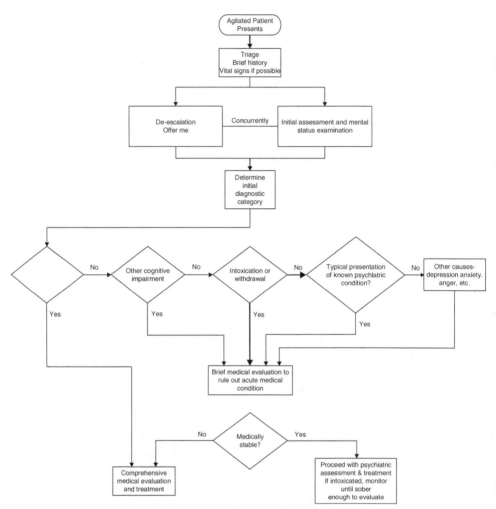

Figure 2.2. Psychiatric evaluation assessment of the agitated patient[41]

reticence to risk stratification based primarily on demographics. Generally, basic demographics are poorly predictive of violence at any given moment; as such, clinicians must use other tools.

Violence rarely erupts without warning signals. Behavioral cues are dynamic risk factors that are particularly predictive. Signs of an agitated mental state include anger, confusion, excitement, uncooperativeness, impulsivity, and confusion.[35,42,57] Physical signs of agitation include a clenched jaw, flared nostrils, flushed face, and clenched or gripping hands that are associated with impending violence.[57] Behavioral cues can be stratified into three categories: speech, posture, and motor activity.[45] Loud and hostile speech, and verbal threats, are obvious cues. Sitting tensely at the edge of a chair, gripping the arm rest, is a postural sign of agitation. Motor activity including pacing or an inability to sit still is an often ignored but important cue to impending violence.

Kapur and Fink describe the "prodrome of violence" in three phases: anxiety, defensiveness, and physical aggression.[58] In the anxiety phase, the patient may exhibit postural,

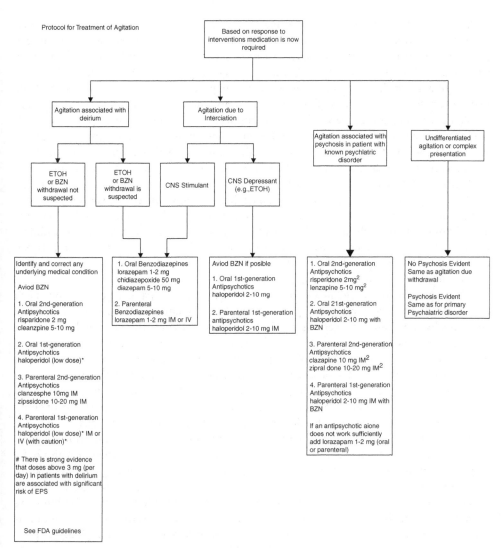

Protocol for Treatment of Agitation

Figure 2.3. Protocol for treatment of agitation[37]

behavioral, and speech cues. A restless appearance, persistent questioning, and pressured speech are all signals of escalating anxiety. Defensiveness is the next prodromic phase of violent behavior. The patient may become verbally abusive and exhibit other signs of hostile and volatile behavior. Verbal assaults may include attacks on staff's weight, gender, or other demographic features. If allowed to escalate, the third phase may be physical aggression. Once the patient has become physically aggressive, he or she has lost control and will likely require some physical intervention to reestablish a safe environment. Overall, a prodromal construct is useful in structuring graded responses to early warning signs. This construct does have its limitations, as there are occasions when there may be a non-linear progression of violence. For example, a patient who initially presents with increasing anxiety may appear temporarily pacified before erupting into severe agitation and violence. While behavioral cues can be viewed as part of a temporal continuum, each should also be interpreted individually.

The clinician must synthesize, as available, the combination of risk factors, contextual history, behavioral cues, and collaborative information into a global assessment of the patient's level of risk. Collaborative information should be obtained from family, friends, paramedics, clinicians, and medical records, wherever possible. As expected, the more information utilized, the greater the accuracy. In practice, where information available may be very limited, clinicians often must make rapid decisions using their best judgment.

Validated tools are available that grade the level of risk into a numerical score.[59–66] However, many of these tools are cumbersome and of limited utility in the emergent setting. Anderson et al. describe a risk stratification system that is simple, yet robust.[42] The patient's risk is categorized into one of three levels: potential, imminent, or emergent. "Potential" patients have been identified through risk assessment but are not currently displaying high risk signs. "Imminent" patients display many concerning signs for violence and are at very high risk of conversion to emergent violence. "Emergently" violent patients are exhibiting signs of physical violence and require immediate intervention. The intuitive comprehensibility of these categories promotes clear and concise communication between different health care specialties and allied fields. Moreover, each classification allows for specific approaches and targeted responses.

The approach to the agitated patient must begin prior to patient presentation. Each institution should have policies and protocols in place to manage staff response to violence. Additionally, a tracking and alert system should exist for patients with prior violence and/or high risk of violence. Staff should be well versed in procedures for activating security. Security personnel should have robust procedures to properly respond and secure all clinical areas. Security staff should also be appropriately trained in techniques for the safe restraint and management of violent patients. A culture of safety should be promulgated, with particular institutional support for staff concerns about safety hazards and ongoing quality improvement initiatives to identify and mitigate dangerous conditions.

For the patient expressing minor to moderate agitation and a "potential" for violence, verbal de-escalation techniques can be successful. Redirection can be achieved with polite, respectful, professional behavior. The establishment of rapport through the validation of feelings, empathy, and courtesy can help reduce anxiety and prevent further escalation. Offering the patient food, if appropriate, can strongly contribute to rapport by implying a deeper concern about the patient's welfare, and can engender positive behavior modification. Additionally, speaking in soft and calm tones, especially when engaging loud patients, encourages a similar effect and patients may often become increasingly calm and reduce their volumes in turn. Notably, the converse is also true; displaying signs of agitation, brusque movements, or anxiety, may trigger a comparable reaction in the patient.

Patients presenting with a potential risk of violence can be provided a "choice" by clinicians with clear and simple but firm and enforceable limits. Reasonable choices help empower the patient and can create a feeling of positive reward for good behavior. For example, in the management of a patient in a waiting room being verbally abusive to staff, a clinician can provide an intuitive choice, "Mrs. J., we are eager to take care of you and really want to treat your pain, but we can only do so if you stop using disrespectful language to our staff. Will you follow our rules and allow us to take care of you?" Generally, it is better to imply consequences in this early stage.

For a patient at an "imminent" risk categorization, if verbal communication is attempted at all, it must be with clear listing of consequences that are readily enforceable. For example, a show of force with security guards may be appropriate when providing

Table 2.1. Ten domains of de-escalation[40]

1. Respect personal space

2. Do not be provocative

3. Establish verbal contact

4. Be concise

5. Identify wants and feelings

6. Listen closely to what the patient is saying

7. Agree or agree to disagree

8. Lay down the law and set clear limits

9. Offer choices and optimism

10. Debrief the patients and staff

this choice, "Ms. J, please sit down and stop yelling or you cannot remain in this area." If compliance is obtained, then it may be appropriate to display a positive gesture. "Ms. J, thank you for following the rules, let me explain why you cannot be in this area and see if I can help expedite your care." Often, agitated patients may develop positive rapport with a particular individual. It is appropriate to exploit that relationship to reduce the patient's risk of violence. Conversely, staff members who appear to inflame or aggravate patients should limit their interaction with the patient if possible.

Efforts to use communication to modify behavior can be challenging and likely emotionally demanding. However, when properly utilized in disruptive and threatening patients, it can be a powerful tool in preventing escalation to physical violence.

Staff response to severely agitated or violent patients should focus both on the patient and the immediate environment.[42,45,58] Establishing a safe environment while managing others must be a priority. Some basic pointers should be kept in mind. Never turn your back on a hostile or potentially hostile patient; avoid approaching the agitated patient from behind; and maintain a safe distance, about an arm's length away, from the agitated patient. If possible, interviews and communication with severely agitated persons should always take place in a quiet area, away from other patients and general staff. Bystanders may inadvertently worsen the situation, and the very presence of others may amplify a need for the patient to grandstand, reducing the possibility of de-escalation. Ideally, interviews and communication with severely agitated persons should take place in pre-identified safe and quiet areas. Staff should have a very low threshold for activating security to escort the patient to a safe environment and ensuring a close security presence throughout the initial assessment. The presence of a security force, even without any overt actions, conveys an implicit boundary and can help motivate patients to be compliant with behavioral limits. Moreover, security personnel can be critical in preventing injury to clinical staff. (Please see Table 2.1 regarding the "Ten domains of de-escalation" as originally published by the Project BETA group.)

"Seclusion" and safe rooms for patients should be utilized for the management of patients with emergent violence and possibly for those with imminent violence as well. These rooms or areas should be large enough to allow the entrance of multiple security personnel, should emergent physical restraint be necessary. The room should have minimal furniture, and any furniture should be solid and difficult to move or overturn. There should be no loose objects that could easily become projectiles. This includes sharp objects, pencils/pens, or items easily branded as weapons. A path of egress should always be available and the patient should never be allowed to obstruct the doorway. The safe room door should always be open during an interview. If security is not immediately at hand, alarm technology or other signals to promptly activate an immediate security presence should be readily available.

Patients in the emergent violence phase have very limited response to verbal negotiations. In such situations, it is imperative that full engagement of the patient occurs in a safe zone, as described above, and that the patient is quickly and appropriately restrained. But it is still important, even as the patient is being restrained, to maintain appropriate professional demeanor and offer a verbal choice to encourage behavioral compliance. Before initiation of restraints, there must be sufficient numbers of appropriately trained personnel available. In most cases, five people are required for full restraints: one person per limb and another person to stabilize the head.[67,68] All staff involved in restraining patients should undergo suitable training and have ongoing skill assessments.

Restraints with padding are the most frequently used.[45,58,67,68] Vests and other tools aimed at torso immobilization are also useful. A simple mask can help prevent spitting. (A soft collar to the neck can help prevent dangerous head turning and biting, but caution and careful observation must be used if any restraint device is placed on or near the neck.) The use of restraints does pose a risk of injury to the patient and as such, the need should be carefully balanced against the risks.[68–77] There are multiple reports of asphyxia and death after restraints[72,74,75] and there is increasing debate discouraging the use of prone restraints.[75–77] Seclusion or isolation, as compared to restraints, may be more effective in some situations as it allows for greater freedom of movement. Seclusion rooms should have strong walls that are not easily damaged. Caution should also be exercised when utilizing seclusion in young or very strong patients who may be at risk of self injury.[78]

Restraints and seclusion are tightly regulated and should be. The balance between safety and patient autonomy must be carefully considered. The Joint Commission offers strict guidelines and standards for the use of restraints; the guiding principle is that these interventions should be used as a last resort and for as brief a period as possible.[79] Any patient who requires restraint or seclusion should have close monitoring and frequent assessments at least every 15 minutes. Assessments should include signs of injury associated with application of restraints and seclusion, nutrition and hydration, circulation and range of motion in extremities, vital signs, hygiene and elimination, physical status and comfort, and readiness for discontinuation of restraint or seclusion.[79] Clinical staff are encouraged to be as thorough and circumspect as appropriate. The Joint Commission does recognize that frequent checks may aggravate an agitated patient and allows for the use of visual checks in certain circumstances.

Currently, the Joint Commission limits the use of restraints or seclusion orders to four hours for adults, two hours for children and adolescents aged 9 to 17 years, and one hour for children less than 9 years of age. The orders are renewable but should not exceed a maximum of 24 hours.[79] State law and individual hospitals may have even more restrictive requirements. Familiarity with your local policies and procedures are essential. (See Figure 2.4 for the algorithm of the use of seclusion and restraints as originally published by the Project BETA group.)

Physical restraints and seclusion are valuable initial tools. But these interventions should be judiciously applied and their use should be as temporary as possible. Chemical sedation

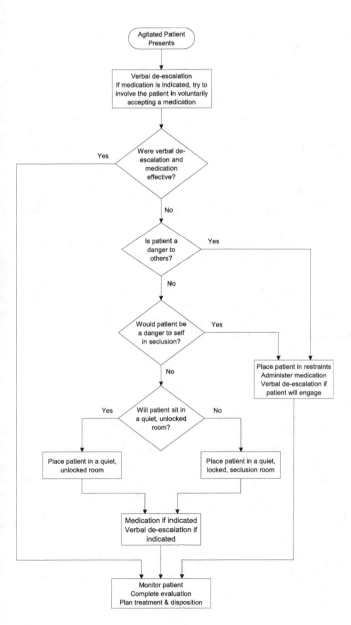

Figure 2.4. Use of seclusion and restraint[39]

is often a useful and necessary adjunct. Medications should be employed at the lowest dose appropriate to calm the patient and allow for safe clinical assessment, without necessarily inducing sleep. Benzodiazepines and antipsychotics are the most frequently utilized pharmacologic adjuncts for behavioral sedation.[80] Intramuscular administration is the preferred route.[81] Placement of intravenous access in patients who are not compliant is strongly discouraged, because of the risk of injury to both patient and provider.

Haloperidol is still the most frequently utilized antipsychotic.[80] It has a rapid onset of action and can be administered intramuscularly. Wilson et al., in a consensus statement for the American Association of Emergency Psychiatry, recommend haloperidol as a medication of choice in patients with agitation due to a psychiatric illness and alcohol intoxication.[37] Haloperidol does have significant side effects, including extra-pyramidal effects, which can be minimized with the use of anticholinergics.[82–84] Huf et al., in a Cochrane review, support the regimen of haloperidol and promethezine over haloperidol alone or benzodiazepines alone in the management of psychosis-induced aggression.[83] Haloperidol's other potential adverse effects include hypotension and dysrhythmias, like QT prolongation, Torsades de pointes, and sudden death. These risks are significantly increased with intravenous administration of haloperidol, which is accordingly discouraged. Additionally haloperidol should generally be avoided in elderly patients, patients with underlying cardiac abnormities, patients on medications that potentially prolong QT, or patients with the presence of significant electrolyte abnormalities. Notably, droperidol, a first-generation antipsychotic in class with haloperidol, which historically had been frequently used for acute agitation, is now much less utilized as it carries a black box warning, the strongest proscription from the FDA, relating to its risk of QTc prolongation and Torsades de pointes.

Second-generation antipsychotics are increasingly accessible and in some studies boast a reduced risk of acute extrapyramidal symptoms as compared to haloperidol alone.[83–86] Olanzapine, in particular, is well regarded by experts, appears efficacious, and has a duration of action considered shorter as compared to haloperidol.[80,83,85] However, second-generation agents generally have been poorly studied, especially in regards to adjunctive usage or relating to targeted causes of agitation, like intoxication. As such, further research and clinical experience is needed to clearly define the role of newer-generation agents in the management of acutely agitated patients.[37,84,86]

Benzodiazepines generally have an excellent sedative profile. However, respiratory depression is a significant adverse effect which limits their usage in patients with potential airway issues. Additionally, benzodiazepines may also cause paradoxical excitatory reactions. These paradoxical reactions are unpredictable and can manifest as an emotional release, excessive movement, and possibly even hostility and rage.[87,88] Several predisposing risk factors have been identified including a possible genetic link, extremes of age, alcoholism and psychiatric disorders.[87] These reactions can be generally managed supportively, although in extreme cases flumazenil may be administered.

Benzodiazepines are frequently used alone or in combination with antipsychotics.[80,89] Initially, some evidence suggested a trend towards improved sedation and decreased extra-pyramidal side effects when haloperidol was used in combination with lorazepam.[89,90] However, a Cochrane review by Gillies et al. on the use of benzodiazepines with or without antipsychotics revealed insufficient evidence to support or refute its use in such patients.[91] In another study, Lonergen et al. found no significant evidence in support of benzodiazepines for the treatment of acute delirium in hospital patients.[92] Benzodiazepines are still the preferred medication for the acute management of major alcohol withdrawal. Benzodiazepine usage is also favored by expert consensus, particularly as a first line agent in cases where little information is available and in patients who may exhibit violent tendencies related to stimulant intoxicants or alcohol.[80,93–97] Midazolam is increasingly displacing lorazepam as the benzodiazepine of choice.[80] Midazolam has a faster onset and a shorter half-life when compared to haloperidol and lorazepam.[83,95]

Successful restraint and sedation of an emergently violent patient should be coupled with an etiologic investigation as to the underlying cause of agitation and violence. However, such examinations should only be completed when safety of both patient and provider can be ensured. Collaborative information through pre-hospital providers, family, and other resources are often invaluable. Blanchard et al. suggest a classification that separates causes into organic versus functional causes.[17] (Also see Chapter 5.) Organic etiologies are classically viewed as having an underlying medical cause that explains the behavior change while functional causes are generally considered psychiatric in nature. Another classification system based on the use of diagnostic groups is recommended by Dubin et al. and is arguably more useful.[45] Broadly, the categories are: toxidromes and withdrawal states, seizure and postictal states, endocrine disorders, organic brain syndromes, acute psychosis, and paranoid and personality disorders. These diagnostic groups help focus the clinical evaluation in a manner that encourages specific corrective treatment.

Summary

Overall the management of the violent or agitated patient is multifaceted. It often begins with a risk factor review, based on as much information as available. The risk assessment, which includes an emphasis on early warning signs, incorporates risk factors and other social and behavioral cues and ultimately allows for patient risk categorization into emergent, imminent, and potential violence classes. Verbal negotiation is a valuable de-escalation tool that can be effective in patients with imminent and potential risk of violence. However, for patients who are emergently violent, the need for restraint and possible sedation may be necessary to protect the patient, staff, and the clinical functioning of the unit. All patients who require physical intervention for behavioral control should have close observation and frequent assessments. Moreover, there should be a care plan in place that allows the discontinuation of the restraints when appropriate. Instituting and adhering to a well planned protocol for the management of violent or agitated patients is important in the appropriate care for patients and to ensure a safe working environments for clinicians.

References

1. US Department of Health and Human Services – *National Institute of Occupational Safety and Health*. Violence in the Workplace. Available at http://www.cdc.gov/niosh/violcont.html

2. Goodman RA, Jenkins EL, Mercy JA. Workplace-related homicide among health care workers in the United States, 1980 through 1990. *JAMA*. 1994;272(21):1686–1688.

3. *Annual survey of occupational injuries and illnesses*. Washington, DC: U.S. Department of Labor, Bureau of Labor Statistics, 1994.

4. Campbell JC, Messing JT, Kub J, et al. Workplace violence: prevalence and risk factors in the safe at work study. *J Occup Environ Med*. 2011; 53(1):82–89.

5. McKenna BG, Poole SJ, Smith NA, Coverdale JH, Gale CK. A survey of threats and violent behaviour by patients against registered nurses in their first year of practice. *Int J Ment Health Nurs*. 2003;12 (1):56–63.

6. Gacki-Smith J, Juarez AM, Boyett L, Homeyer C, Robinson L, MacLean SL. Violence against nurses working in US emergency departments. *J Nurs Adm*. 2009;39(7–8):340–349.

7. Crilly J, Chaboyer W, Creedy D. Violence towards emergency department nurses by patients. *Accid Emerg Nurs*. 2004 Apr;12 (2):67–73.

8. Petzäll K, Tällberg J, Lundin T, Suserud BO. Threats and violence in the Swedish pre-hospital emergency care. *Int Emerg Nurs*. 2011;19(1): 5–11.

9. Chapman R, Styles I. An epidemic of abuse and violence: nurse on the front line. *Accid Emerg Nurs.* 2006;**14**(4):245–249.

10. Kwok RP, Law YK, Li KE, et al. Prevalence of workplace violence against nurses in Hong Kong. *Hong Kong Med J.* 2006;**12**(1):6–9.

11. Shiao JS, Tseng Y, Hsieh YT, Hou JY, Cheng Y, Guo YL. Assaults against nurses of general and psychiatric hospitals in Taiwan. *Int Arch Occup Environ Health.* 2010;**83**(7):823–832.

12. Camerino D, Estryn-Behar M, Conway PM, van Der Heijden BI, Hasselhorn HM. Work-related factors and violence among nursing staff in the European NEXT study: a longitudinal cohort study. *Int J Nurs Stud.* 2008;**45**(1):35–50.

13. King LA, McInerney PA. Hospital workplace experiences of registered nurses that have contributed to their resignation in the Durban metropolitan area. *Curationis.* 2006;**29**(4):70–81.

14. Anderson C, Parish M. Report of workplace violence by Hispanic nurses. *J Transcult Nurs.* 2003;**14**(3):237–243.

15. Lin YH, Liu HE. The impact of workplace violence on nurses in South Taiwan. *Int J Nurs Stud.* 2005;**42**(7):773–778.

16. Boz B, Acar K, Ergin A, et al. Violence toward health care workers in emergency departments in Denizli, Turkey. *Adv Ther.* 2006;**23**(2):364–369.

17. Blanchard JC, Curtis KM. Violence in the emergency department. *Emerg Med Clin North Am.* 1999;**17**(3):717–731.

18. Behnam M, Tillotson RD, Davis SM, Hobbs GR. Violence in the emergency department: a national survey of emergency medicine residents and attending physicians. *J Emerg Med.* 2011;**40**(5):565–579.

19. McAneney CM, Shaw KN. Violence in the pediatric emergency department. *Ann Emerg Med.* 1994;**23**(6):1248–1251.

20. Kowalenko T, Walters BL, Khare RK, Compton S. Michigan College of Emergency Physicians Workplace Violence Task Force. Workplace violence: a survey of emergency physicians in the state of Michigan. *Ann Emerg Med.* 2005;**46**(2):142–147.

21. Kansagra SM, Rao SR, Sullivan AF, et al. A survey of workplace violence across 65 U.S. emergency departments. *Acad Emerg Med.* 2008;**15**(12):1268–1274.

22. Fernandes CM, Bouthillette F, Raboud JM, et al. Violence in the emergency department: a survey of health care workers. *CMAJ.* 1999;**161**(10):1245–1248.

23. Anglin D, Kyriacou DN, Hutson HR. Residents' perspectives on violence and personal safety in the emergency department. *Ann Emerg Med.* 1994;**23**(5):1082–1084.

24. Jankowiak B, Kowalczuk K, Krajewska-Kułak E, Sierakowska M, Lewko J, Klimaszewska K. Exposure of doctors to aggression in the workplace. *Adv Med Sci.* 2007;**52**(Suppl 1):89–92.

25. Arimatsu M, Wada K, Yoshikawa T, et al. An epidemiological study of work-related violence experienced by physicians who graduated from a medical school in Japan. *J Occup Health.* 2008;**50**(4):357–361.

26. Fernandes CM, Raboud JM, Christenson JM, et al. The effect of an education program on violence in the emergency department. Violence in the Emergency Department Study (VITES) Group. *Ann Emerg Med.* 2002;**39**(1):47–55.

27. Arnetz JE, Arnetz BB. Implementation and evaluation of a practical intervention programme for dealing with violence towards health care workers. *J Adv Nurs.* 2000;**31**(3):668–680.

28. Holloman GH Jr, Zeller SL. Overview of Project BETA: Best practices in Evaluation and Treatment of Agitation. *West J Emerg Med.* 2012;**13**(1):1–2.

29. Simon HK, Khan NS, Delgado CA. Weapons detection at two urban hospitals. *Pediatr Emerg Care.* 2003;**19**(4):248–251.

30. Mattox EA, Wright SW, Bracikowski AC. Metal detectors in the pediatric emergency department: patron attitudes and national

prevalence. *Pediatr Emerg Care.* 2000;**16** (3):163–165.

31. Meyer T, Wrenn K, Wright SW, Glaser J, Slovis CM. Attitudes toward the use of a metal detector in an urban emergency department. *Ann Emerg Med.* 1997;**29** (5):621–624.

32. McNamara R, Yu D, Kelly JJ. Public perception of safety and metal detectors in an urban emergency department. *Am J Emerg Med.* 1997;**15**:40–42.

33. Rustin TA. Reducing contraband in a psychiatric hospital through the use of a metal detector. *Tex Med.* 2007;**103**(5): 51–56.

34. Rankins RC, Hendey GW. Effect of a security system on violent incidents and hidden weapons in the emergency department. *Ann Emerg Med.* 1999;**33** (6):676–679.

35. McNeil DE, Binder RL. Patients who bring weapons to the psychiatric emergency room. *J Clin Psychiatry.* 1987;**48**:230–233.

36. Rankins RC, Hendey CW. Effect of a security system on violent incidents and hidden weapons in the emergency department. *Ann Emerg Med.* 1999;**33**:676–679.

37. Wilson MP, Pepper D, Currier GW, Holloman GH Jr, Feifel D. The psychopharmacology of agitation: consensus statement of the American Association for Emergency Psychiatry project Beta psychopharmacology workgroup. *West J Emerg Med.* 2012;**13** (1):26–34.

38. Nordstrom K, Zun L, Wilson MP, et al., Medical evaluation and triage of the agitated patient: consensus statement of the American Association for Emergency Psychiatry Project BETA Medical Evaluation Workgroup. *West J Emerg Med.* 2012;**13**(1):3–10.

39. Use and avoidance of seclusion and restraint: consensus statement of the American Association for Emergency Psychiatry Project BETA Seclusion and Restraint Workgroup. *West J Emerg Med.* 2012;**13**(1): 35–40.

40. Verbal de-escalation of the agitated patient: consensus statement of the American Association for Emergency Psychiatry Project BETA De-escalation Workgroup. *West J Emerg Med.* 2012;**13**(1):17–25.

41. Stowell KR, Florence P, Harman HJ, Glick RL. Psychiatric evaluation of the agitated patient: Consensus statement of the American Association for Emergency Psychiatry Project BETA Psychiatric Evaluation Workgroup. *West J Emerg Med.* 2012;**13**(1):11–16.

42. Anderson TR, Bell CC, Powell TE, Williamson JL, Blount MA Jr. Assessing psychiatric patients for violence. *Community Ment Health J.* 2004;**40** (4):379–399.

43. Monahan J, Steadman HJ. *Violence and Mental Disorder: Developments in Risk Assessment.* Chicago, IL: The University of Chicago Press, 1994.

44. Johnson BR. Assessing the risk for violence. In Bell C (Ed.), *Psychiatric Aspects of Violence: Issues in Prevention and Treatment.* San Francisco, CA: Jossey-Bass, 2000.

45. Dubin WR. Evaluating and managing the violent patient. *Ann Emerg Med.* 1981;**10** (9):481–484.

46. Rao H, Luty J, Trathen B. Characteristics of patients who are violent to staff and towards other people from a community mental health service in South East England. *J Psychiatr Ment Health Nurs.* 2007;**14**(8):753–757.

47. Elbogen EB, Johnson SC. The intricate link between violence and mental disorder: results from the National Epidemiologic Survey on Alcohol and Related Conditions. *Arch Gen Psychiatry.* 2009;**66**(2):152–161.

48. Fazel S, Långström N, Hjern A, Grann M, Lichtenstein P. Schizophrenia, substance abuse, and violent crime. *JAMA.* 2009;**301** (19):2016–2023.

49. Hahn S, Muller M, Needham I, Dassen T, Kok G, Halfens RJG. Patient and visitor violence in general hospitals: a systematic review of the literature. *Aggression and Violent Behavior.* 2008;**13**:431–441.

50. Hazlett SB, McCarthy ML, Londner MS, Onyike CU. Epidemiology of adult psychiatric visits to US emergency departments. *Acad Emerg Med.* 2004;**11**(2):193–195.

51. Amore M, Menchetti M, Tonti C, et al. Predictors of violent behavior among acute psychiatric patients: clinical study. *Psychiatry Clin Neurosci.* 2008;**62**(3): 247–255.

52. Swanson JW, Holzer CE, Ganzu VK, et al. Violence and psychiatric disorder in the community: evidence from the epidemiological catchment area surveys. *Hosp Community Psych.* 1990;**41**:761–770.

53. Shetgiri R, Kataoka S, Ponce N, Flores G, Chung PJ. Adolescent fighting: racial/ ethnic disparities and the importance of families and schools. *Acad Pediatr.* 2010;**10**(5):323–329.

54. Sampson RJ, Morenoff JD, Raudenbush S. Social anatomy of racial and ethnic disparities in violence. *Am J Public Health.* 2005;**95**(2):224–232.

55. Otto R. Assessing and managing violence risk in outpatient settings. *J Clin Psychol.* 2000;**56**(10):1239–1262.

56. Cotten NU, Resnick J, Browne DC, Martin SL, McCarraher DR, Woods J. Aggression and fighting behavior among African-American adolescents: individual and family factors. *Am J Public Health.* 1994;**84**(4):618–622.

57. Berg A, Bell CC, Tupin J. Clinician safety: assessing and managing the violent patient. In Bell C (Ed.), *Psychiatric Aspects of Violence: Issues in Prevention and Treatment.* San Francisco, CA: Jossey-Bass, 2000.

58. Tintinalli JE, Stapczynski JS, Ma OJ, Cline DM, Cydulka RK, Meckler GD (Eds.), *Emergency Medicine: A Comprehensive Study Guide.* 7th ed. New York, NY: McGraw-Hill, 2011.

59. Zeller SL, Rhoades RW. Systematic reviews of assessment measures and pharmacologic treatments for agitation. *Clin Ther.* 2010;**32**(3):403–425.

60. Dolan M, Doyle M. Violence risk prediction. Clinical and actuarial measures and the role of the Psychopathy Checklist. *Br J Psychiatry.* 2000;**177**:303–311.

61. Snowden RJ, Gray NS, Taylor J, Fitzgerald S. Assessing risk of future violence among forensic psychiatric inpatients with the Classification of Violence Risk (COVR). *Psychiatr Serv.* 2009;**60**(11):1522–1526.

62. Woods P, Almvik R. The Brøset violence checklist (BVC). *Acta Psychiatr Scand Suppl.* 2002;**412**:103–105.

63. Almvik R, Woods P, Rasmussen K. Assessing risk for imminent violence in the elderly: the Brøset Violence Checklist. *Int J Geriatr Psychiatry.* 2007;**22**(9):862–867.

64. Downey LV, Zun LS. Violence prediction in the Emergency Department. *J Emerg Med.* 2007;**33**(3):307–312.

65. Abderhalden C, Needham I, Miserez B, et al. Predicting inpatient violence in acute psychiatric wards using the Brøset-Violence-Checklist: a multicentre prospective cohort study. *J Psychiatr Ment Health Nurs.* 2004;**11**(4):422–427.

66. Lam LC, Chui HF, Ng J. Aggressive behaviour in the Chinese elderly – validation of the Chinese version of the rating scale for aggressive behaviour in the elderly (RAGE) in hospital and nursing home settings. *Int J Geriatr Psychiatry.* 1997;**12**(6):678–681.

67. Coburn VA, Mycyk MB. Physical and chemical restraints. *Emerg Med Clin North Am.* 2009;**27**(4):655–667.

68. Dorfman DH. The use of physical and chemical restraints in the pediatric emergency department. *Pediatr Emerg Care.* 2000;**16**(5):355–360; quiz 362–3.

69. Zun LS. A prospective study of the complication rate of use of patient restraint in the emergency department. *Emerg Med.* 2003;**24**(2):119–124.

70. Rubin BS, Dube AH, Mitchell EK. Asphyxial deaths due to physical restraint. A case series. *Arch Fam Med.* 1993;**2**(4):405–408.

71. Nunno MA, Holden MJ, Tollar A. Learning from tragedy: a survey of child and adolescent restraint fatalities. *Child Abuse Negl.* 2006;**30**(12):1333–1342.

72. Karger B, Fracasso T, Pfeiffer H. Fatalities related to medical restraint devices – asphyxia is a common finding. *Forensic Sci Int.* 2008;**178**(2–3): 178–184.

73. Retsas AP, Crabbe H. Breaking loose. Use of physical restraints in nursing homes in Queensland, Australia. *Collegian.* 1997;**4** (4):14–21.

74. Miles SH, Irvine P. Deaths caused by physical restraints. *Gerontologist.* 1992;**32** (6):762–766.

75. O'Halloran RL, Frank JG. Asphyxial death during prone restraint revisited: a report of 21 cases. *Am J Forensic Med Pathol.* 2000;**21**(1):39–52.

76. Chan TC, Vilke GM, Neuman T, Clausen JL. Restraint position and positional asphyxia. *Ann Emerg Med.* 1997;**30** (5):578–586.

77. Vilke GM, Chan TC, Neuman T, Clausen JL. Spirometry in normal subjects in sitting, prone, and supine positions. *Respir Care.* 2000;**45**(4):407–410.

78. American Academy of Child and Adolescent Psychiatry. Practice parameter for the prevention and management of aggressive behavior in child and adolescent psychiatric institutions, with special reference to seclusion and restraint. *J Am Acad Child Adolesc Psychiatry.* 2002;**42**:4S–45S.

79. Restraint and Seclusion for Hospitals that Use the Joint Commission for Deemed Status Purposes. Updated 2009. Available at http://www.jointcommission.org/ standards_information/jcfaqdetails.aspx? StandardsFaqId=260&ProgramId=1. Accessed Aug 2011.

80. Allen MH, Currier GW, Carpenter D, Ross RW, Docherty JP. Expert Consensus Panel for Behavioral Emergencies 2005. The expert consensus guideline series. Treatment of behavioral emergencies 2005. *J Psychiatr Pract.* 2005;**11** (Suppl 1):5–108.

81. Zimbroff DL. Pharmacological control of acute agitation: focus on intramuscular preparations. *CNS Drugs.* 2008;**22** (3):199–212.

82. Battaglia J. Pharmacological management of acute agitation. *Drugs.* 2005;**65**(9):1207–1222.

83. Huf G, Alexander J, Allen MH, Raveendran NS. Haloperidol plus promethazine for psychosis-induced aggression. *Cochrane Database Syst Rev.* 2009;**8**(3):CD005146.

84. Krakowski MI, Czobor P, Citrome L, Bark N, Cooper TB. Atypical antipsychotic agents in the treatment of violent patients with schizophrenia and schizoaffective disorder. *Arch Gen Psychiatry.* 2006;**63**(6):622–629.

85. Belgamwar RB, Fenton M. Olanzapine IM or velotab for acutely disturbed/agitated people with suspected serious mental illnesses. *Cochrane Database Syst Rev.* 2005;**18**(2):CD003729.

86. Satterthwaite TD, Wolf DH, Rosenheck RA, Gur RE, Caroff SN. A meta-analysis of the risk of acute extrapyramidal symptoms with intramuscular antipsychotics for the treatment of agitation. *J Clin Psychiatry.* 2008;**69**(12):1869–1879.

87. Mancuso CE, Tanzi MG, Gabay M. Paradoxical reactions to benzodiazepines: literature review and treatment options. *Pharmacotherapy.* 2004;**24**(9):1177–1185.

88. Hall RW, Zisook S. Paradoxical reactions to benzodiazepines. *Br J Clin Pharmacol* 1981;**11**:99S–104S.

89. Battaglia J, Moss S, Rush J, et al. Haloperidol, lorazepam, or both for psychotic agitation? A multicenter prospective, double-blind emergency department study. *Am J Emerg Med.* 1997;**15**:335–340.

90. Bieniek SA, Ownby RL, Penalver A, Dominguez RA. A double-blind study of lorazepam versus the combination of haloperidol and lorazepam in managing agitation. *Pharmacotherapy.* 1998;**18** (1):57–62.

91. Gillies D, Beck A, McCloud A, Rathbone J, Gillies D. Benzodiazepines alone or in combination with antipsychotic drugs for acute psychosis. *Cochrane Database Syst Rev.* 2005;**19**(4):CD003079.

92. Lonergan E, Luxenberg J, Areosa Sastre A. Benzodiazepines for delirium. *Cochrane Database Syst Rev.* 2009;(4):CD006379.

93. Rund DA, Ewing JD, Mitzel K, Votolato N. The use of intramuscular benzodiazepines and antipsychotic agents in the treatment of acute agitation or violence in the emergency department. *J Emerg Med.* 2006;**31**(3):317–324.

94. Mayo-Smith MF, Beecher LH, Fischer TL, Gorelick DA, Guillaume JL, et al. Management of alcohol withdrawal delirium. An evidence-based practice guideline. *Arch Intern Med.* 2004;**164**(13):1405–1412.

95. Nobay F, Simon BC, Levitt MA, Dresden GM. A prospective, double-blind, randomized trial of midazolam versus haloperidol versus lorazepam in the chemical restraint of violent and severely agitated patients. *Acad Emerg Med.* 2004;**11**(7):744–749.

96. Shoptaw SJ, Kao U, Ling WW. Treatment for amphetamine psychosis. *Cochrane Database Syst Rev.* 2008;**8**(4):CD003026.

97. Jackson KC, Lipman AG. Drug therapy for delirium in terminally ill patients. *Cochrane Database Syst Rev.* 2004;(**2**):CD004770.

Chapter

3

Suicide assessments

Holly C. Wilcox, Annette L. Beautrais,
and Gregory Luke Larkin

Acknowledgements:
The authors wish to thank Dr. J. Raymond DePaulo for his helpful comments and
suggestions.

Background and introduction

Worldwide each year approximately 1,000,000 people die by suicide.[1] Using the most recent
national data, in 2008 in the US, over 36,000 people died by suicide. [CDC, WISQARS,
2011] In the US in 2009, the number of emergency department (ED) presentations for self-
harm was 374,486.[2] Suicide, which has tripled among young males in the US since the
1950s,[3] is the third leading cause of death among 10 to 24 year olds and accounts for 12%
of all deaths amongst 15 to 24 year olds.[4] Completed suicides "represent only the tip of
the public health iceberg."[5] Rates of suicidal ideation and suicide attempts are significantly
higher than suicide rates,[4,6] with an estimated 10–200 suicide attempts for each completed
suicide.[4] However, these numbers may be even higher. Suicide rates are likely underesti-
mated due to state or religious sanctions on reporting, insurance considerations, family
and community sensitivity, the variation in professions and qualifications of individuals
entrusted with the delineation of suicide, and issues involving how to define suicide.[7]

Patients with mental health-related admissions are the fastest growing subgroup of ED
patients.[8] Between 1992 and 2001, ED visits specific for suicide attempts and self-injury
increased from 0.8 to 1.5 visits per 100 US population, a 47% increase, and mental health-
related visits increased 27.5%, from 17.1 to 23.6 per 1000.[9,10] EDs now have an increasing
role in the mental health care of patients whether insured or uninsured due to the following:
the Emergency Medical Treatment and Active Labor Act (EMTALA) legislation, mental
health insurance carve outs, and changes in mental health and primary care service
accessibility (closure of psychiatric inpatient facilities, limitations in accessibility of some
outpatient mental health facilities, limited number of practitioners in some areas, reductions
in inpatient psychiatric beds, and increased costs of general practitioner visits).[11,12] The ED is
now the *de facto* immediate health care option for suicidal patients.[13] Suicide attempts
account for 2–3% of all ED visits with rates as high as 5.4%.[14] However, suicidal thoughts
are prevalent among patients who present to EDs for non-psychiatric reasons. Claassen and
Larkin (2005) reported that, when questioned in the ED specifically about suicidal ideation,
11% of patients presenting for non-psychiatric reasons reported passive suicidal ideation
and 8% thought actively about killing themselves;[15] many of these patients would not have

---

Emergency Psychiatry, ed. Arjun Chanmugam, Patrick Triplett, and Gabor Kelen. Published by
Cambridge University Press. © Cambridge University Press 2013.

spontaneously disclosed suicidal ideation.[16] Similarly, Ilgen and colleagues (2009), found that of 5641 patients seeking routine, non-suicide-related care in an inner-city ED, approximately 8% reported some form of suicidal ideation within the previous two weeks.[17]

The existence of a subgroup of patients who repeatedly are seen in the ED with suicide ideation and attempts reflects the need for the medical community to adequately address the distress and improve the coping skills of these patients. A 10-year longitudinal study found that after an index suicide attempt, 28.1% were readmitted for a further non-fatal attempt and 4.6% died by suicide.[18] Risk for suicide among suicide attempters seen in EDs is highest in the days and weeks immediately after discharge. Crandall and colleagues (2006) found that suicide rates among those seen in an ED for suicide attempt or ideation, self-harm, or overdose were approximately six times higher than in ED patients with non-suicide-related visits.[19] ED visits provide a window of opportunity for assessment and intervention for patients at risk for suicide who may not be seen in other sites such as primary care or outpatient psychiatric services.[20] One challenge in working with suicide attempters is to find innovative ways to enhance engagement with mental health services in post-ED referrals, and thereby minimize management failure visits to the ED.[11]

Current standards of care in EDs for suicidal patients

The needs of psychiatric patients, especially those expressing suicidal thoughts and behaviors, are inconsistent with the fast-paced contemporary operations of most US EDs, which are designed for rapid, effective responses to patients with highly acute medical conditions such as acute coronary syndromes, strokes, sepsis, and severe traumatic physical injuries. Patients with primary psychiatric presentations not only don't fit this model, but may even "get in the way" of staff trying to care more efficiently for the patients that do fit the model.

Currently, no US-developed evidence-based standards exist for ED management of suicidal patients, with the exception of proposed guidelines for adolescents.[21] As a result, the approach to detecting and managing suicidal individuals varies widely throughout the US and sometimes even within individual departments. At least four problems may contribute to the lack of standardization.

(1) Some feel that emergency physicians training in the assessment and management of patients with suicide risk is limited because rotation(s) on a psychiatry service is not a specific education requirement of the Accreditation Council for Graduate Medical Education, the residency certifying body. However, there is no evidence that residency trained, board certified, emergency physicians have any failings greater than psychiatrists in this regard.

(2) Others feel that many patients with elevated risk do not receive appropriate care in the ED, or at follow-up. Again, this has not been specifically shown, but rather is inferred by lack of time and resources in both ED and outpatient referral settings.

(3) EDs expend substantial resources providing services to ED patients presenting with suicidal thoughts who may be at minimal risk of suicide; there are no guidelines to help distinguish suicidal patients who are at high risk from those with minimal risk. As a result EDs expend substantial resources providing services to all ED patients presenting with suicidal thoughts even though only a tiny fraction are at serious risk. Further, in emergency settings, there is a zero tolerance among the public and medical field for discharging a patient who ultimately makes an attempt soon after. Unfortunately, the risk factors (discussed below), and high sensitivity but poor specificity even in the hands

of highly experienced practitioners (psychiatrists, psychologists, social work counselors, and emergency physicians) compel acute care providers to be comprehensive in the evaluation of any patient who presents with suicidal ideation.

(4) There are approximately 4000 general EDs in the US, of which only 4% house psychiatric specific areas (also known as psych EDs). Thus, the vast majority of patients with suicide-related issues will be seen in general EDs,[22] yet many general EDs do not have ready access to mental health services and, in many communities, there is a shortage of outpatient mental health services.[12,23,24]

An efficient and effective method to assess and intervene with suicidal ED patients is needed.[25] ED-based strategies involving assessment and brief interventions are especially important when mental health services are not available in EDs or in the community. National mental health associations have called for self-harm care pathway protocols and algorithms that improve the standard and continuity of care for individuals at risk for suicide following discharge from EDs.[26] The idea of establishing a "chain of care" in terms of guidelines for the psychosocial follow-up and care for suicidal individuals after ED or psychiatric hospital discharge shows promise for reducing suicide.[27,28] Increasing communication between secondary and primary care following an ED admission is one obvious way to improve the chain of care for patients discharged from EDs.[29]

Risk and protective factors for suicide

A previous suicide attempt is one of the most powerful predictors of likelihood of subsequent completed suicide[30–32] as 1% of those with an attempt will go on to die by suicide in the next 12 months.[33] Patients who present with self-harm are at high risk for future suicide with 50 to 100 times increased risk for suicide within the first year, compared to the risk in the general population.[33–35] In Britain, Gairin and colleagues found that 39% of those who die by suicide had visited an ED in the previous 12 months, with more than one third of these visits for self-harm.[36]

Another well-established risk factor for suicide is suicide intent. Indicators include wanting to die, premeditation, avoiding discovery at the time of attempt, and suicide plans. Suicide intent at the time of self-harm is associated with short-term (within 12 months) risk of subsequent suicide.[37] In one UK study almost 80% of women and two thirds of men who went on to die by suicide had high suicide intent scores at the ED assessment following their index attempt.[37] The lethality of the method used in an index attempt (medical seriousness of the attempt as assessed by a physician) is the strongest predictor of suicide risk.[38]

Studies that use standardized interviews at the time of ED presentation consistently find that 90% of patients who present with self-harm have psychiatric disorders including alcohol and substance dependence. The association with risk of suicide is strongest for depression.[39,40]

A family history of suicide or suicidal behavior is associated with increased risk for suicide.[30,41] Trait aggression and impulsivity are well-known risk factors and together comprise a candidate endophenotype for suicidal behaviors.[42] Childhood trauma, including childhood physical or sexual abuse, severe enough to meet criteria for PTSD, is an important risk factor for suicidal behaviors.[30,43,44] Access to lethal means of suicide such as firearms are important as up to 50–70% of suicides in the US are associated with such weapons.[45,46] Recent losses and acute psychosocial stressors such as job loss, the deterioration of physical health, marital dissolution, and other interpersonal losses are all important risk factors for suicide.[47–49]

Military personnel and veterans are two other groups with special needs who have an elevated risk for suicide. There also has been increased awareness that in Veterans Health Administration settings, people with traumatic brain injury (TBI) are at greater risk for suicide, compared with those without TBI.[50] Male veterans with bipolar disorder and female veterans with substance use disorders are at particularly high risk of suicide.[51] Caucasian white males over age 85 have the highest suicide rates in the United States.[3] Those who die by suicide are more likely than those who survive an attempt to be older, male, living alone, or physically ill.[52] Patients with this profile who present to the ED need to be carefully assessed and referred in view of their suicide potential. Young females aged 15–19 are the demographic group seen most frequently in EDs with non-fatal suicide attempts. These attempts made by young females are typically of low suicide intent and low medical lethality.[53] However, while their risk of suicide is lower than that of older white males, a small fraction of these young female attempters will make future lethal attempts. Since it is difficult to predict with any certainty which of these young females are most at risk of further attempts, careful evaluation is also needed in this population.

Compared to factors associated with increased suicide risk, there is less evidence about factors potentially protective for suicide, and some debate about whether nominated protective factors are merely the obverse of risk factors.[54] Beyond good physical and mental health, limited data suggest protection is offered by social connectedness,[45] personal resilience and good problem-solving skills,[55] the early identification and appropriate treatment of psychiatric illness,[32] religious or cultural beliefs opposed to suicide,[56,57] and lack of access to guns.[45,58] Table 3.1 summarizes factors which may increase suicide risk and those that may confer some protection against suicide.

Suicide screening in EDs

All patients, including those who apparently need only evaluation for suicidal behavior (defined here as suicide ideation or attempt), require a medical evaluation. The approach and extent required are discussed in Chapter 1, and will not be repeated here. There are currently no evidence-based practices for the systematic assessment of suicide risk in ED patients. Unique aspects of many ED settings (i.e., busy, pressured, crowded, under-resourced) require that assessment be brief, cost-effective, easy to understand, and capable of being rapidly scored and assisting ED staff in making a disposition decision.[59] Appropriate identification of people at risk for a suicide re-attempt is a key objective of assessing suicide risk. Patients who present to the ED with suicidal ideation, suicide plans, or suicide attempts require specific measures for self-protection.[52] Any items that could be used in a suicide attempt must be removed from the patient's possession as well as the treatment room. The patient must remain under the supervision of a staff member or a reliable family member at all times. Some EDs have patient monitors or members of the security staff available to provide supervision for suicidal patients. Wait times should be minimized for patients with suicidal ideation, and these individuals should not be allowed to leave the ED before a psychiatric evaluation is completed.[52]

Unfortunately, accurate prediction of suicide following self-harm is restricted by a low base rate and by the low positive predictive power of strongly associated factors. Two cohort

Table 3.1. Risk and protective factors for suicide

Factors	May increase suicide risk	May lessen suicide risk
Social factors		
Sex	Male	Female
Age	<19, >65 years	Middle-aged adult
Marital status	Widowed, divorced, separated (especially recent separation)	Married
Living arrangements	Lives alone	Lives with family, partner
Children	No children	Children, especially dependent and aged <18 years
Work	Unemployed	Employed
Relationships	Conflict laden	Stable
	Socially isolated, without good support	Supportive social relationships
Life events	Stressful life events especially recent, shameful	No recent life events
Health		
Physical	Chronic illness	Healthy
	Degenerative illness	
Mental	Depression	
	Schizophrenia	
	Alcohol and drug dependence	
	Panic disorder	
	Personality disorder especially borderline, narcissistic, antisocial	
	Aggressive, violent behavior	
Suicidal behavior		
Suicide attempt	Previous attempt	
	Recent	
	Multiple	Single or no suicidal history
	Planned	Impulsive
	Rescue unlikely	Likely to be found and rescued
	Lethal method	Less lethal method
	Regrets surviving	Relieved to survive
	Clearly states determination to make another attempt to die	Large attention, appeal component
Suicidal ideation	Pervasive	Fleeting
	Intense	Mild
	Has a clear plan with method and has access to method	Lacks clear plan
Cognitive factors and symptoms		
	Hopelessness	Some optimism
	Not future oriented	Some plans for the future
	Few reasons for living	Numerous, strong reasons for living
	Unstable affect	Appropriate affect
	Anhedonia	
	Insomnia	No sleep disturbance

Table 3.1. (cont.)

Factors	May increase suicide risk	May lessen suicide risk
	Inability to focus and concentrate Psychomotor agitation	Can focus
Relationship with health professional		
	Lacks insight	Insight
	Lacks rapport	Rapport
Contextual factors		
	Access to lethal means	

Adapted from: Goldney RD, Beautrais AL. Suicide and suicidal behaviour. In Bloch S, Singh BS (Eds.), *Foundations of Clinical Psychiatry*. Melbourne: Melbourne University Press, 2007.

studies have followed large samples of attempters. In a cohort of approximately 8000 people with self-harm who presented to EDs in northern England, suicide risk was highest in the first six months after self-harm, suggesting that interventions initiated in the ED or implemented immediately after ED presentations might be helpful.[35] Subsequent suicide after an ED presentation was associated with not living with a close relative, avoiding discovery at the time of the index self-harm, alcohol misuse, previous psychiatric treatment, and physical health problems. Tidemalm and colleagues (2008), using Swedish registry data, studied the impact of co-existent psychiatric morbidity on risk of suicide after hospitalization for a suicide attempt in almost 40,000 people.[60] Death from suicide was more common in the first years after the suicide attempt, especially in those with schizophrenia and bipolar or unipolar depression. These findings underlie the need for suicide risk screening to be closely linked to focused aftercare during the first two years after suicide attempt, especially for those with existing mental disorders.

Although there are well over 20 suicide risk scales, a "gold standard" suicide risk assessment tool does not currently exist.[61] The goal of any risk assessment framework is categorization and linkage to decision-making.[25] Evaluating risk and risk stratification are critical to maximizing the effectiveness of existing services and for identifying and reducing service gaps. Risk stratification models are used in ED settings to improve clinical care for many medical conditions with the potential for adverse outcomes such as pneumonia, pulmonary embolus, syncope, and acute coronary syndrome,[62] yet such strategies have not been well developed for suicide risk. Suicidal ED patients have a continuum of risk.[63] Psychosocial assessment of personal circumstances, social context, mental state, and suicide risk is central to the clinical management of self-harm.[64,65]

Managing patients with complex clinical presentations, especially those with a history of self-harm without a clear history of psychiatric disorder or suicidal intent, can be challenging.[64] Some of that challenge may be due to difficult behavior at presentation, failure to cooperate with physical exam and physical treatment, physical aggression, agitation and self-discharge.[66] Self-discharge (leaving the ED without a completed exam or psychiatric assessment) is a particular concern as these patients are often at increased risk of repeat attempt and suicide.[66]

Screening: Screening for suicide risk is a cost-effective mechanism for identifying those requiring evaluation and treatment as indicated. Because many EDs do not have staff with specialized mental health training, screening tools to guide ED staff in the rapid and accurate detection of risk for suicide and the improved care and management of ED patients at risk for suicide are important.[6] The goal of screening is to increase the proportion of at-risk individuals receiving appropriate and effective mental health services and to correctly identify those at lower risk that may not need a psychiatric evaluation and referral. Screening programs are usually conducted in two stages: (1) screen for suicide risk; (2) assess those who screen positive for suicide risk with a more comprehensive approach. Screening can identify people who are developing symptoms before the symptoms become severe and lead to a suicide attempt that may be fatal, and can quantify the level of suicide risk in order to guide appropriate referral.

Screening instruments should be accurate (sensitive and specific), practical, easy to administer, not burdensome to ED staff or to the patients screened, adaptable to a variety of ED settings, and with clear linkage between level of risk and available referral resources. The fast pace of ED settings is not conducive to suicide risk screening using many of the established instruments, which are time-consuming to administer,[67] designed to be administered only by clinicians, and require cumbersome calculation and review by trained mental health professionals.[6] Brief and easy-to-administer scales that have been used in ED settings are the SAD PERSONS scale,[68] the Risk Assessment Matrix (RAM), used mainly in the UK,[67] and the Risk of Suicide Questionnaire (RSQ), which has been used with adolescent ED patients.[6] Many scales have moderate to high sensitivity, but provide many false-positive results indicating poor specificity (i.e., they incorrectly identify ED patients as being at high risk), which could increase the burden on scarce psychiatric resources. However, this is strongly preferable to low sensitivity (i.e., missing those at risk). Screening programs have rarely been evaluated but could have value as part of a comprehensive approach to suicide prevention.

Using a risk stratification model, Cooper and colleagues reported that four questions used as a brief screening tool (any history of self-harm, prior psychiatric treatment, benzodiazepine use in index attempt, and any current psychiatric treatment) correctly identified 94% of patients who repeated self-harm in the next six months. However, specificity was 25%.[69] In a pediatric population, Horowitz and colleagues found that current and past suicidal behavior, past self-destructive behavior, and current stressors yielded the highest sensitivity.[6]

A rapid and automated suicide risk assessment that is available at all times in the ED would provide ED staff with a valuable tool for the evaluation of these complex clinical situations and increase the opportunity to successfully intervene.[66] Computerized self screening of all non-trauma ED patients might be an efficient and feasible way to help identify those at risk of suicide.[15] As psychopathology in the ED population in general is greater than that found in the general public, a comprehensive approach needs to extend beyond those who present with mental health problems.[11]

Despite the difficulties in predicting suicide risk,[70] all patients with mental health-related ED visits should be assessed for such risk. The modified SAD PERSONS scale (MSPS) (Table 3.2) is a widely used suicide risk assessment for ED providers.[71] It is based on the first letters of 10 evidence-based suicide risk factors.

These letters underlined in the table represent 10 areas of assessment. There is a summed scoring approach for the modified SAD PERSONS: a score of $>=6$ on the weighted-MSPS had a sensitivity of 94% and a specificity of 71% in identifying patients requiring hospitalization. A score of $<=5$ had a negative predictive value for hospitalization of 95%.

Table 3.2. Modified SAD PERSONS scale

Risk factor	Criteria	Scoring
Sex	Male	1
Age	Less than 19, greater than 45	1
Depression or hopelessness	Patient admits to depression or decreased concentration, appetite, sleep, or libido	2
Previous suicide attempts or psychiatric care	Previous suicide attempt; or inpatient or outpatient psychiatric care	1
Excessive alcohol or drug use	Stigmata of chronic addiction or recent frequent use	1
Rational thinking loss	Organic brain syndrome or psychosis	2
Separated, divorced, or widowed		1
Organized or serious attempt	Well thought out plan or "life-threatening" presentation	2
No social supports	No close family, friends, job, or active religious affiliation	1
Stated future intent	Determined to repeat attempt or ambivalent	2

The modified SAD PERSONS scale includes recommendations for disposition and is relatively easy to use. However, predicting risk for suicide is much more complex than risk assessments suggest at face value. The modified SAD PERSONS risk assessment assigns risk level based on empirically derived weighting whereas the original SAD PERSONS scale assigned risk on the basis of a point system which assumes that the 10 factors are equally weighted.[68] It may be challenging for ED staff to remember all 10 factors from memory. However, in the age of personal digital assistants, electronic patient records, and ready access to internet and intranets, lack of ready access to any helpful medical instruments is unlikely in most settings.

The SAD PERSONS scale has been adapted for use with children and adolescents (Adapted-SAD PERSONS Scale; A-SPS).[72] The child and adolescent specific risk factors addressed in the A-SPS are sex; age; depression or affective disorder; previous attempt; ethanol/drug abuse; rational thinking loss; social supports lacking; organized plan; negligent parenting, significant family stressors or suicidal modeling by parents or siblings; and school problems.

The SAD PERSONS scale is useful in helping non-psychiatrists to quickly and easily obtain the objective information necessary to make an initial assessment of risk for suicide but should not be used in isolation.[73] No high quality validation studies of the assessment have been published to date. This assessment has limitations but is a significant improvement over a less structured approach. The American Psychiatric Association and the workgroups involved in version 5 revisions of the *Diagnostic and Statistical Manual of Mental Disorders* have created and are field testing a clinician-rated suicide risk assessment scale which appears to show improvements over existing suicide risk assessment measures.

Interventions delivered in ED settings

Traditionally, suicidal patients in ED settings have been referred to a psychiatric ED, inpatient hospitalization, or for outpatient treatment in their community. However, changes in mental health infrastructure make this model outmoded.[22] Controlled trials which have evaluated interventions conducted in the ED to reduce suicidal behavior are rare. Of those conducted, most focus on pediatric or adolescent populations.[72] Effective interventions for all populations are greatly needed.

There have been a few promising interventions identified. For example, an ED-based intervention for treating suicidal adolescents designed to improve ED care and outcomes (through training of ED staff on compassionate, non-judgmental techniques, an educational videotape, family treatment sessions with a crisis counselor) combined with free access to brief family-based cognitive behavioral therapy (CBT) was shown to be associated with improved treatment adherence, reduced depression levels, and less severe suicidal ideation, with some gains maintained over an 18-month follow-up period.[74,75] A multisite randomized trial of a brief information session combined with systematic long-term contact/follow-up among suicide attempters identified in EDs was part of the Multisite Intervention Study on Suicidal Behaviors (SUPRE-MISS) project launched by the World Health Organization in 2000.[76–78] This study applied the same intervention protocol to 1867 attempters in five countries. The dropout rate at 18 months was only 9%. The "Brief Intervention and Contact" (BIC) treatment, in addition to Treatment as Usual (TAU), involved a one-hour protocolized individual information session emphasizing that suicidal behavior is a sign of psychological/social distress. The BIC program also reviewed participants' risk and protective factors for suicide, basic epidemiology, risk for repetition, alternatives to suicidal behavior, coping strategies regarding treatment, and referral options. If the project staff determined that the patient needed more intensive treatment, a referral was made. As close to the time of discharge as possible and, up to 18 months post-ED discharge, nine follow-up contacts (phone calls or visits) at 1, 2, 4, 7 and 11 week(s) and 4, 6, 12 and 18 months were made by project staff with clinical experience (doctor, nurse, psychologist). Significantly, fewer deaths from suicide (0.2%) occurred amongst the BIC population compared to the TAU group (2.2%). An advantage of this study was that the BIC program required little training, in contrast to more sophisticated psychotherapeutic approaches (e.g., cognitive behavioral therapy).[78] This intervention can be carried out with limited resources of space, equipment and personnel, although the feasibility of such a program in low-resource community hospitals needs to be fully examined. Another intervention that has shown some success in children involves teaching parents. EDs provide a forum for "teachable moment" opportunities to recommend such important measures as removal of access to firearms as means of suicide. Education provided to parents in the ED resulted in action taken to limit access to handguns and other means that could be used by children and adolescents in a lethal suicide attempt.[79,80]

Larkin and colleagues have suggested that an approach used for alcohol intervention could be modified to deliver ED screening and brief safety intervention for suicidal behaviors. One of these is the Alcohol Screening, Brief Intervention and Referral to Treatment (ED SBIRT) to classify patients according to alcohol use and dependence as means to identify those at risk of related illness and injury.[81] In this approach, ED patients are quickly screened. Subsequently, staff deliver brief interventions (BI) to those deemed at risk using motivational interviewing techniques to increase patient awareness and motivation to change, and make facilitated referrals to longer-term treatment.[82] Staff are also trained to deliver interventions that are more comprehensive than BI alone and include assessment, patient education, teaching problem solving and coping skills, facilitating patient referrals to long-term care, and encouraging patients to develop a supportive social environment.[59]

The *Emergency Department Safety Assessment and Follow-up Evaluation Trial* (ED-SAFE) funded in 2009 by the National Institute of Mental Health is underway and expected to enroll nearly 1440 participants (half with ideation only and half with attempts) over five years in eight US EDs. This effectiveness study will: (1) design and test a standardized approach to universally screening ED patients for suicide risk that could be feasibly integrated into routine ED care yet maintain potency; (2) refine and test an ED-initiated intervention to reduce suicidal behavior among people who self-identify or screen positive for suicidal ideation; and (3) conduct an economic costs analysis.[83]

There is an ongoing Veterans Administration-funded clinical demonstration project called Suicide Assessment and Follow-up Engagement: Veteran Emergency Treatment Project (SAFE VET). This project includes an ED-based clinical intervention (safety planning, described below) and telephone follow-up care after ED discharge to maintain the patients' safety during the transition to outpatient care. At six months follow-up, veterans who received the SAFE VET intervention, as compared to controls, were at least twice as likely to be linked to mental health and substance abuse treatment (80% as compared to 10–40%) and the frequency of visits attended was higher in the intervention group. The next step of the project is to study the impact of the intervention on suicide-related outcomes.

Safety plans can be used as a brief ED intervention with suicidal patients. Ideally, safety plans should be developed following a comprehensive suicide risk assessment. A safety plan involves a prioritized written list of coping strategies and sources of support that patients can use during or preceding suicidal crises.[84] It provides patients with something more than just a referral and is useful when the opportunity or circumstance for longer-term care is limited. Components of a stepwise enacted personal safety plan include:

Steps	Coping strategies and sources of support
Step 1	Recognition of warning signs that may trigger a suicidal crisis
Step 2	Identification and employment of internal coping strategies without needing to contact another person
Step 3	Utilization of contacts with people as a means of distraction from suicidal thoughts and urges
Step 4	Contact with family members or friends who may help to resolve a crisis
Step 5	Contact with mental health professionals or agencies
Step 6	Reduction of the potential for use of lethal means (ie restrict access to lethal means)

Patients are instructed first to recognize when they are in crisis (step 1), and if suicidal ideation is not sufficiently decreased, then each subsequent step is enacted as outlined in the plan until the step that adequately decreases the level of suicide risk, as perceived by the individual and provider, is reached.[84]

The combination of a brief supportive informational session emphasizing adherence to treatment recommendations after ED discharge coupled with follow-up contact appears to be a cost-effective, practical, sustainable, ED intervention approach for adolescents and adults at risk for suicidal behaviors.

The quality of interactions with ED staff affects adherence to treatment.[85] ED interactions appear to be related to the rate at which adolescent suicide attempters keep their first follow-up appointment, although more studies are needed to better quantify the extent of that impact.[74]

Interventions delivered after ED or psychiatric hospital discharge

A series of interventions delivered after ED discharge may reduce the risk of further suicidal behavior. Multisystemic Therapy (MST),[86] an intensive family and community-based treatment that mobilizes resources and support, has been shown to reduce rates of subsequent suicide attempts and improve adjustment among youth in psychiatric crisis. MST was significantly more effective than emergency hospitalization at decreasing suicide attempt rates at a one-year follow-up.[86]

A randomized controlled trial of four sessions of a domiciliary psychodynamic interpersonal intervention,[87,88] designed to address interpersonal problems in ED patients after deliberate self harm, reduced suicide ideation and self-reported suicide attempts at six months follow-up.[89] However, this intervention is intensive and expensive and therefore not feasible in most settings or for broad implementation.

Intervention approaches that have focused on maintaining contact with suicidal individuals after ED-discharge have begun to show promise in reducing self-harm. A study that involved sending letters to patients who were discharged after hospitalization for depression or suicidal thoughts or behaviors resulted in a lower suicide rate in the contact group during the first two years after discharge compared to a group without contact.[90] Two other studies built on this concept by sending personally written postcards over a 12-month period.[86,87] The authors emphasize the value of an ED service model that emphasizes respect for the patient, high quality medical and psychiatric management, and follow-up. Many of the authors of these intervention trials suggest that the mechanism of intervention action is social connectedness for people lacking social support.

Telephone contact with psychiatrists who have experience in managing suicidal crises, one month after attempted suicide by deliberate self-poisoning, may help reduce the proportion of people who reattempt suicide by these means.[91] Telephone contact enables the detection of people at high risk of further suicide attempts and timely referral for emergency care. However, the timing of the contact is important as a delay of contact of three months appears to have no effect. It is hypothesized that the patient's motivation to change may also be greater just after the suicide attempt, which may provide for the optimal window of opportunity. Telephone contact is inexpensive and is generally acceptable to participants that have telephones.

Summary and recommendations

This chapter highlights the need for focused attention regarding patients who engage or contemplate self-harm including the need for more research and education, care models, and appropriate resources. Recent innovative programs have helped patients and are extremely important, but are just the beginning of what is needed. A sizeable number of individuals who have attempted suicide or who present with suicidal ideation or plans for suicide present initially to general EDs. Standard effective screening instruments do not yet exist. There are no accepted best practices for further evaluation of high-risk individuals and no practice standards for facilitating appropriate referrals for follow-up care.

Interventions that form a "chain of care" in which identification, assessment and interventions are integrated to improve patient outcomes appear to offer a model for best practice.[28,92] Ultimately, these approaches should be practical and feasible to implement widely within existing delivery and financing systems. In order to move toward forming a chain of care, the following priority areas need to be strengthened: (1) development of interventions that establish a strong bridge from ED referral to follow-up care; (2) identifying best-practice approaches for special high-risk populations (e.g., adolescents, elderly males, patients with schizophrenia or depression).

The risk for suicide death among attempters seen in EDs is clearly highest in the days and weeks immediately after discharge. Thus, it is essential to improve referral mechanisms to effective post-discharge suicide prevention services. Given the absence of evidence-based ED practices for the assessment and treatment of suicidal behaviors, this is an area of great research opportunity. Interventions that focus on enhancing engagement and adherence to follow-up mental health treatment are needed. An important goal is to help ED patients to recognize the necessity of post-ED visit access to mental health services.[21] ED services for suicidal patients need to be tailored for different demographic and age groups. Adolescent females have the highest rate of ED self-harm presentations, yet adolescents are often excluded from ED interventions.[89] Two other groups of concern are adult males and older adults whose risk is accentuated with certain associated factors or conditions. Unique strategies are needed for adolescents and elderly individuals that are more family-focused as these age groups have legal guardians or may rely on family members for practical or financial support. Also, these two subpopulations may have more obstacles in getting to follow-up care appointments. Veterans, especially those with traumatic brain injury, are also at higher risk and more investigation on ED and post-ED interventions are needed. Finally, research is needed that addresses the cost effectiveness of all ED-based and ED-initiated suicide prevention approaches.

References

1. Krug EG, Dahlberg L, Mercy J, Zwi A, Lozano R. *World Report on Violence and Health*. Geneva: World Health Organization, 2002.

2. Pitts SR, Niska RW, Xu J, Burt CW. National Hospital Ambulatory Medical Care Survey: 2006 emergency department summary. *Natl Health Stat Report*. 2008;(7):1–38.

3. Goldsmith SK, Pellmar TC, Kleinman AM, Bunny WE (Eds.). Institute of Medicine. *Reducing Suicide: A National Imperative*. Washington, DC: The National Academies Press, 2002.

4. Centers for Disease Control and Prevention. Youth Risk Behaviors Survey 2010. Available at http://www.cdc.gov/HealthyYouth/yrbs/data/index.htm.

5. Frankenfield DL, Keyl PM, Gielen A, et al. Adolescent patients – healthy or hurting? Missed opportunities to screen for suicide risk in the primary care setting. *Arch Ped Adolesc Med*. 2000;**154**(2): 162–168.

6. Horowitz LM, Wang PS, Koocher GP, et al. Detecting suicide risk in a pediatric emergency department: development of a brief screening tool. *Pediatrics*. 2001;**107**(5):1133–1137.

7. Goldney RD. A note on the reliability and validity of suicide statistics. *Psychiatry, Psychology and Law.* 2010;**17**(1):52–56.

8. Larkin GL, Beautrais AL. The epidemiology of emergency department visits for suicide attempts in the South Pacific: New Zealand, 1997–2006. *Ann Emerg Med.* 2008;**51**(4):554–555.

9. Larkin GL, Beautrais AL, Gibb SJ, Laing S. The epidemiology of presentations for suicidal ideation to the Emergency Department. *Academic Emerg Med* 2008;**15**(5 Suppl 1):S208–S209.

10. Larkin GL, Claassen CA, Emond JA, Pelletier AJ, Camargo CA. Trends in U.S. emergency department visits for mental health conditions, 1992 to 2001. *Psychiatr Serv.* 2005;**56**(6):671–677.

11. Larkin GL, Beautrais AL. Emergency departments are underutilized sites for suicide prevention. *Crisis.* 2010;**31**(1):1–6.

12. Baraff LJ. A mental health crisis in emergency care. Emergency departments lack adequate in-house and community resources to care for suicidal patients. *Behavioral Healthcare.* 2006;**26**(11):39–40.

13. Fields WW, Asplin BR, Larkin GL, et al. The Emergency Medical Treatment and Labor Act as a federal health care safety net program. *Academic Emerg Med.* 2001;**8**(11):1064–1069.

14. Hazlett SB, McCarthy ML, Londner MS, Onyike CU. Epidemiology of adult psychiatric visits to US emergency departments. *Academic Emerg Med.* 2004;**11**(2):193–195.

15. Claassen CA, Larkin GL. Occult suicidality in an emergency department population. *Br J Psychiatry.* 2005;**186**:352–353.

16. Kemball RS, Gasgarth R, Johnson B, Patil M, Houry D. Unrecognized suicidal ideation in ED patients: are we missing an opportunity? *Am J Emerg Med.* 2008;**26**(6):701–705.

17. Ilgen MA, Walton MA, Cunningham RM, et al. Recent suicidal ideation among patients in an inner city emergency department. *Suicide Life Threat Behav.* 2009;**39**(5):508–517.

18. Gibb SJ, Beautrais AL, Fergusson DM. Mortality and further suicidal behaviour after an index suicide attempt: a 10-year study. *Aus New Zeal J Psychiatry.* 2005;**39**(1–2):95–100.

19. Crandall C, Fullerton-Gleason L, Aguero R, LaValley J. Subsequent suicide mortality among emergency department patients seen for suicidal behavior. *Academic Emerg Med.* 2006;**13**(4):435–442.

20. Asarnow Jr, Baraff LJ, Berk M. Pediatric emergency department suicidal patients: two-site evaluation of suicide ideators, single attempters, and repeat attempters. *J Am Acad Child Adolesc Psychiatry.* 2008;**47**(8):958–966.

21. Kennedy SP, Baraff LJ, Suddath RL, Asarnow JR. Emergency department management of suicidal adolescents. *Ann Emerg Med.* 2004;**43**(4):452–460.

22. Larkin GL, Beautrais A, Spirito A, et al. Mental health and emergency medicine: a research agenda. *Acad Emerg Med.* 2009;**16**:1110–1119.

23. Baraff LJ, Janowicz N, Asarnow JR. Survey of California Emergency Departments about practices for management of suicidal patients and resources available for their care. *Annals Emerg Med.* 2006;**48**(4):452–458.

24. Menchine MD, Baraff LJ. On-call specialists and higher level of care transfers in California emergency departments. *Acad Emerg Med.* 2008;**15**(4):329–336.

25. Wingate LR, Joiner TE, Jr., Walker RL, Rudd MD, Jobes DA. Empirically informed approaches to topics in suicide risk assessment. *Behav Sci Law.* 2004;**22**(5):651–665.

26. Parks J, Radke A, Mazade N. Measurement of Health Status for People with Serious Mental Illnesses. 2008. Available at http://www.nasmhpd.org/general_files/publications/med_directors_pubs/NASMHPD%20Medical%20Directors%20Health%20Indicators%20Report%2011-19-08.pdf.

27. Mehlum L, Mork E, Reinholdt NP, Fadum EA, Rossow I. Quality of psychosocial care of suicide attempters at general hospitals in

Norway – a longitudinal nationwide study. *Arch Suicide Res.* 2010;**14**(2):146–157.

28. Rossow I, Mehlum L, Gjertsen F, Moller B. Chain of care for patients with intentional self-harm: an effective strategy to reduce suicide rates? *Suicide Life Threat Behav.* 2009;**39**(6):614–622.

29. Lilley R, Owens D, Horrocks J, et al. Hospital care and repetition following self-harm: multicentre comparison of self-poisoning and self-injury. *Br J Psychiatry.* 2008;**192**(6):440–445.

30. Beautrais AL, Joyce PR, Mulder RT. Psychiatric illness in a New Zealand sample of young people making serious suicide attempts. *New Zealand Med J.* 1998;**111** (1060):44–48.

31. Brent DA, Perper JA, Moritz G, et al. Psychiatric risk factors for adolescent suicide: a case-control study. *J Am Acad Child Adolesc Psychiatry.* 1993;**32** (3):521–529.

32. Goldney RD. Suicide prevention is possible: a review of recent studies. *Arch Suicide Res.* 1998;**4**:329–339.

33. Hawton K, Fagg J. Suicide, and other causes of death, following attempted suicide. *Br J Psychiatry.* 1988;**152**:359–366.

34. Owens D, Horrocks J, House A. Fatal and non-fatal repetition of self-harm. Systematic review. *Br J Psychiatry.* 2002;**181**:193–199.

35. Cooper J, Kapur N, Webb R, et al. Suicide after deliberate self-harm: a 4-year cohort study. *Am J Psychiatry.* 2005;**162** (2):297–303.

36. Gairin I, House A, Owens D. Attendance at the accident and emergency department in the year before suicide: retrospective study. *Br J Psychiatry.* 2003;**183**(1):28–33.

37. Harriss L, Hawton K, Zahl D. Value of measuring suicidal intent in the assessment of people attending hospital following self-poisoning or self-injury. *Br J Psychiatry.* 2005;**186**:60–66.

38. Cooper JB, Lawlor MP, Hiroeh U, Kapur N, Appleby L. Factors that influence emergency department doctors' assessment of suicide risk in deliberate self-harm patients. *Eur J Emerg Med.* 2003;**10** (4):283–287.

39. Haw C, Hawton K, Houston K, Townsend E. Psychiatric and personality disorders in deliberate self-harm patients. *Br J Psychiatry.* 2001;**178**:48–54.

40. Harris EC, Barraclough B. Suicide as an outcome for mental disorders. *Br J Psychiatry.* 1997;**170**:205–228.

41. Wilcox HC, Kuramoto SJ, Lichtenstein P, et al. Psychiatric morbidity, violent crime, and suicide among children and adolescents exposed to parental death. *J Am Acad Child Adolesc Psychiatry.* 2010;**49** (5):514–523; quiz 30.

42. Mann JJ, Arango VA, Avenevoli S, et al. Candidate endophenotypes for genetic studies of suicidal behavior. *Biol Psychiatry.* 2009;**65**(7):556–563.

43. Wilcox HC, Storr CL, Breslau N. Posttraumatic stress disorder and suicide attempts in a community sample of urban American young adults. *Arch Gen Psych.* 2009;**66**(3):305–311.

44. Wilcox HC, Arria AM, Caldeira KM, et al. Prevalence and predictors of persistent suicide ideation, plans, and attempts during college. *J Affect Dis.* 2010;**127**(1):287–294.

45. Resnick MD, Bearman PS, Blum WR, et al. Protecting adolescents from harm: findings from the National Longitudinal Study on adolescent health. *JAMA.* 1997;**278**(10):823–832.

46. Centers for Disease Control. Source of firearms used by students in school-associated violent deaths – United States, 1992–1999. *Morbidity and Mortality Weekly Report.* 2003;**289**(13):1626–1627.

47. Goldney RD, Beautrais AL. Suicide and suicidal behaviour. In Bloch S, Singh BS (Eds.), *Foundations of Clinical Psychiatry.* Melbourne, Australia: Melbourne University Press, 2007.

48. Mann JJ. Neurobiology of suicidal behaviour. *Nature Rev Neuroscience.* 2003;**4**:819–828.

49. Cavanagh JT, Owens DG, Johnstone EC. Life events in suicide and undetermined death in south-east Scotland: a case-control

study using the method of psychological autopsy. *Social Psychiatry & Psychiatric Epidemiology*. 1999;**34**(12):645–650.

50. Brenner LA, Ignacio RV, Blow FC. Suicide and traumatic brain injury among individuals seeking Veterans Health Administration services. *J Head Trauma Rehab*. 2011;**26**(4):257–264.

51. Ilgen MA, Bohnert AS, Ignacio RV, et al. Psychiatric diagnoses and risk of suicide in veterans. *Arch Gen Psychiatry*. 2010;**67**(11):1152–1158.

52. Larkin GL, Beautrais AL. Behavioral disorders. In Tintinalli JE (Ed.), *Emergency Medicine*. In press.

53. Centers for Disease Control and Prevention. 2010. Available at http://www.cdc.gov/nchs/fastats/ervisits.htm.

54. Fergusson DM, Beautrais AL, Horwood LJ. Vulnerability and resiliency to suicidal behaviours in young people. *Psychol Med*. 2003;**33**:61–73.

55. Frederico M, Davis C. *Gatekeeper Training and Youth Suicide Prevention*. Canberra: Australian Catholic University, 1996.

56. Stack S. Marriage, family, religion, and suicide. In Maris RW, Berman AL, Maltsberger JT, Yusif RI (Eds.), *Assessment and Prediction of Suicide*. New York, NY: Guilford Press, 1992.

57. Stack S, Lester D. The effect of religion on suicide ideation. *Social Psychiatry & Psychiatric Epidemiology*. 1991;**26**:168–170.

58. Brent DA. Firearms and suicide. *Ann N Y Acad Sci*. 2001;**932**:225–239.

59. Larkin GL, Beautrais AL, Spirito A, et al. Mental health and emergency medicine: a research agenda. *Acad Emerg Med*. 2009;**16**(11):1110–9.

60. Tidemalm D, Elofsson S, Stefansson C-G, Waern M, Runeson BS. Predictors of suicide in a community-based cohort of individuals with severe mental disorder. *Social Psychiatry & Psychiatric Epidemiology*. 2005;**40**(8):595–600.

61. Patel AS, Harrison A, Bruce-Jones W. Evaluation of the risk assessment matrix: a mental health triage tool. *EMJ*. 2009;**26**(1):11–14.

62. Goldman L, Cook EF, Brand DA, et al. A computer protocol to predict myocardial infarction in emergency department patients with chest pain. *N Engl J Med*. 1988;**318**(13):797–803.

63. Asarnow JR, Baraff LJ, Berk M, et al. Pediatric emergency department suicidal patients: two-site evaluation of suicide ideators, single attempters, and repeat attempters. *J Am Acad Child Adoles Psychiatry*. 2008;**47**(8):958–966.

64. Kapur N, Murphy E, Cooper J, et al. Psychosocial assessment following self-harm: results from the Multi-Centre Monitoring of Self-Harm Project. *J Affect Disord*. 2008;**106**(3):285–293.

65. Jacobs DG. *Guide to Suicide Assessment and Intervention*. San Francisco: HC Printing, 1999.

66. Hickey L, Hawton K, Fagg J, Weitzel H. Deliberate self-harm patients who leave the accident and emergency department without a psychiatric assessment. *J Psychosomatic Res*. 2001;**50**:87–93.

67. Hart C, Colley R, Harrison A. Using a risk assessment matrix with mental health patients in emergency departments. *Emerg Nurse*. 2005;**12**(9):21–28.

68. Patterson WM, Dohn HH, Bird J, Patterson GA. Evaluation of suicidal patients: the SAD PERSONS scale. *Psychosomatics*. 1983;**24**(4):343–5.

69. Cooper J, Kapur N, Dunning J, et al. A clinical tool for assessing risk after self-harm. *Ann Emerg Med*. 2006;**48**(4):459–466.

70. Goldney RD. Prediction of suicide and attempted suicide. In Hawton K, van Heeringen K (Eds.), *The International Handbook of Suicide and Attempted Suicide*. New York, NY: John Wiley & Sons, 2000.

71. Hockberger RS, Rothstein RJ. Assessment of suicide potential by nonpsychiatrists using the sad persons score. *J Emerg Med*. 1988;**6**(2):99–107.

72. Juhnke G. The adapted-SAD PERSONS: a suicide assessment scale designed for use with children. *Elementary School Guidance & Counseling*. 1996;**30**(4):252–258.

73. Khan MM. Travellers on a dark journey: caring for a patient with chronic psychiatric illness. *Psychiatr Bull.* 2008;**32**:26–27.

74. Rotheram-Borus MJ, Piacentini J, van Rossem R, et al. Enhancing treatment adherence with a specialized emergency room program for adolescent suicide attempters. *J Am Acad Child Adolesc Psychiatry.* 1996;**35**(5):654–663.

75. Rotheram-Borus MJ, Piacentini J, Cantwell C, Belin TR, Song J. The 18-month impact of an emergency room intervention for adolescent female suicide attempters. *J Consulting Clin Psychol.* 2000;**68**(6):1081–1093.

76. Bertolote JM, Fleischmann A, DeLeo D, et al. Suicide attempts, plans, and ideation in culturally diverse sites: the WHO SUPRE-MISS community survey. *Psychol Med.* 2005;**35**:1457–1465.

77. Fleischmann A, Bertolote JM, De Leo D, et al. Characteristics of attempted suicides seen in emergency-care settings of general hospitals in either low- and middle-income countries. *Psychol Med.* 2005;**35**:1467–74.

78. Fleischmann A, Bertolote JM, Wasserman D, et al. *Brief intervention and ongoing contact for suicide attempters decreases subsequent deaths from suicide: a randomized controlled trial in Brazil, China, India, the Islamic Republic of Iran, and Sri Lanka.* Bulletin World Health Organization. 2008.

79. Kruesi MJ, Grossman J, Pennington JM, et al. Suicide and violence prevention: parent education in the emergency department. *J Am Acad Child Adoles Psychiatry.* 1999;**38**(3):250–255.

80. Larkin GL. Screening for adolescent firearms-carrying: one more way to save a life. *Ann Emerg Med.* 2003;**42**(6):808–810.

81. Academic ED SBIRT Collaborative. The impact of screening, brief intervention, and referral for treatment on emergency department patients' alcohol use. *Annals Emerg Med.* 2007;**50**(6):699–710.e6.

82. http://sbirt.samhsa.gov/documents/ SBIRT_guide_Sep07.pdf.

83. http://clinicaltrials.gov/show/ NCT01150994.

84. Stanley B, Brown G. *Safety Plan Treatment Manual to Reduce Suicide Risk: Veteran's Version.* Washington, DC: Veterans Health Administration, 2008.

85. Spirito A, Boergers J, Donaldson D, Bishop D, Lewander W. An intervention trial to improve adherence to community treatment by adolescents after a suicide attempt. *J Am Acad Child Adolesc Psychiatry.* 2002;**41**(4):435–442.

86. Huey SJ, Jr., Henggeler SW, Rowland MD, et al. Multisystemic therapy effects on attempted suicide by youths presenting psychiatric emergencies. *J Am Acad Child Adolesc Psychiatry.* 2004;**43**(2):183–90.

87. Shapiro D, Startup M. *Raters' Manual for the Sheffield Psychotherapy Rating Scale.* Leeds, England: Psychological Therapies Research Centre, University of Leeds, 1990.

88. Hobson R. *Forms of Feeling: The Heart of Psychotherapy.* London: Tavistock Publications, 1985.

89. Guthrie E, Kapur N, Mackway-Jones K, et al. Randomised controlled trial of brief psychological intervention after deliberate self poisoning. *BMJ.* 2001;**323**(7305):135–138.

90. Motto JA, Bostrom AG. A randomized controlled trial of postcrisis suicide prevention. *Psychiatric Services.* 2001;**52**(6):828–833.

91. Vaiva G, Ducrocq F, Meyer P, et al. Effect of telephone contact on further suicide attempts in patients discharged from an emergency department: randomised controlled study. *BMJ* 2006;**332**(7552):1241–1245.

92. Mehlum L, Mork E, Fadum EA, Reinholdt NP, Rossow I (Eds.). Is it possible to make hospitals and local communities collaborate better in the follow-up care for deliberate self harm patients? Evaluating the Norwegian national strategy for suicide prevention. XXIV World Congress – IASP, 2007.

Chapter 4

Managing substance abuse in the acute setting

Arjun Chanmugam, Dave Milzman, Curtis Bone, and Hahn Soe-Lin

Introduction

Substance abuse emergencies represent a unique set of challenges for physicians working in acute care settings. Patients presenting acutely with substance abuse issues often suffer from other psychiatric disorders, medical disorders, or frequently a combination of both. Furthermore, many patients who abuse alcohol, prescription drugs, or illicit drugs will present without revealing this fact at all. The prevalence of serious mental health disorders in patients with a history of substance abuse has been estimated to be over 25%.[1] Medical emergencies associated with substance abuse have been estimated to be 2 million visits per year according the Drug Abuse Warning Network (DAWN).[2]

Another challenge with substance abuse patients is the presence of "altered mental status" (delirium or stupor) associated with acute and subacute ingestions, which frequently confounds a provider's ability to obtain an accurate medical and psychiatric history and can obscure aspects of the examination. Furthermore, clinical presentations from different substance exposures and withdrawal states share common signs, potentially causing delays in definitive diagnoses. Finally, screening and detection through the utilization of toxicological analysis remains an imperfect and still developing technology. All of these challenges associated with substance abuse, in combination with potentially obscured medical and psychiatric comorbidities, often compel the clinician to make critical diagnostic and therapeutic decisions with incomplete information.

The prevalence of substance abuse in the general population is about 9%,[2,3] and in the Emergency Department (ED), the number of drug-related visits has increased by over 70% from 2004 through 2008. Substance dependence, as distinct from substance abuse, is a maladaptive pattern of use which is manifested by the following: (1) tolerance to the substance (need for increasing amounts or diminished effect with continued use), (2) withdrawal symptoms, or (3) frequent consumption beyond what is intended. Dependence is also manifested by (4) a persistent desire for the substance or by efforts to cut down or stop, (5) by excessive time spent in acquiring the substances, reduction of important social, occupational, or recreational activities related to the acquisition or consumption of the substance, or (6) the continued use despite persistent problems which the patient knows are related to the substance.[4] A significant number of patients who frequently abuse a substance will likely become dependent if they survive and continue to have access to the substance. Given that the percentage of patients suffering from both substance abuse and substance dependence is significant (see Figure 4.1), providers in acute care settings should be aware that

Emergency Psychiatry, ed. Arjun Chanmugam, Patrick Triplett, and Gabor Kelen. Published by Cambridge University Press. © Cambridge University Press 2013.

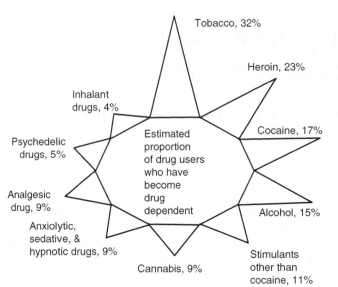

Tobacco, 32%

Heroin, 23%

Inhalant drugs, 4%

Psychedelic drugs, 5%

Cocaine, 17%

Estimated proportion of drug users who have become drug dependent

Analgesic drug, 9%

Anxiolytic, sedative, & hypnotic drugs, 9%

Alcohol, 15%

Cannabis, 9%

Stimulants other than cocaine, 11%

Figure 4.1. Estimated probability of drug dependence among drug users, by drug group. With permission from Anthony JC, Warner LA, Kessler RC. Comparative epidemiology of dependence on tobacco, alcohol, controlled substances, and inhalants: basic findings from the National Comorbidity Survey. *Exp Clin Psychopharmacol.* 1994;**2**:244–268.

substance dependence is a diagnostic entity that needs to be addressed in an appropriate setting. In some cases, acute intervention and specific management may be necessary, which may include an admission to an inpatient unit. All ED patients require outpatient follow-up. Understanding the issues that are associated with substance abuse can help the acute care provider make the most appropriate disposition and referral recommendations.

An examination of whether addiction is better regarded as a disease or as a behavior has manifestly practical implications for clinicians. According to the American Psychiatric Association, drug dependence is a chronic, relapsing disorder in which drug-seeking and drug-taking behaviors persist despite serious negative consequences. While there are common brain processes associated with most forms of dependence, these same systems also appear to be associated with addiction behavior.

The mesocorticolimbic system, which projects from the cortical area and the amygdala, has also been implicated. The dopaminergic subreceptor families of D1 and D2 appear to influence at least some addiction phenotypes.[5] Additional studies with highly selective D3 receptor antagonists indicate that the central D3 receptor may play a role in drug-induced reward and other drug-seeking behaviors.[6] This evolving understanding of the central pathways involved in dependence may help to provide novel substance abuse treatment modalities. It is likely that in the future, more specific therapies will be devised that target dopamine subreceptors as part of a more comprehensive management strategy.

The issue of whether we regard addiction as a disease or as behavior may be somewhat contentious but remains important. Both explanatory constructs have some virtue. It is pretty easy to see that in the dependent patient the decision to consume alcohol or heroin is not an unfettered free choice, but it is also true that most patients who successfully become abstinent have done so with great personal effort and choice. The application of the disease model makes the diagnosis less stigmatizing and serves to remind the physician that the prognosis is likely to be a long and possibly relapsing chronic condition. The application of the behavior model serves to remind that addiction can be viewed as a learned condition response and with the right interventions the patient can be motivated to make better decisions regarding their substance abuse.

In the acute care setting, the effects of drug addiction will certainly impact management decisions. However, the extent of that impact will vary depending on the individual, their past medical and psychiatric history, their current disease burden, the types and duration of substances abused and most importantly, the patient's commitment to substance abuse cessation. The medical and psychiatric management of substance abuse is complex because of the associated comorbidities (which often take precedence over immediate substance abuse issues), and the short- and long-term complications of substance abuse itself. The acute medical management of patients with substance abuse should involve a careful review of both medical and psychiatric illness, including a thorough physical examination and a mental status examination that includes an estimation of the degree of intoxication or drug effect.

When managing a patient with possible substance abuse, the following issues are worthy of consideration:

1. Estimates of substance abuse are thought to be underreported among ED patients. Alcohol is the leading substance of abuse in ED patients and has been responsible for nearly 68.8 million ED visits between 1992 and 2000. In addition to the visits due to alcohol abuse, there were 1.74 million ED visits in 2006 for other substances. Of these, 31% were for illicit drugs, 28% for abuse of prescription drugs, and 41% for a combination of alcohol and drugs.[7]

   Because substance abuse among ED patients is very common, a probing social history should be routinely sought, even in cases with an initial low suspicion. In addition, cultural stereotypes should be ignored. Patients who present to the ED tend to have higher rates of alcohol and substance abuse than the general population[3]; however, the problem is pervasive in all segments of society. Various screening tools, some associated with brief (acute setting) interventions, are being developed to help providers uncover abuse in certain populations.[8,9]

2. By definition, patients with a history of substance abuse are considered to have risky health behavior. Many of these patients will have more than one risky health behavior, including unsafe sexual practices. In conjunction with the high-risk profile and the direct effects of the substances abused, these individuals also tend to have more injuries than the general population. In particular, increased alcohol consumption tends to be associated with an increased risk of injuries, mainly those associated with motor vehicles.[10] In 2006, 32% of all motor vehicle fatalities involved alcohol intoxication.[11] Many of these cases involved individuals with prior alcohol-related vehicle collisions or those who had a history of significant alcohol addiction. In a recent meta-analysis, the amount of alcohol consumed was shown to increase the odds of injury.[9] Among traumatic brain injury (TBI) patients, 42% had a history of being heavy drinkers prior to injury, and 35–81% were alcohol intoxicated at the time of injury.[11] A high degree of suspicion of injury, especially the possibility of TBI, should be maintained when managing a patient with suspected substance abuse.

3. When patients with substance abuse present to the ED, there may be opportunities to mitigate their health risk through brief interventions.[12] As mentioned previously, several screening tools and brief ED-based interventions have been explored, but it appears that a multidisciplinary approach is needed. Acute care visits, although limited

by time constraints and resources, represent an important opportunity to engage at-risk patients towards better health care behaviors. The use of prescription and illicit drugs is among the most modifiable of health risks.

4. Sexual violence and substance abuse have been shown to be associated. Sexual abuse is a complex issue; patients with a history of substance abuse are vulnerable to sexual violence[13] and in nearly one third of sexual assault cases, the perpetrator was intoxicated with either alcohol or other drugs.[14] In addition, more than half of sexual assault cases are committed by someone known to the victim. Drug-related sexual assault is underreported and a growing concern, especially on college campuses, and is often associated with voluntary alcohol consumption.[15]

5. Patients who present with combative behavior and have a history of recent substance abuse may be at risk for excited delirium. This condition occurs in settings of significant physical exertion and is often associated with physical restraint, which can result in unexpected death.[16] These patients are often found to be in the custody of police.[17] The pathogenesis of this syndrome is not well understood, but is thought to be multifactorial, with drug toxicity, positional asphyxia, and catecholamine release all playing a role. Stimulants, including cocaine, methamphetamines, PCP and LSD, are the drug class most often related to excited delirium.[18]

6. Patients with a history of substance abuse or those with substance dependence are at a higher risk for suicidal thoughts and behaviors. A wide range of substances has been associated with completed suicide, suicide activity, and suicide ideation. Patients who present to an acute care environment should be carefully screened for suicide ideation or attempts.[19]

Patients with a dual diagnosis, that is, both mental illness and substance abuse, are not only at increased risk of suicide or self injury, but also at higher risk for drug abuse, poor medical compliance, and overall poor health.[20] Furthermore, patients with substance abuse who have comorbidities are likely to suffer further consequences because of their substance abuse. These can include, but are not limited to: loss of efficacy of medications, medical non-compliance, or exacerbation of organ dysfunction.[21] Management of patients with substance abuse, especially those with frequent ED visits, should involve examination of three domains: substance abuse, medical comorbidities, and mental health. While it is difficult to address every issue in each domain in the acute setting, priority should be placed on identifying the issues for each patient. In terms of successful planning to reduce substance abuse, intervention targets should include supportive housing, detoxification, rehabilitation, transition planning, and post-discharge patient support.[22]

While the full spectrum of ingested substances is beyond the scope of this chapter, the following is a brief overview of commonly presenting acute presentations related to substances of abuse, including clues to initial diagnosis and management. Although the acute ingestion of many substances of abuse in non-lethal amounts does not require sophisticated interventions, the underlying medical and/or psychiatric problems (including addiction), host stability, and other concurrent injuries can complicate management. For these reasons, patients who suffer from acute ingestion of substances of abuse require vigilance from care providers, including careful observation over time and consideration of possible complications that may not be evident on initial assessment.

Alcohol

Alcohol is one of the oldest and most prevalent substances of abuse. The global burden of ethanol intoxication is staggering, with an estimated 3.8% of global deaths and 4.6% of global disability-adjusted life years attributable to its abuse.[23] Alcohol also contributes to the calculable disease burden of numerous chronic conditions including neuropsychiatric disorders, cancer, diabetes mellitus, and more relevant to the acute setting, both unintentional and intentional injury.[24] In the US, mean annual consumption of alcohol was estimated at over 8 liters of pure ethanol per person, and ED visits attributable to alcohol occurred at a rate of 29 per 1000 US population.[25] Furthermore, alcohol-related disease was a comorbid component in up to 40% of hospital admissions.

The quantity and severity of acute alcohol intoxication symptoms are attributable to a variety of factors related to the person's body weight, tolerance level, time frame, and volume of alcohol consumed. The measurement of blood alcohol concentration (BAC) can yield a few dose-dependent generalizations. Clinically significant symptom onset occurs at concentrations as low as 50 mg/dl. Progressive increases in ataxia, dysarthria, and amnesia correlate with increasing BAC. There is increased risk of respiratory depression above 300 mg/dl, and death (without supportive management) generally occurs at concentrations in excess of 500 mg/dl,[26] but may occur at lower levels in alcohol naïve individuals.

It should be noted that ethanol intoxication occurs not only from alcoholic beverages, but also from a variety of common household substances that are present in the environments of both pediatric and adult populations. Substances such as mouthwash, cough syrup, and antifreeze contain additional chemical contaminants, such as phenol, antihistamines, methanol, and ethylene glycol, which present with comorbid toxidromes.[27]

The overall treatment of acute alcohol toxicity is supportive, with airway management, intravenous fluids, glucose, folic acid, and thiamine repletion as cornerstones of initial therapy.[28] However, it should be noted that vitamin repletion strategies have not been supported by evidence.[29]

Acutely, central respiratory depression leading to respiratory compromise is one of the major risks of severe alcohol intoxication. Aspiration due to emesis/reflux/regurgitation and an inability to protect one's airway secondary to depressed level of consciousness can contribute to respiratory compromise. Additionally, intentional or accidental head trauma, and in particular, occult TBIs associated with acute ETOH ingestion can contribute to central respiratory depression.[30] Once an individual's airway is secured, any patient presenting with possible head injury, impaired consciousness, poor recall or inability to provide a reliable history should receive a standard trauma survey and consideration for a timely head CT to exclude a potentially catastrophic intracranial hemorrhage.

Many intoxicated patients in acute care settings are observed and become ambulatory, often without a measured BAC. Measuring BAC accomplishes two important measures in a busy ED. First, it establishes a timeline for patient recovery and second, it provides evidence of whether alcohol intoxication is a reasonable explanation for the patient's depressed level of consciousness. If the BAC is lower than explanatory, then other causes such as head trauma or metabolic derangement must be explored. A positive BAC, however, does not rule out the existence of concomitant conditions such as TBI. For example, if the rate of mental status recovery is not within the expected rate, and aggressive search for alternate explanations must be undertaken. The practitioner must keep on guard for serious life-threatening emergencies in patients thought to be "severely intoxicated."

For most occasional users, BAC in the range of the legal limit of 80–100 mg/dl typically leads to some impaired judgment and memory and initial coordination deficits. Due to their high tolerance, it would not be unusual for a well-appearing chronic alcoholic to have BACs > 200 mg/dl. In contrast, many occasional drinkers may appear obtunded at this level. It is noteworthy that a BAC > 400 mg/dl has been fatal in 50% of adults mostly due to respiratory depression and airway compromise in the poorly monitored patient in the hospital or in the unmonitored out-of hospital setting.[31] Although breath analyzers do not directly measure BAC and are not appropriate for legal readings when administered in the ED, they do provide a rapid, reliable estimate of BAC.

Altered mental status is common in patients with acute intoxication and may persist in individuals acutely experiencing alcohol withdrawal. Severe memory disturbances, disorientation to people, place and time, and waxing levels of consciousness can be early signs of withdrawal. In some patients suffering from alcoholism, tremors may occur as quickly as within hours after a last drink. In addition, seizures, atrial fibrillation, or more serious ventricular arrhythmias can develop. Other acute perturbations of consciousness can be the result of a rapid progression to fever or electrolyte abnormality. Delirium tremens, which is a severe form of alcohol withdrawal involving significant central nervous system dysfunction, can occur within 72 hours after the last drink. Delirium tremens may occur up to 7–10 days after the last drink, and is a life threatening and occasionally fatal disease even in the modern era.

Although most acutely intoxicated patients do not require any acute medications, many EDs administer intravenous fluids. Additional vitamin supplements are often added when the intoxicated patient is believed to be a chronic alcoholic, and thus presumed thiamine, magnesium, and folate deficient. However, benefits to this approach remain unproven. Added supplements such as folic acid are given either PO, IM, or SC in doses of 0.4–1.0 mg daily. Magnesium sulfate may be given for hypomagnesemia PO, IM, or IV. The usual dose of thiamine is 100 mg intravenously administered once daily and is traditionally recommended prior to glucose administration in order to prevent the development of Wernicke encephalopathy (WE). WE is caused by acute thiamine deficiency and is generally underdiagnosed. WE may have variable neuropsychiatric presentations but presenting signs and symptoms often include gait and balance disorders, classic eye movement disorders (ophthalmoplegias), and altered consciousness, some of which can be closely mimicked by signs seen in ethanol intoxication.[32,33] It is important to treat clinically decompensating intoxicated patients with parenteral thiamine repletion. Permanent neurologic injury such as Korsakoff psychosis (a syndrome that can vary in its presentation but is often marked by short-term memory deficits, difficulty with learning new information, personality change, confabulation, and lack of insight into the problem) can occur. There are no laboratory values that are confirmatory and radiographic imaging with CT and MRI has produced few sensitive findings to aid diagnosis.

Brief motivational interventions

Given the significant medical and economic burden of alcohol intoxication and abuse on the general population, attention has more recently been focused on screening and intervention strategies to prevent recurrent abuse. Equally important is the recognition that an ED visit as a result of intoxication represents an important opportunity to provide meaningful alcohol counseling. Patients are often remorseful during the ED visit, because of the resultant self injury or inadvertent injury to others related to the alcohol abuse. As a result, patients may be more receptive to advice about alcohol and substance abuse issues during this time. This "teachable moment" represents an opportunity for intervention which could have long-term implications.

The use of alcohol screening tools in EDs continues to be a subject of research. An important distinction to note is that most of the available screening tools are designed for general screening as opposed to the individual who presents to the ED as a result of alcohol-related misadventure. In the latter case, the individual is already identified to be at risk for alcohol abuse and dependence, and additional screening may be unnecessary and possibly counterproductive.

A comprehensive strategy of Screening, Brief Motivational Intervention, and Referral to Treatment (SBIRT) has gained support from the National Institute of Alcohol Abuse and Alcoholism (NIAAA) and others for implementation in both emergency departments and primary care settings.[34] The functional implementation of such screening and intervention, however, remains in question, as evidenced by the variety of screening questionnaires, many of which are too long and cumbersome for realistic use in an acute care setting.

The four-question CAGE questionnaire is recommended by the NIAAA Physician's Guide B and referenced by the American College of Emergency Physicians.[35] More recently, comprehensive questionnaires that screen not only for alcohol but also tobacco and substance abuse have been in development. An example is the World Health Organization sponsored effort known as the Alcohol, Smoking, and Substance Involvement Screening Test (ASSIST) questionnaire. While also too cumbersome for emergency department use, this questionnaire is currently being modified by the National Institute on Drug Abuse (NIDA) in its recently developed NIDAMED questionnaire. The feasibility and efficacy of this recently developed tool in stratifying at-risk alcohol, tobacco, and substance abusers remains to be determined.[36,37]

Opioid abuse

Opioid abuse can take a variety of forms. Opioids may be smoked as opium, injected in the form of morphine or heroin, prescribed in pill form as codeine, hydrocodone, or hydromorphone, as a transdermal patch (fentanyl) or even as a lollipop (fentanyl). The signs and symptoms of abuse vary greatly with different modes of use, although the signs of withdrawal are all similar. Those that utilize parenteral forms of opioids or other injectable drugs place themselves at great risk for blood-borne diseases including HIV, HCV, HBV, bacterial endocarditis, and abscess formation as well as sepsis. Among IV drug user populations, the increased risk of contracting chronic and often fatal infectious diseases such as hepatitis C and HIV has been reported to be as high as 60% and 10% respectively.[38]

There continues to be a rapid rise in the number of people seeking or requiring medical care for opioid-related substance abuse. In the 2008 Drug Abuse Warning Network report, an estimated 200,000 visits to the ED were related to heroin abuse and more than 350,000 visits were related to non-medical use of opioid pain relievers.[39]

Acccording to the CDC, there is currently a growing, deadly epidemic of prescription painkiller abuse with nearly three out of four prescription drug overdoses caused by prescription opioid pain relievers. There has been a 300% increase in overdose deaths since 1999, which reflects the sale of these strong painkillers. These drugs were involved in 14,800 overdose deaths in 2008, more than cocaine and heroin combined.[40]

Decades of public health interventions and treatment methods have produced little progress; from 2004 to 2008 the number of ED visits has more than doubled for most pharmaceutical-grade opioid products.[2] Clinicians working in the emergency setting need to understand the varied effects of opioids and have the ability to recognize and treat acute intoxication-related problems as well as withdrawal conditions. Endogenous peptides from naturally occurring opioids, such as enkaphalins (Met and Leu), endorphins, and dynorphins, play a significant role in effects of opioids. Endorphins that bind G-protein coupled opioid receptors (GPCR mu, kappa and delta),[41] are most notably tied to cAMP signaling and perception of pain.[42] Both exogenous and synthetic opioids, like endogenous peptides, will trigger downstream signaling pathways via mu receptors that result in euphoria, analgesia, decreased respiratory drive, and GI stasis.[42] Synthetic modifications to morphine create substances with extended half-lives and increased potencies. Fentanyl, one of these synthetic narcotics, is an estimated 80–100 times more potent than morphine.[43] The problem many physicians have with the synthetic morphine derivatives is that their high potency makes them potentially dangerous in non-monitored settings because of their high rates of associated morbidity, mortality, and high abuse potential. Nearly 50% of heroin and other highly potent narcotics users experience a non-fatal overdose at some point in their lives and thousands of individuals die from opioid overdose annually.[44] Reports link the near doubling of overdose deaths from 1996 to 2006 to an increase in narcotic abuse.[45]

Common findings of opioid intoxication include respiratory and mental status depression, analgesia, and pupil constriction (miosis). The classic slowing of respiratory drive from narcotic overdosage results in carbon dioxide retention (respiratory acidosis) and hypoxia. Often the expected miosis is not present and specific opioids (such as meperidine) do not induce miosis. Situations can occur where drug combinations (e.g., atropine-like effects) may mask this finding. In sufficient doses, opioids will cause depressed respiratory drive and a decreased level of consciousness to the extent that airway management may be needed and empiric treatment with an opioid antagonist is indicated.[46]

Naloxone is the medication of choice for most opioid overdoses. Intravenous administration is the preferred route. If intravenous administration is not possible or not preferred, then intramuscular or subcutaneous administration are possible in both children and adults. Intranasal administration is gaining attention, especially as it avoids establishing intravenous access in patients who otherwise do not need it.

The safety of naloxone is well established in the pre-hospital setting,[47] but very rare episodes of rapid immersion from opioid toxicity have been associated with ventricular tachycardia and sudden death.[48] Naloxone can be safely administered intravenously at starting doses of 0.4–0.8 mg, which can be advanced to 2.0 mg as needed. For some long-acting narcotics, close observation and repeat dosing of naloxone at defined intervals may be required.[49] Naloxone's short half-life of 20 to 40 minutes makes it possible for patients to experience rebound toxicity, and without vigilance and further intervention, significant respiratory depression can occur, leading to death.[49] Approximately 1 mg of naloxone should counteract 25 mg of heroin. However, information about the type or quantity of opiate used is rarely available or reliable, however, when it is, this knowledge may be helpful in choosing an initial dose. The best measure is a trial dose based on response to treatment, with usual improvement seen within 1–2 minutes. If symptoms, especially hypoventilation, fail to improve, then increased doses of the naloxone should be administered. Some drugs with opioid effects such as propoxyphene may require as much as 10 mg of naloxone before reversal is accomplished.

The therapeutic administration of naloxone is normally considered safe, but it does carry some risks, including possible aspiration from GI upset and from vomiting. In addition, too much naloxone can induce acute withdrawal syndrome with catecholamine surges, resulting in hypertension, tachycardia, and arrhythmia.[50] Since the response is dose dependent, it is best to titrate naloxone to prevent sudden inducement of withdrawal with associated effects, such as severe vomiting. In most situations, careful administration of naloxone titrated for an adequate respiratory drive can help prevent significant withdrawal manifestations.

Although extremely uncomfortable, opioid withdrawal is not considered a medical emergency except among some patients with underlying comorbidities (i.e., coronary artery disease).[51] Maintenance therapies (clonidine, methadone, and buprenorphine) have been associated with decreased drug use, crime, overdose, and infectious disease.[50] Acute care providers should be familiar with the opioid withdrawal syndrome (OWS) and the commonly used therapeutics (see below). In addition, providers should be aware of the institutional, local, state, and federal policies and credentialing requirements related to prescribing of these medications.[52]

The opioid withdrawal syndrome is characterized by rhinorrhea, lacrimation, pilo-erection, yawning, cramping of intestines and extremities, dilated pupils, vomiting, and diarrhea.[53] Although not life threatening in itself, these patients are at increased risk for complications from inadequate monitoring or insufficient supportive treatment. Simple resuscitative measures include intravenous fluid starting at 20–30 cc/kg or 2–3 L of normal saline or lactated Ringers in adult patients, and anti-emetics as needed to correct losses from emesis and diarrhea. The peak and duration of these symptoms varies with the type of opioid used and its specific half-life. For heroin users, withdrawal symptoms begin after four to six hours of last use, peak at one to three days, and can last one to two weeks. For methadone users, onset of withdrawal symptoms typically begins at 36 hours, peaks at three to five days, and may last three to four weeks, based on prior exposures.[54]

Clonidine, a centrally-acting alpha 2 agonist, is an anti-hypertensive with additional activity in the locus ceruleus which can help to alleviate symptoms associated with the opioid withdrawal syndrome.[55] The known side effects of clonidine include dry mouth and sedation, which may be useful to a patient going through the withdrawal syndrome.[56] Clonidine dosing for withdrawal syndrome can begin at 0.2 mg of oral medications, with repeat doses at 1–2 hours, and can be adjusted to match the symptom severity.[56]

Methadone and buprenorphine for long-term addiction treatment

Methadone has nearly a century of use in addiction treatment with demonstrated efficacy in reducing heroin-related deaths, HIV infection, and hepatitis infections.[57] Since its introduction in 2002, buprenorphine has been used in the treatment of acute withdrawal and maintenance, but at this time while methadone still predominates as part of long-term maintenance programs, the utility of buprenorphine is in the short and intermediate time frame.

Methadone, when used for analgesia, is started at doses of 2.5–10 mg. Chronic users may require upwards of 60–80 mg every 6–8 hours with close initial observations for level of consciousness and respiratory depression. In acute opioid withdrawal, dosing should be determined based on severity of symptoms, as higher doses (20–80 mg) may be required for appropriate effect.[57] In accordance with local and federal requirements, only credentialed providers should be prescribing methadone for this indication. Recent awareness of methadone's potential to prolong the QT interval and induce Torsades des pointes has raised appropriate concerns on universal use.[58,59] Although this evidence only comes from case reports and series, the FDA has issued a black box warning for cardiac and respiratory depression, and clinicians should remain aware of this potential complication.

Buprenorphine, as compared to methadone, has a different mechanism with both a partial mu agonist and a kappa antagonist, and thus places a "ceiling effect" (about 16 mg) on the medication dosing.[41,42,60] Important to note is that low doses provide relief from withdrawal while high doses may induce a withdrawal syndrome.[61] Furthermore, it is believed that the kappa antagonist property of buprenorphine mitigates the level of respiratory depression experienced from the medication, which greatly limits its toxicity. As a result, death from overdose of buprenorphine is rare, especially compared to methadone.[62,63]

Cocaine/crack

Cocaine and its derivatives have long been substances of abuse in the US. A 2008 National Survey on Drug Use and Health (NSDUH) estimated 1.9 million (0.7% US population) current (within past 30 days) users, and of these, 18% were crack users.[64] Cocaine abuse leading to cocaine dependence involves increasing amounts of substance use for longer periods of time with unsuccessful attempts to stop or reduce dependency.[65] It should be noted that the development of cocaine dependence follows a somewhat different pattern compared to alcohol, benzodiazepines (BZDs), or opiates.

Cocaine, or benzoyl-methylecgonine, is a crystalline tropane alkaloid found in the chewable plant leaf erythroxylon cocoa.[66] The purified form is available as a white powder, typically a salt of alkaloid hydrochloride, or in its basic "freebase" form. The term "crack" comes from the sound heard when heating the freebase forms, as a chemical reaction occurs during this process, which produces additional byproducts such as methylecgonidine and accounts for different and deleterious effects of crack as compared with the cocaine salt.[67]

Blood testing for the presence of cocaine or its metabolites is typically not indicated, as symptoms do not correlate with plasma concentrations, and testing may be positive up to three days post-use. Similarly, urine testing, which is somewhat pH-dependent, may be positive for up to four days, and metabolites can be detected as late as a week after heavy use. The metabolite benzoylecgonine may be present in urine for as long as three weeks.[68] The ratio of benzoylecgonine to cocaine found in the urine can be used to assess recent ingestions; if the ratio is less than 100:1, then either the cocaine was ingested within 10 hours or less before sample collection or ongoing liberation of cocaine is occurring from a body package.[69]

Repeated cocaine or amphetamine use can lead to acute psychosis which is often characterized by delusions and hallucinations.[70] Agitated delirium, also known as excited delirium, is a fatal condition that can occur and is often marked by four phases, elevated temperature, severe agitation, respiratory depression, and death. It can occur as a result of cocaine toxicity, although other drugs have been implicated.[71] If the patient is acutely intoxicated, it is best to have the patient avoid excessive physical exertion. Although the mechanism causing death has yet to be elucidated, one explanation is that in excited delirium, there are varied adrenergic drivers that exacerbate cardiac arrhythmia and conduction abnormalities.[72]

Cocaine intoxication can generate ECG changes such as non-specific t-wave changes, and possibly QRS widening with/without tachyarrhythmia. Depending on pre-existing injuries to the heart and the effect cocaine has on the patient's myocardium, ECG findings can also include bundle branch blocks, bradyarrhythmias, ST elevations, and ventricular arrhythmias including ventricular tachycardia and fibrillation, thereby causing sudden death.[73]

The acute presentation of cocaine abuse is varied and involves the spectrum of short-lived autonomic arousal to sudden collapse and cardiac death. Second only to ethanol, cocaine and its derivatives now account for a significant number of ED visits and deaths.[73] It is common for cocaine to be found in patients who use other illicit substances. Many patients with acute cocaine intoxication will present with symptoms and signs of a significant adrenergic toxidrome, including some or all of the following findings: chest pain, tachycardia, hyper-dynamic precordium, hypertension, diaphoresis, myadriasis, agitation, and delirium as well as a drug-induced psychosis that can mimic schizophrenia symptoms.[74,75] Cocaine abuse is also associated with suicidal ideation and suicide attempts.

The standard approach to cocaine-induced chest pain is similar to the approach of acute coronary syndrome (ACS). The method includes administration of aspirin, nitroglycerin, and consideration of percutaneous coronary intervention in the face of ST elevation myocardial infarction (STEMI). However, two significant differences between the approaches is the strong recommendation not to use beta-blockers, and the consideration of BZDs, as they are a class I recommendation for ACS with considerable evidence for effectiveness specific to "cocaine chest pain."[75] Beta blockers should be avoided in patients who present with a history of cocaine use within the past 12–24 hours, as it is felt that unopposed alpha effects can cause severe hypertension and exacerbate myocardial ischemia.[76] Labetalol, which is one of the few beta blockers that is non-cardioselective, has an alpha to beta blocking ratio of 1:7 in parenteral form, and approximately a 1:3 ratio in oral drug formulation. Nevertheless, most sources discourage the use of medications with beta blocking activity in the acute setting.[77]

BZDs are the mainstay for treatment of tachycardia and hypertension associated with cocaine abuse as well as for cocaine-induced seizures. Since lorazepam has no active metabolites, there are some pharmacological advantages of using lorazepam over diazepam, such as a shorter onset and shorter but more effective duration.[78]

Benzodiazepines

BZDs are part of the sedative hypnotic class of medications. Therapeutic uses for BZDs include insomnia, muscle relaxation, anxiety, and in some cases, seizure prophylaxis. In the acute setting, BZDs are used primarily for seizure control, sedation, procedural sedation anesthetic adjunct, and acute alcohol withdrawal. BZDs have also led to a decrease in mortality rates when used as prophylaxis for alcohol withdrawal. Other acute care uses include the treatment of mania, psychosis, and sedation for agitated patients. Some patients are maintained on long-term BZD therapy, with the downside of a significant abuse potential for this class of medication.[79,80]

Since BZDs affect the GABA receptor, they share some commonalities with alcohol and are a mainstay in the treatment of alcohol withdrawal. BZDs mainly act on the central

GABA receptor, can produce respiratory depression and can result in hypoventilation and death, especially when used in combination with other sedative hypnotics such as alcohol.[81] Acute intoxication with BZDs causes slurred speech, disequilibrium, ataxia, amnesia, behavior changes, mood lability, psychosis, stupor, and coma.[82] As seen in alcohol withdrawal, abrupt cessation of long-term BZD abuse can result in seizures and possibly death. Safe and effective BZD withdrawal treatment often requires inpatient care, involving close observation, monitoring, and control of adrenergic side-effects.[83]

Chronic use of BZDs leads to the development of tolerance and dependence. Tolerance becomes highly problematic as the diminished pharmacological effect develops relatively quickly to the sedative, hypnotic, anticonvulsant, and muscle relaxant actions.[84] Developing tolerance to the anti-anxiety effects of BZD takes place more slowly. There is minimal effectiveness beyond four to six months of continued use[85] and there is a possibility that anxiety may worsen with long-term use.[85] Partial tolerance to the amnestic effects may develop, yet some reports have found that "the memory impairment is limited to a narrow window within 90 minutes after each dose."[86]

BZDs should never be abruptly stopped or severely reduced in dose without consideration for rebound and withdrawal. Even after a relatively short course of treatment (three to four weeks), rebound symptoms can occur. These may be symptoms that were present before treatment, and can sometimes be more severe than the initial symptoms. Withdrawal symptoms are the new symptoms that occur when BZD usage is stopped and are a reflection of physical dependence.[86]

The abrupt or rapid cessation of BZDs can create alcohol-like withdrawal symptoms, including seizures and delirium tremens, all of which can be fatal. Common withdrawal symptoms include insomnia, irritability, sweating, and hypersensitivity to stimuli. Psychiatric symptoms include de-personalization, de-realization, and more serious problems such as depression, suicidal behavior, and psychosis.[87,88]

Even gradual reduction can precipitate withdrawal symptoms; protracted symptoms can occur in approximately 10% of chronic BZD users, but symptoms gradually lessen over time, eventually disappearing altogether.[89] A slow and gradual withdrawal customized to the individual and psychological support (if indicated) is the most effective way of managing the withdrawal. A goal of less than six months has been suggested,[90] but specific dosing regimens and patient-specific conditions and needs may require exceedingly slow dose tapering over 6–12 months.[85,91] Optimal treatment for withdrawal is to begin the patient on a longer acting BZD, such as diazepam or chlordiazepoxide, since these two benzodiazepines have the longest half-life and are metabolized into long-acting active metabolites. The ability to fractionally reduce dose is aided by cutting pills or even using liquid formulations for more reliable and accurate dose reductions.

Phencyclidine (PCP)

Phencyclidine (phenylcyclohexyl piperidine, or PCP), as well as ketamine and dextromethorphan, are structurally related drugs that have been abused for their dissociative properties. PCP use can be found in all age groups, and unfortunately the popularity of these drugs has increased greatly in the past 10–15 years.[92] The psychotomimetic effects of these agents include euphoria, occasional violent behavior (made more dangerous from the drug's anesthetic effects), delirium and manic like states, as well as hyperthermia, rhabdomyolysis, metabolic acidosis and more lethal side effects of coma, seizures, and even cardiogenic shock.[93] Medical treatment is usually supportive, but if chemical restraints are required, haloperidol, ziprasidone, and benzodiazepines may be useful. Close monitoring, including ECG and respiratory status, is necessary to watch for significant metabolic derangements or other changes in a patient's condition.

The past 50 years have seen significant rises and falls in PCP abuse with a very recent rise again in PCP use. PCP was first developed as an induction anesthetic agent in the late 1950s and was found to produce agitation and dysphoria in the post-operative period, thereby leading to the discontinuation of commercial production and distribution in 1979. The abuse of PCP was first noted as a hallucinogen in the 1960s and later peaked as an abused substance in the 1970s. The most recent rise has occurred in the past decade, as it is often smoked together with marijuana and creates diagnostic confusion on initial presentation to many EDs.[94,95]

PCP is most often illegally sold as a powder, and dextromethorphan is commonly obtained from widely available over-the-counter cough and cold medicines. Due to its easy accessibility, dextromethorphan is more popular in younger to mid-teens.[96] Ketamine is not usually produced illegally but rather is stolen from pharmacies or veterinary sources for abuse.

PCP and its related pharmaceutical cousins produce psychotomimetic effects by antagonizing the N-methyl-d-aspartate (NMDA) receptors in both the limbic and cortical structures, which inhibits release of neuro-excitatory amino acid transmitters.[97] These agents also produce dose-dependent reuptake blockade of dopamine, serotonin, and norepinephrine, which creates the psychomotor, sympathomimetic, and psychotomimetic effects whereby patients feel fearless, supremely strong, and anesthetic to pain.[98] These dissociative effects, in addition to the common "out- of-body experience," render patients dangerous to themselves and others.

PCP is a lipophilic, weak base that is rapidly absorbed after almost all routes of ingestion, including oral, nasal, IV, and inhalation (smoking).[97] Usual onset of effects is dependent on the mode of ingestion; for instance, smoking produces effects within 2 minutes and oral intake brings upon effects within 30–60 minutes. Acute toxicity may peak within 6 hours and will fully resolve within 48 hours.[93]

PCP has an atypical predominance within the enterogastric circulation where significant amounts of the drug are found in the gut, with gastric fluid concentrations 50 times that found in the serum. The slightly acidic cerebral spinal fluid (CSF) increases trapping of PCP and creates CSF concentrations of the drug nine times greater than serum. As a result, the drug may take a longer time to clear.[98] PCP ingested orally has a large volume of distribution and is metabolized in the liver, with a significant first pass effect. Smoking and parenteral use do not clear via this method, as metabolites created from smoking PCP persist for up to one week and chronic abusers may maintain positive metabolites for up to one month.[98]

Horizontal, vertical, or rotary nystagmus is the classic neurologic finding to occur in over half of all intoxicated patients. Additional pupillary findings include meiosis and rapid reactivity. Due to the dissociative and anesthetic effects, patients are often unaware (or unconcerned) of even serious injuries.[93,99]

It is important to realize that, although rare, death does occur from PCP. A condition referred to as excited delirium occasionally occurs when violent patients aggressively exert themselves. Excited delirium usually results after these patients resist physical restraints. Furthermore, these patients can develop dangerous levels of rhabdomyolysis and rapidly worsening metabolic acidosis, hyperthermia, and sudden shock associated with cardiovascular collapse.

In order to reduce complications arising from rhabdomyolysis and metabolic acidosis, early and aggressive use of pharmacologic restraints is favored over physical restraints. Concern over non-productive attempts to restrain the patient or continued patient attempts to free themselves should prompt use of pharmacologic agents. However, physical restraint may be necessary initially to administer appropriate pharmacologic agents. Unlike other abused substances, there has been little reported success in "talking down" PCP intoxicated patients because persistent attempts could easily lead to violent outbursts. In addition to violent, aggressive behavior, prominent psychiatric effects of PCP include mania, catatonia, and visual hallucinations. Long-term PCP abuse is associated with diminished abstract thought and incidental memory.

PCP intoxication is usually an empiric diagnosis. Acute intoxication can usually be treated with an intramuscular injection of a BZD (usually lorazepam), of which starting doses range from 1.0–2.0 mg for adults. Lorazepam has a faster onset and offset than diazepam (starting dose 5–10 mg IM/IV). Midazolam, which has the shortest onset, is too fast acting and has too short a half-life to be effective in most patients (starting dose 2–4 mg IM/IV in adults). Ideally, the administration should be done by an experienced member of staff, especially with patients in need of physical restraint. Additional control has been achieved with haloperidol starting at 5.0–10.0 mg IM/IV, and escalating the dose as needed can occur but caution should be exercised. There has been excellent experience with combination therapy of an antipsychotic and a sedative, although the patient must be carefully monitored. Older protocols have used chlorpromazine, which has too low a therapeutic side effect spectrum and although the formerly new and popular ziprasidone had been exceedingly successful and well tolerated, there is now a black box warning. Starting doses for ziprasidone are 10 mg IM (not available for IV administration) in adult patients, but further dosing should be carefully titrated.[100]

There have been reports of success for chemical restraints with haloperidol and other antipsychotic medications, but the presence or potential development of metabolic acidosis, intravascular volume collapse, and hyperthermia make the use of chemical restraints occasionally problematic. The need for adequate fluid hydration is extremely important at preventing complications, such as rhabdomyolysis and the rare neuroleptic malignant syndrome. Clinicians should remain vigilant for electrolyte disturbances, metabolic acidosis, dehydration, and renal insufficiency.

MDMA (ecstasy)

Methamphetamines have a high abuse potential. The class of non-catechol sympathomimetic amines, or more specifically amphetamines, methamphetamines, and methylenedioxymethamphetamine (MDMA or ecstasy) have both acute and chronic abuse potential. (For example, the synthetic amphetamine-like substance, "bath salts," which is mephedrone based, has caused difficulty for law enforcement and hospitals as the numbers of patients and deaths have risen dramatically.) Usual routes of ingestion include oral, nasal insufflation, inhalation by smoking, and intravenous injection. A recent NIDA study in the US reported that over 14 million persons over age 12 had tried MDMA. Usage appears to be increasing, as 1.1 million Americans reported using MDMA for the first time in 2008, which was over a 20% increase from the 2007 first-time user rate.[101,102]

Amphetamines are weak bases with only limited renal excretion, so attempts at urine acidification are not recommended. It may actually cause untoward sequelae from resultant acute kidney injury.[103] Gastro-enteral clearance with activated charcoal is only indicated for large ingestions, usually reserved for body packers. MDMA popularity may be associated with its ability to increase alertness, cause euphoria, and give feelings of increased physical and mental capabilities. With repeated use, there is most likely a down-regulation effect of postsynaptic receptors as well as depletion of presynaptic stores of neurotransmitters in chronic abusers, thus requiring increased doses to obtain the same effect.[104,105] The acute use of the drug is associated with prolonged anorexia and insomnia. This is often followed by a recovery phase, which is associated with excessive recovery sleep and severe hunger.[105]

Prolonged use often results in depression and significant problems at home, work, and school, with the inability to complete assignments and uphold the previous responsible lifestyle.[106] Clinical findings of acute toxicity on exam include anxiety, visual and auditory hallucinations, hyper-vigilance, and paranoia.[104,107] The clinical presentation often includes chest pain, nausea/vomiting, anhedonia, headache, tachycardia, and elevated blood pressure. Less commonly, patients may have intra-cerebral hemorrhage, tachyarrhythmias, hemoptysis, or trismus. Many patients will have dilated pupils (sympathomimetic effect), skin lesions from self-mutilation, severe dental decay, and gingivitis (meth mouth).[110] Short and long-term memory loss may not return to baseline even after long periods of drug cessation. Laboratory findings may include hyponatremia and elevated serum creatine phosphokinase. Obtaining a liver function screening and a CK-MB and/or ECG testing (if cardiac involvement is suspected) is also highly recommended.[103,108]

There is little established evidence to guide treatment success. The typical agitation and "revved up" acute catecholamine surge symptoms appear to be best managed with BZDs and judicious use of rate controlling and blood pressure agents. Unlike cocaine, there is no absolute contraindication for beta blockade, but in the absence of proven safety, their use cannot be generally recommended except in critical hemodynamic emergencies that fail to control with other agents. Both droperidol and haloperidol have been found to better control the associated psychosis than BZDs.[109] (However, the increased sedation and possible respiratory depression along with the potential risk of QTc widening make these drugs potentially risky.) Careful monitoring of electrolytes is most important, as hyponatremia can easily occur because patient attempts at rehydration with free water worsen sodium levels and exacerbate already low levels.[110] Hepatic toxicity is well reported and concern over acute kidney injury also requires close monitoring.

The best care is supportive with sedation as needed as well as vigorous IV balanced salt solution administration (0.9% saline or lactated Ringers) to maintain good urine output of 1 ml/kg/hr. Caution with regards to attempting pharmacologic modification of heart rate may result in hemodynamic collapse. Antipyretics may induce serious uncoupling at the metabolic level and should be reserved for fever $> 39°C$.[118] New reports have found success with dantrolene for severe toxicities associated with high fever and onset of rhabdomyolysis.[111]

Summary

Substance abuse and dependence affects a great number of people, and as a result, acute care providers are likely to encounter such patients. Managing substance abuse and dependence requires an understanding that any patient, regardless of age and background, may be affected and that these patients may also suffer from medical and psychiatric comorbidities. A systematic and multidisciplinary approach that focuses on their medical conditions, the psychiatric disorders, and their social situation, as well as the specific substances of abuse will be useful in helping patients get the treatments they need. In some cases, such as those situations involving depression, anxiety, or suicidal ideation, the issues may be obscured, and thus careful evaluation is required to identify these situations. Helping patients to confront their substance abuse and related issues in the ED or other acute care settings may be difficult, but it is an important step in their journey towards improved health.

References

1. New Freedom Commission on Mental Health. *Achieving the Promise: Transforming Mental Health Care in America. DHHS, Final Report, Publication no. SMA-03-3832.* Rockville, MD: DHHS, 2003.

2. Substance Abuse and Mental Health Services Administration, Center for Behavioral Health Statistics and Quality (2011). Drug Abuse Warning Network, 2008. *National Estimates of Drug-Related Emergency Department Visits. HHS Publication No. SMA 11-4618.* Rockville, MD: HHS, 2011

3. http://www.cdc.gov/nchs/fastats/druguse. htm. Accessed September, 2011.

4. American Psychiatric Association. *Diagnostic and Statistical Manual of Mental Disorders, Fourth Edition, Text Revision (DSM- IV-TR).* Arlington, VA: American Psychiatric Association, 2000.

5. Le Foll B, Gallo, A, Le Strat, Y, Lu L. Gorwood P. Genetics of dopamine receptors and drug addiction: a comprehensive review. *Behav Pharmacol.* 2009;20(1):1–17.

6. Heidbreder CA, Gardner EL, Xi ZX, et al. The role of central dopamine D3 receptors in drug addiction: a review of pharmacological evidence. *Brain Res Rev.* 2005;49(1):77–105.

7. Bernstein SL. The clinical impact of health behaviors on emergency department visits. *Acad Emerg Med.* 2009;16(11):1054–1059.

8. Newton AS, Gokiert R, Mabood N, et al. Instruments to detect alcohol and other drug misuse in the emergency department: a systematic review. *Pediatrics.* 2011;128(1): e180–e192.

9. Vaca F, Winn D, Anderson C, Kim D, Arcila M. Feasibility of emergency department bilingual computerized alcohol screening, brief intervention, and referral to treatment. *Subst Abus.* 2010;31 (4):264–269.

10. Taylor B, Irving HM, Kanteres F, et al. The more you drink, the harder you fall: a systematic review and meta-analysis of how acute alcohol consumption and injury or collision risk increase together. *Drug Alcohol Depend.* 2010;110(1–2):108–116.

11. Opreanu RC, Kuhn D, Basson MD. Influence of alcohol on mortality in traumatic brain injury. *J Am Coll Surg.* 2010;210(6):997–1007.

12. Academic ED SBIRT Research Collaborative. The impact of screening, brief intervention, and referral for treatment on emergency department patients' alcohol use. *Ann Emerg Med.* 2007;50(6):699–710.

13. Luce H, Schrager S, Gilchrist V. Sexual assault of women. *Am Fam Physician.* 2010;81(4):489–495.

14. http://www.rainn.org/get-information/ statistics/sexual-assault-offenders. Accessed October, 2011.

15. Du Mont J, Macdonald S, Rotbard N, Asllani E, Bainbridge D, Cohen MM. Factors associated with suspected drug-facilitated sexual assault. *CMAJ.* 2009;180 (5):513–519.

16. Otahbachi M, Cevik C, Bagdure S, Nugent K. Excited delirium, restraints, and unexpected death: a review of pathogenesis. *Am J Forensic Med Pathol.* 2010;31(2):107–112.

17. Pollanen MS, Chiasson DA, Cairns JT, Young JG. Unexpected death related to

restraint for excited delirium: a retrospective study of deaths in police custody and in the community. *CMAJ.* 1998;**158**(12):1603–1607.

18. Takeuchi A, Ahern TL, Henderson SO. Excited delirium. *West J Emerg Med.* 2011;**12**(1):77–83.

19. Vaszari JM, Bradford S, O'Leary CC, Arbi BA, Cottler LB. Risk factors for suicidal ideation in a population of community-recruited female cocaine users. *Compr Psychiatry.* 2011;**52**(3):238–246.

20. Buckley PF. Prevalence and consequences of the dual diagnosis of substance abuse and severe mental illness. *J Clin Psychiatry.* 2006;**67** (Suppl 7):5–9.

21. Khalsa JH, Treisman G, McCance-Katz E, Tedaldi E. Medical consequences of drug abuse and co-occurring infections: research at the National Institute on Drug Abuse. *Subst Abus.* 2008;**29**(3):5–16.

22. Raven MC, Carrier ER, Lee J, Billings JC, Marr M, Gourevitch MN. Substance use treatment barriers for patients with frequent hospital admissions. *J Subst Abuse Treat.* 2010;**38**(1):22–30.

23. Vonghia L, Leggio L, Ferrulli A, et al. Acute alcohol intoxication. *Eur J Intern Med.* 2008;**19**:561.

24. Pletcher MJ, Maselli J, Gonzales R. Uncomplicated alcohol intoxication in the emergency department: an analysis of the National Hospital Ambulatory Medical Care Survey. *Am J Med* 2004; **117**:863.

25. LaVallee RA, Williams GD, Yi H. Alcohol Epidemiologic Data System. *Surveillance Report #87: Apparent Per Capita Alcohol Consumption: National, State, and Regional Trends, 1970–2007.* Bethesda, MD: National Institute on Alcohol Abuse and Alcoholism, Division of Epidemiology and Prevention Research, 2009.

26. Marco CA, Kelen GD. Acute intoxication. *Emerg Med Clin North Am.* 1990;**8**:731.

27. Yost DA. Acute care for alcohol intoxication. Be prepared to consider clinical dilemmas. *Postgrad Med.* 2002;**112**:14.

28. Boba A. Management of acute alcoholic intoxication. *Am J Emerg Med.* 1999;**17**:431.

29. Morse RM, Flavin DK. The definition of alcoholism. The Joint Committee of the National Council on Alcoholism and Drug Dependence and the American Society of Addiction Medicine to Study the Definition and Criteria for the Diagnosis of Alcoholism. *JAMA.* 1992;**268**:1012.

30. Hasin DS, Stinson FS, Ogburn E, Grant BF. Prevalence, correlates, disability, and comorbidity of DSM-IV alcohol abuse and dependence in the United States: results from the National Epidemiologic Survey on Alcohol and Related Conditions. *Arch Gen Psychiatry.* 2007;**64**:830.

31. Eckardt M, Harford T, Kaelber C. Health hazards associated with alcohol consumption. *JAMA.* 1981;**246**(6): 648–666.

32. O'Connor PG, Schottenfeld RS. Patients with alcohol problems. *N Engl J Med.* 1998;**338**:592.

33. Gilbertson R, Ceballos NA, Prather R, Nixon SJ. Effects of acute alcohol consumption in older and younger adults: perceived impairment versus psychomotor performance. *J Stud Alcohol Drugs.* 2009;**70**:242.

34. National Institute on Alcohol Abuse and Alcoholism. *Helping Patients Who Drink Too Much: A Clinician's Guide.* Bethesda, MD: National Institute on Alcohol Abuse and Alcoholism, 2005.

35. D'Onofrio G, Bernstein E, Bernstein J, et al. Patients with alcohol problems in the emergency department. Part 1: Improving detection. *Acad Emerg Med.* 1998;**5**:1200–1209.

36. Academic ED SBIRT Research Collaborative. The impact of screening, brief intervention, and referral for treatment on emergency department patients' alcohol use. *Ann Emerg Med.* 2007 Dec;**50**(6):699–710.

37. Newton AS, Gokiert R, Mabood N, et al. Instruments to detect alcohol and other drug misuse in the emergency department:

a systematic review. *Pediatrics.* 2011;**128** (1):e180–e192.

38. Pilon R, Leonard L, Kim J, et al. Transmission patterns of HIV and hepatitis C virus among networks of people who inject drugs. *PLoS One.* 2011;**6**(7):e22245.

39. Degenhardt L, Bucello C, Mathers B, et al. Mortality among regular or dependent users of heroin and other opioids: a systematic review and meta-analysis of cohort studies. *Addiction.* 2011;**106** (1):32–51.

40. CDC. Vital signs: Overdoses of prescription opioid pain relievers – United States, 1999–2008. *MMWR* 2011;**60**:1–6.

41. Harrison LM, Kastin AJ, Zadina JE. Opiate tolerance and dependence: receptors, G-proteins, and antiopiates. *Peptides.* 1998;**19**(9):1603–1630.

42. Waldhoer M, Bartlett SE, Whistler JL. Opioid receptors. *Annu Rev Biochem.* 2004;**73**:953.

43. Stanley TH. The history and development of the fentanyl series. *J Pain Symptom Manage.* 1992;**7**(3 Suppl):S3–S7.

44. Centers for Disease Control and Prevention. Overdose deaths involving prescription opioids among Medicaid enrollees – Washington 2004–2007. *MMWR* 2009;**58**(42): 1171–1175.

45. Sporer KA. Acute heroin overdose. *Ann Intern Med.* 1999;**130**(7):584–590.

46. Chamberlin JM, Klein BL. A comprehensive review of naloxone for the emergency physician. *Am J Emerg Med.* 1994;**12**(6):650–660.

47. Buajordet I, Naess AC, Jacobsen D, Brørs O. Adverse events after naloxone treatment of episodes of suspected acute opioid. *Eur J Emerg Med.* 2004;**11**(1):19–23.

48. Andree RA. Sudden death following naloxone administration. *Anesth Analg.* 1980;**59**(10):782–784.

49. van Dorp EL, Yassen A, Dahan A. Naloxone treatment in opioid addiction: the risks and benefits. *Expert Opin Drug Saf.* 2007;**6**(2): 125–132.

50. No authors listed. Effective medical treatment of opiate addiction. National Consensus Development. *JAMA.* 1998;**280** (22):1936–1943.

51. Zealberg JJ, Brady KT. Substance abuse and emergency psychiatry. *Psychiatr Clin North Am.* 1999;**22**(4):803–817.

52. Joranson D, Gilson A. Policy issues and imperatives in the use of opioids to treat pain in substance abusers. *J Law Med Ethics.* 1994:**22**(3):215–223.

53. Jaffe JH, O'Keeffe C. From morphine clinics to buprenorphine: regulating opioid agonist treatment of addiction in the United States. *Drug Alcohol Depend.* 2003;**70**(2 Suppl):S3–S11.

54. McKeown Nathaniel TA. Withdrawal syndromes clinical presentation. http:// emedicine.medscape.com/article/819502-clinical.

55. Brunton L, Parker K (Eds.). *Goodman and Gilman's The Pharmacologic Basis of Therapeutics.* 11th ed. New York, NY: McGraw-Hill, 2006.

56. Gold MS, Pottash AL, Extein I, Kleber HD. Clonidine and opiate withdrawal. *Lancet.* 1980;**2**(8203):1078–1079.

57. Connrock M, Juarez-Garcia A, Jowett S, et al. Methadone and buprenorphine for the management of opioid dependence: a systematic. *Health Technol Assess.* 2007;**11** (9):1–171.

58. Krantz MJ, Kutinshy IB, Robertson AD, Mehler PS. Dose-related effects of methadone on QT prolongation in a series of patients with torsade de pointes. *Pharmacotherapy.* 2003;**23**(6):802–805.

59. Nordt SP, Zilberstein J, Gold B. Methadone-induced torsade de pointes. *Am J Emerg Med.* 2011;**29**(4):1.

60. Sporer, KA. Buprenorphine: a primer for emergency physicians. *Ann Emerg Med.* 2004;**43**(5):580–584.

61. Maremmani I, Gerra G. Buprenorphine-based regimens and methadone for the medical management of opioid dependence: selecting the appropriate drug for treatment. *Am J Addict.* 2010;**19** (6):557–568.

62. No authors listed. Buprenorphine replacement therapy: a confirmed benefit. *Prescrire Int.* 2006;**15**(82):64–70.

63. Reynaud M, Petit G, Poterd D, Courty P. Six deaths linked to concomitant use of buprenorphine and benzodiazepines. *Addiction.* 1998;**93**(9):1385–1392.

64. 2008 National Survey on Drug Use and Health (NSDUH). http://www.drugabuse. gov/infofacts/cocaine.html. http://www. drugabuse.gov/PDF/RRCocaine.pdf.

65. Massachusetts Poison Control System. Cocaine poisoning: an update. *Clin Toxicol Rev.* 1995;**17**:1–3.

66. Robins RJ, Abraham TW, Parr AJ, Eagles J, Walton NJ. The biosynthesis of tropane alkaloids in datura stramonium: the identity of the intermediates between N-methylpyrrolinium salt and tropinone. *J Am Chem Soc.* 1997;**119** (45):109.

67. Hiestand BC, Smith SW. Cocaine chest pain: between a (crack) rock and a hard place… *Acad Emerg Med.* 2011;**18**(1):68–71.

68. Leete E, Bjorklund JA, Kim SH. The biosynthesis of the benzoyl moiety of cocaine. *Phytochemistry.* 1988;**27**(8):255.

69. Mandava N, Chang RS, Wang JH, et al. Establishment of a definitive protocol for the diagnosis and management of body packers (drug mules). *Emerg Med J.* 2011;**28**(2):98–101.

70. Vorspan F, Bloch V, Brousse G, et al. Prospective assessment of transient cocaine-induced psychotic symptoms in a clinical setting. *Am J Addict.* 2011;**20** (6):535–537.

71. Pozner CN, Levine M, Zane R. The cardiovascular effects of cocaine. *J Emerg Med.* 2005;**29**(2):173–178.

72. Lange RA, Hillis LD. Cardiovascular complications of cocaine use. *N Engl J Med* 2001;**345**:351–358.

73. Hillis L, Lange RA. Sudden death in cocaine abusers. *Eur Heart J* 2010; **31** (3):271–273.

74. Virmani R, Robinowitz M, Smialek JE, Smyth DF. Cardiovascular effects of cocaine: an autopsy study of 40 patients. *Am Heart J.* 1988;**115**:1068–1076.

75. Chang AM, Walsh KM, Shofer FS, McCusker CM, Litt HI, Hollander JE. Relationship between cocaine use and coronary artery disease in patients with symptoms consistent with an acute coronary syndrome. *Acad Emerg Med.* 2011;**18**(1):1–9.

76. American Heart Association. Toxicology in emergency cardiovascular care. In Field JM. *Advanced Cardiovascular Life Support Resource Text for Instructors and Experienced Providers.* AHA, Dallas. 2008.

77. Riva E, Mennini T, Latini R. The alpha- and beta-adrenoceptor blocking activities of labetalol and its RR-SR (50:50) stereoisomers. *Br J Pharmacol.* 1991;**104** (4):823–828.

78. McCord J, Jneid H, Hollander JE, et al. Management of cocaine-associated chest pain and myocardial infarction: a scientific statement from the American Heart Association Acute Cardiac Care Committee of the Council on Clinical Cardiology. *Circulation.* 2008;**117** (14):1897–1907.

79. Stevens JC, Pollack MH. Benzodiazepines in clinical practice: consideration of their long-term use and alternative agents. *J Clin Psych* 2005;**66**(Suppl 2):21–27.

80. Devlin, JW, Roberts RJ. Pharmacology of commonly used analgesics and sedatives in the ICU: benzodiazepines, propofol, and opioids. *Crit Care Clin.* 2009;**25**(3):431–449.

81. Ashton CH. Protracted withdrawal syndromes from benzodiazepines. *J Subst Abuse Treat.* 1991;**8**(1–2):19–28.

82. Ebell MH. Benzodiazepines for alcohol withdrawal. *Am Fam Phys.* 2006; **73**(7):1191.

83. Harrison PC, Gelder MG, Cowen P. The misuse of alcohol and drugs. In *Shorter Oxford Textbook of Psychiatry.* 5th ed. Oxford: Oxford University Press, 2006.

84. Longo LP, Johnson B. Addiction: Part I. Benzodiazepines – side effects, abuse risk and alternatives. *American Family Physician* 2000;**61**(7):2121–2128.

85. Fraser AD. Use and abuse of the benzodiazepines. *Ther Drug Monit.* 1998;**20**(5):481–489.

86. Lader M, Tylee A, Donoghue J. Withdrawing benzodiazepines in primary care. *CNS Drugs.* 2009;**23**(1): 19–34.

87. Ashton CH. The diagnosis and management of benzodiazepine dependence. *Curr Opin Psychiatry.* 2005;**18**(3):249–255.

88. Mattila-Evendon M, Franck J, Bergman U. A study of benzodiazepine users claiming drug-induced psychiatric morbidity. *Nord J Psychiatry.* 2001; **55**(4):271–278.

89. McIntosh A, Semple D, Smyth R, Burns J, Darjee R. Depressants. In *Oxford Handbook of Psychiatry.* 1st ed. Oxford: Oxford University Press, 2004.

90. Charlson F, Degenhardt L, McLaren J, Hall W, Lynskey M. A systematic review of research examining benzodiazepine-related mortality. *Pharmacoepidemiol Drug Saf.* 2009;**18**(2):93–103.

91. Chouinard G. Issues in the clinical use of benzodiazepines: potency, withdrawal, and rebound. *J Clin Psychiatry.* 2004;**65** (Suppl 5):7–12.

92. National Institute on Drug Abuse. NIDA InfoFacts: Hallucinogens – LSD, Peyote, Psilocybin, and PCP. DrugAbuse.gov.

93. Caravatti EM. Hallucinogenic drugs. In: Dart RC, Caravatti EM, McGuigan MA, et al (Eds.). *Medical toxicology.* 3rd ed. Philadelphia, PA: Lippincott, Williams, and Wilkins, 2004.

94. Holland J, Nelson L, Ravikumar P. Embalming-fluid soaked marijuana: a new high or new guise for PCP? *J Psychoactive Drugs.* 1998;**30**:215–219.

95. Litovitz T, Klein-Schwartz W, Caravati E. 2002 Annual report of the American Association of Poison Control Centers toxic exposure surveillance system. *Am J Emerg Med.* 2003;**22**:517–575.

96. Boyer E, Quang L, Woolf A, Shannon M, Magnani B. Dextromethorphan and ecstasy pills. *JAMA* 2001;**285**:409–410.

97. Misra A, Pontani R, Bartolomeo J. Persistence of phencyclidine and metabolites in brain and adipose tissue and implications for long-lasting behavioral effects. *Pharmacol.* 1979; **24**:431–435.

98. Liang I, Boyer E. Dissociative agents. In *Haddad and Winchester's Clinical Management of Poisoning and Drug Overdose.* 4th ed. Philadelphia, PA: Saunders Elsevier, 2007.

99. Carls KA. Ruehter Vl evaluation of PCP psychosis. *Am J Drug Alcohol Abuse.* 2006;**32**:673.

100. Giannini AJ, Eighan MS, Loiselle RH, Giannini MC. Comparison of haloperidol and chlorpromazine in the treatment of phencyclidine psychosis. *J Clin Pharmacol.* 1984;**24**(4):202–204.

101. National Institute on Drug Abuse. *MDMA (Ecstasy) Research Report Series. Electronic Version.* http://nida.nih.gov/Research Reports/MDMA/.

102. Drug Abuse Warning Network (DAWN) Reports 2005. http://dawninfo.samhsa.gov/. Accessed June 8, 2008.

103. Fahal IH, Sallomi DF, Yaqoob M, Bell GM. Acute renal failure after ecstasy. *BMJ.* 1992;**305**(6844):29.

104. Burgess C, O'Donohoe A, Gill M. Agony and ecstasy: a review of MDMA effects and toxicity. *Eur Psychiatry.* 2000;**15** (5):287–294.

105. Christophersen AS. Amphetamine designer drugs – an overview and epidemiology. *Toxicol Lett.* 2000;**112–113**:127–31.

106. Schwartz RH, Miller NS. MDMA (ecstasy) and the rave: a review. *Pediatrics.* 1997;**100** (4):705–708.

107. Reneman L, Booij J, Schmand B, van den Brink W, Gunning B. Memory disturbances in "Ecstasy" users are correlated with an altered brain serotonin neurotransmission. *Psychopharmacology (Berl).* 2000;**148**(3):322–324.

108. Andreu V, Mas A, Bruguera M, et al. Ecstasy: a common cause of severe acute hepatotoxicity. *J Hepatol.* 1998;**29** (3):394–397.

109. Maxwell DL, Polkey MI, Henry JA. Hyponatraemia and catatonic stupor after taking "ecstasy". *BMJ*. 1993;**307** (6916):1399.

110. Dafters RI, Lynch E. Persistent loss of thermo-regulation in the rate induced by 3,4-methylene-dioxymethamphetamine (MDMA or "Ecstasy") but not by fenfluramine. *Psychopharmacology*. 1998;**138**:207–212.

111. Grunau BE, Wiens MO, Brubacher JR. Dantrolene in the treatment of MDMA-related hyperpyrexia: a systematic review. *CJEM*. 2010;**12**(5):435–442.

Psychosis

Paul P. Rega

Introduction

The *Diagnostic and Statistical Manual of Mental Disorders* (DSM-IV-TR) acknowledges that the term "psychosis" has been redefined a number of times, no version of which has achieved universal acceptance. Psychosis will be defined here as a disturbance in the perception of reality characterized by the presence of hallucinations and/or delusions. Hallucinations are sensory perceptions (visual, auditory, gustatory, olfactory, tactile) in the absence of external stimuli. Delusions are fixed, false, idiosyncratic beliefs which may occur with or without hallucinations. Illusions are another type of false perception in which a person misperceives real objects (e.g., a coat on a chair in a dark room is perceived as someone sitting there), but these are not classed as a psychotic symptom. Hallucinations and delusions should be thought of as symptoms, not a diagnosis. The pathophysiology and etiology underlying the symptoms may be due to a single process, could be the result of multiple issues, or could be unknown. New-onset psychosis merits thorough examination and thoughtful treatment planning. Patients with psychosis should be monitored closely during the course of their evaluation to ensure that all acute medical conditions are addressed appropriately while a careful search for any acute, potentially reversible causes of their symptoms is pursued.

Assessment of psychosis may be complicated by clouded sensorium as seen in delirium, disordered thought, or the so-called "negative symptoms" seen in some psychotic conditions.* Psychosis is often complicated by other symptoms, including agitation. Although some patients with psychosis may be agitated, not all patients with psychosis are prone to violence. Nevertheless, it is prudent for all patients with pyschosis to have close monitoring while they undergo a careful evaluation.

---

*Negative symptoms include Bleuler's famous "four As": Affect, Ambivalence, Autism, and Associations. Affect: inappropriate or flattened affect, diminished emotional response to stimuli. Autism: social withdrawal, loss of awareness of external events. Ambivalence: an apparent inability to make decisions. Associations: loosening of thought association, leading to disordered pattern of thought and speech.

McNally K. "Eugene Bleuler's Four As." *History Of Psychology* 2009;12(2):43–59., PsycAR-TICLES, EBSCOhost, viewed December 30, 2011.

Emergency Psychiatry, ed. Arjun Chanmugam, Patrick Triplett, and Gabor Kelen. Published by Cambridge University Press. © Cambridge University Press 2013.

Acute psychosis may arise from a number of conditions (Table 5.1). Depending on the underlying condition, psychosis may manifest as disorganized speech, catatonic behavior, or it may present with other mental and physical impairments which can significantly interfere with normal life activities. This effect on ability to function, combined with the patient's impaired reality testing, may put these individuals at high risk for danger to themselves and others. Thus, as stated previously, all patients with psychosis should be assessed as rapidly and safely as possible.

A consideration for delirium (see also Chapter 6) should always be kept in mind when assessing psychosis. Delirium is a state of global cerebral dysfunction that produces a waxing and waning level of consciousness. This distortion may be subtle, depending on the underlying condition and course of disease. Delirium is described in this chapter because it may manifest with the symptoms of psychosis. Accurate identification of delirium is important because delirium is associated with a poor medical prognosis and high rates of mortality.

When examining an at-risk patient who appears to manifest psychotic symptoms, consider the following four diagnostic categories: (1) confusional-delirious state – this category implies that the patient's symptoms have one or multiple medical causes, (2) psychoses associated with focal or multifocal cerebral lesions, (3) affective disorders (bipolar and depressive psychoses), and (4) schizophrenia and schizophreniform disorders. Although categorizing patients with psychosis into one of these four groups is helpful, the main theme in this chapter is that any presentation of psychosis should prompt an immediate evaluation and thorough search for reversible causes. The following cases illustrate this point and represent the variety of patients that can be seen with a diagnosis of psychosis.

Patient #1: A 15-year-old discovered wandering downtown in his underwear having visual hallucinations; pupils are markedly dilated. Diagnosis: jimsonweed intoxication.

Patient #2: An octogenarian who normally completes the *New York Times* crossword in one hour has been staring out the window and mumbling incoherently since she woke up this morning. Diagnosis: left lower lobe pneumonia.

Patient #3: A 45-year-old schizophrenic on parole and unable to afford his medications believes his newborn nephew is Beelzebub. His family escorts him to the local emergency department (ED) for evaluation. In the ED, he becomes anxious and frustrated. He states that he wants to leave the ED and nothing is wrong with him. He becomes loud and displays threatening behavior. Diagnosis: exacerbation of chronic schizophrenia and medication non-compliance.

Patient #4: A 34-year-old, formerly obese male with no previous psychiatric history, who had gastric bypass surgery two months earlier. Since the surgery, with his major weight loss and frequent episodes of copious vomiting, he has developed progressive psychiatric symptoms (viz. visual/auditory hallucinations, violent behavior, and disorientation). Diagnosis: Wernicke's encephalopathy due to thiamine deficiency secondary to severe gastric outlet stenosis.[1]

Patients 1, 2, and 4 all represent delirium. They all manifested psychotic symptoms, but when observed long enough they also demonstrated a waxing and waning level of consciousness – all these patients actually suffered from an acute medical condition. In case 3, the patient suffered from a psychiatric illness that impaired his ability to perceive and interact appropriately with the environment, but the presentation would still merit a screening workup for obvious reversible sources. Even with an evaluation that is unrevealing for a medical or reversible cause, his condition may require inpatient treatment.

These presentations reflect the spectrum of disorders that may produce psychosis. It is essential for the emergency physician and other acute care providers to appreciate the complexities of psychosis in order to competently prepare for and respond to life-threatening potentials, not only for the patient, but also for those providing care.

Table 5.1. Diagnoses and conditions that can cause psychosis.[2-14]

A. Delirium (see Chapter 6)

  Causes: An acute/subacute/chronic medical or traumatic condition

    Endogenous

    Exogenous

      Environmental

      Trauma

      Pharmacologic

    Principal characteristics

      Decreased awareness of surrounding environment

      Memory deficit

      Disorientation

      Language disturbance

    Time course: Acute (hours/days)

    Characteristic feature: Severity fluctuates over a brief period of time.

    Reversibility: With prompt recognition of the underlying cause and subsequent medical intervention

    Autonomic system involvement likely

    Manifestations: Subtle to overt

B. Dementia

  Definition: A pervasive disturbance of cognitive function that may involve memory, abstract thinking, judgment, personality, etc.

    Aphasia: Language disturbance

    Apraxia: Impaired motor activity with intact motor function

    Agnosia: Non-recognition of objects

    Anomia: Difficulty naming objects

  Onset: Insidious

  No fluctuation in level of consciousness

  Most common: Alzheimer's disease

    Delusional: 50% of patients

  Time course: Gradual (months-years)

Table 5.1. (cont.)

Reversibility: Possible, but unlikely (~10%)

Autonomic system involvement unlikely

C. Major depression with psychotic overtones

D. Bipolar mania with psychotic overtones

E. Delusional disorder

Psychiatric condition characterized by non-bizarre delusions that may dominate patient's life

Erotomanic

Persecutory

Grandiose

F. Brief psychotic disorder

Sudden onset of an acute psychiatric condition

In response to any major stress

Immediate postpartum period

Loss of a loved one

Combat

Duration: days to one month

G. Schizophrenia/schizophreniform disorder

Definition: A predominance of psychotic symptoms with emphasis on delusions (fixed false beliefs) and/or hallucinations (false sensory perceptions).

Most prevalent form of psychosis

Manifestations

Functional deterioration

Poor self-care

Active phase (positive) symptoms

Hallucinations: Non-existent sensory experience

Delusions: Erroneous beliefs involving a misinterpretation or perceptions or experiences

Disorganized speech

Disorganized behavior

Catatonic behavior

Passive phase (negative) symptoms

Blunted affect

Emotional withdrawal

Lack of spontaneity

Attention deficit

Cognitive impairment

Table 5.1. (cont.)

H. **D**rugs

  Prescribed

    ADHD (attention-deficit/hyperactivity disorder) agents

    Anticholinergics

    Anticonvulsants

    Antidepressants

    Antihistamines

    Antiparkinsonian agents

    Antipsychotics

    Barbiturates

    Benzodiazepines

      Corticosteroids

    Histamine

    H2 blockers

    Lithium

    Opioid analgesics

  Substance use/misuse

    Methamphetamine

    Ketamine

    Cocaine

    PCP

    LSD

    Cannabis

    Jimsonweed

    Mescaline

    Inhalants

    Alcohol

    Ethylene glycol

    Methanol

    Anabolic steroids

    Narcotics

    Benzodiazepines

I. **E**ndocrine/**E**nvironmental

    Hypoglycemia

    Thyroid storm

Table 5.1. (*cont.*)

    Cushing's disease

    Addison's disease

    Parathyroid disease

    Postpartum psychosis

    Sydenham's chorea

    Panhypopituitarism

    Carbon monoxide

    Hypothermia

    Hyperthermia

    Heavy metal exposure

J. **N**eurologic

  Medical

    CVA

    Alzheimer's disease

    Multiple sclerosis

    Neoplasm

    Paraneoplastic encephalopathy

    Normal-pressure hydrocephalus

    Epilepsy

    SAH

    Postictal states

    Hepatic encephalopathy

    Multiple sclerosis

    CNS vasculitis

  Traumatic

    Subdural hematoma

    Concussion

K. **I**nfections/Inflammatory

    Encephalitis

    Generalized sepsis

    Sarcoidosis

    Systemic lupus erythematosus

    Temporal arteritis

    SBE

Table 5.1. (cont.)

RMSF
West Nile Virus encephalopathy
L. **Metabolic**
Electrolyte imbalance
Niacin, thiamine, B12, folate deficiency
Body temperature imbalance
Anemia
Hypoxia
Hypercarbia
Hypercalcemia
Porphyria

Background

There were 53 million mental health-related ED visits between 1992 and 2001, representing an annual jump from 17.1 mental health patients per 1000 visits to 23.6. From another perspective, behavioral disturbances are responsible for up to 6% of all ED visits in the US, of which patients with acute psychosis represent an important subgroup.[5,15] In addition, more than four million people are admitted for emergency treatment annually in the US to control their aggressive and impulsive behavior.[16] (See Chapter 2.) Implicit in this last statement is the potential for random violence.[17] Not all patients with psychosis will become violent. Many of these patients can be managed safely without much difficulty. However, it should be kept in mind that the patient with psychosis will have an impaired sense of reality which can affect their insight and judgment. How the patient responds to this impaired sense of reality could jeopardize the safety and well-being of the clinician, the staff, and the other patients, as well as the patient.[3,6–9,18]

Anticipation of violent activities in patients with psychosis must be part of the management plan. Violence in patients with psychosis is usually preceded by verbal and non-verbal cues that should alert the staff caring for the patient, but violence may also erupt without warning.[19] This is especially true in patients with a medical condition causing or exacerbating their psychosis.[20] No clinician should rely solely on his/her ability to predict violent behavior.[9,18,21] Instead, reliance should be placed on a team approach that utilizes a careful monitoring system based on multiple multidisciplinary evaluations.[9,18,21]

Fundamentally, the immediate approach to the patient with psychosis must address these two questions: is the patient in a safe environment, and does the patient's psychosis represent a medical emergency? Once the safety factor has been satisfactorily addressed, then the etiology of the psychosis must be considered. "Psychosis" is no more diagnostic than "headache" or "abdominal pain." Psychosis should not be considered a psychiatric complaint until medical causes have been ruled out by history, physical examination, and ancillary testing.[3,8,9] Until that point arrives, the evaluation of the psychotic patient should be considered a true medical emergency.

Therefore, when dealing with the patient with psychosis, emergency providers must fulfill multiple roles and responsibilities including: controlling the patient and the environment to allow optimal management and to ensure patient, staff, and visitor safety; diagnosing the root cause of the psychosis; and treating any reversible cause of the psychotic behavior.

This chapter will briefly address the safety issues associated with a patient who manifests psychotic features. (Management of the patient with agitation is covered more comprehensively in Chapter 2.) Secondly, this chapter will discuss assessment and management options associated with the patient with psychosis.

Safety and situational awareness

Safety issues associated with the patient with psychosis should be well planned far in advance of any patient presentation. Protocols for contingencies should be in place for potential patients. Like chess, the success or failure of the endgame is often dictated by the opening gambit. Optimal outcomes cannot be realized if a plan is devised at the time of presentation. In fact, impromptu actions may deteriorate the situation further thereby jeopardizing everyone's safety, the patient's included.

The approach to a patient with psychosis should be an evolving process of planning, preparedness, response, and recovery. Each situation should be discussed, analyzed, and digested in anticipation of the next case.

Employing case-based simulated scenarios can be an effective strategy to highlight strengths and discover deficiencies in current policies and procedures. It has greater resonance when as many of the ED staff as possible are involved. It will encourage the appreciation and timely application of verbal and behavioral techniques to control agitation and violent action. This education could help to avoid the inappropriate administration of physical or chemical restraints which could be injurious to all concerned.[22]

The patient with psychosis: a case-based scenario

A 36-year-old male is brought into the triage area by family with a chief complaint of "hearing voices from the radio." The voices are telling him to kill his mother. He's agitated. He requires familial hand-holding and reassurance. He attempts to walk out. His family tries to exert control, but he becomes increasingly loud, belligerent, angry, and profane.

Questions/considerations to be raised during a tabletop exercise or action steps to be evaluated during a functional exercise:

i.   Was the patient separated safely from the rest of the patients in the waiting room?
ii. How quickly was the patient brought back to the ED?
iii. Was security notified and involved in a timely manner?
iv. Did the triage staff have enough training to manage this type of situation and did they follow an established protocol?
v.   When was the patient brought back to a "safe room"?
vi. Was the "safe room" operational and was there an assessment of its utility for this patient?
vii. Has the staff tasked to manage this patient removed any potentially dangerous equipment, decorations, jewelry, and any other personal items from clothes/uniforms?
viii. Was the rest of the staff alerted?

ix. Did the staff taking care of the patient talk to the patient?

x. Did the staff follow the training protocol for managing patients like this?

In the room, the patient gets into an argument with his sister-in-law. He believes she has been using her lighter to "irradiate" him and he attacks her in self-defense.

xi. Was there enough staff to control the situation all the time?

xii. Does the staff know how to physically restrain such a patient safely?

xiii. Is there a specific or special alert in cases like this?

It is by developing a scenario and working through the process as a team that illuminates issues that can help management of future patients.

Presentation

There are two principal ways a patient with psychosis may present to the ED. Typically in most EDs, the patient is brought by a family member or friend, describing relatively new or worsening concerning behaviors. The patient often has had an acute behavior change for which the physician must evaluate, manage, and arrange proper disposition.

The second presentation is more common in EDs that have designated psychiatric emergency services embedded or associated with the main ED, but can occur in any acute care environment. In these situations, patients are brought for urgent psychiatric evaluation and "medical clearance" (a problematic term; see Chapter 1), either by police, EMS, group home providers or others. Emergency assessment is usually requested for patients with a known psychiatric disorder who have anticipated needs for admission to some facility.[23] The patient is brought to the ED to ensure that there are no medical problems causing or complicating the presumed psychiatric behavior to ensure that admission to a psychiatric venue can occur without interference from any active medical problems. This may be the earliest opportunity to properly recognize the psychotic features as a manifestation of a medical condition. Properly identifying a medical condition posing as a psychiatric condition can be life-saving.

It is not surprising, therefore, that imaging and serological protocols have become standardized in some settings for all such patients regardless of whether they are needed or not. However, much of what has become "The Rule" is also uneconomical, inefficient, and not evidence-based. The American College of Emergency Physicians has taken the position that "medical clearance" testing should be done on a case-by-case basis with targeted diagnostic studies based upon history and presentation.[15,23] In short, for adult patients with primary psychiatric complaints, with normal vital signs, with a non-contributory history and physical examination, routine testing has a "very low yield and need not be performed as part of the ED assessment".[15] However, a high degree of vigilance is still required when evaluating these patients, because many do have significant medical concerns that should be addressed before transfer to a psychiatric facility. Accepting institutions may have protocols that direct certain testing prior to transfer. Psychiatric services are loath to admit patients without a comprehensive medical workup, as many of these services are unable to provide for acute complex medical needs.

There is advocacy to change the concept of "medical clearance" to "medical screening" or "focused medical assessment," which better captures the emergency physician's judgment that the patient's presentation is unrelated to an acute medical condition.[5,24] At the completion of the emergency medical assessment, the emergency physician declares that the

Table 5.2. Features of presentation correlated with specific diagnoses

- Herpes simplex encephalitis is associated with olfactory and gustatory hallucinations.[5]

- In the geriatric population, changes in mental status are frequent with occult pneumonia and urinary tract infections.[5,10,25] Delirium in the elderly is also commonly seen with CHF, MI, ischemic bowel disease, malnutrition, and pain.

- Obtaining a comprehensive travel history may be diagnostic. Exotic diseases with psychotic manifestations: cryptococcus, malaria, etc.[26,27]

- The prevalence of psychosis during an HIV infection ranges from 0.5–15%.[28,29] This may be due to CNS infections, CNS malignancies, and/or medications.[4]

- An immunocompromised patient with new-onset cognitive impairment may have meningitis without fever, meningismus, and headache.

- It is estimated that 14% of elderly ED patients and up to 21% of elderly hospitalizations abuse alcohol.[10,22]

- Withdrawal manifestations are particularly seen with alcohol and the sedative hypnotic abuse.[5]

- Drug/alcohol intoxication and withdrawal are the most common diagnoses in violent ED patients.[24]

- Even one exposure to MDMA (ecstasy) can trigger intense and prolonged psychotic behavior.[30]

- Cocaine and amphetamines are the most commonly abused stimulants in the US.[5]

- Frontal lobe epilepsy is frequently misdiagnosed as a psychiatric problem. Symptoms: sudden screaming, kicking, and/or incontinence.[5]

- Fecal impaction may cause delirium in mental retardation/developmental delay patients.[31]

- While hypoglycemia is a well-recognized condition responsible for mental status changes, hypothyroidism and hyperthyroidism are two of the most common endocrine conditions that cause psychiatric manifestations. Both are easily missed initially.[5]

patient has: (1) no medical condition, or (2) a stable, co-existing medical condition that does not require acute intervention and is not related to the psychiatric issue at hand, or (3) an acute medical condition that has been addressed, allowing for the safe disposition of the patient to a psychiatric venue.[5]

Certain features and symptom complexes point toward specific medical diagnoses. These are shown in Table 5.2.

Geriatrics: special considerations

The number of Americans over 65 years of age with psychiatric conditions reached 7 million by 2000 and is expected to double by 2030.[22] The relationship between this population and psychosis is considerable. Nearly half of those patients with Alzheimer's disease will have a psychotic episode during the course of the illness.[32] Sixteen to 23% of the elderly are diagnosed with "organic psychoses".[22] As comorbidities increase with age, psychotic manifestations will be multifactorial.[4,10] Besides infections, delirium in the elderly is commonly seen with CHF, MI, ischemic bowel disease, malnutrition, and pain.[22]

Determining the underlying medical cause(s) for altered mental status in the elderly can be a complex exercise and may not be readily accomplished in the ED setting. Often, determination of the cause requires time, patience, serial examinations, and sophisticated testing. When dealing with a geriatric patient, the emergency physician should assume a medical etiology in total or in part (see also Chapter 11). Emergency physicians should rule out the life-threatening possibilities, and consider admitting the patient to a medical venue first, before consideration of a psychiatric admission if there is any doubt. A psychiatric evaluation can be done as an adjunctive measure.

The history

Good history-taking and a thorough, targeted physical examination is important in the workup of psychosis. While it is important to attempt to obtain a history from the patient, the psychotic overlay may impede or taint the answers. Therefore, the clinician should seek supplementary information from family or anyone else (EMS, law enforcement, bystanders, etc) who knows the patient or who has accompanied the patient to the ED.[4,6] While most medical questions are standardized (e.g., fever, trauma, new medications, etc.), inquiries should be made for psychiatric-specific questions as well. These include seeking information about mood, affect, suicidal ideation/behavior, social withdrawal, hallucinatory stimuli, delusional thoughts, etc.[24,33] Establishing the patient's baseline function is a critical aspect of the family/friend interview.[5] Obtaining a travel and occupational history when appropriate should not be omitted.

The physical examination

The assessment of a psychotic patient begins with accurate vital signs (including oxygen saturation). Any abnormality must be assiduously investigated. Patients should not be discharged without an explanation of any abnormal vital sign.

Another early step is a mental status examination looking for cognitive impairment.[6] Prior studies have indicated that many physicians and nurses fail both to recognize cases of cognitive impairment and to screen with specific instruments.[4,34] The results of this testing may give an indication of cognitive impairment due to the underlying condition(s) causing psychosis or from pre-existing cognitive impairment; knowledge of the patient's baseline cognitive functioning is important. There are numerous instruments that have been used and validated in a variety of circumstances (see Tables 5.3–5.6). For emergency medicine, the ideal instrument should be:

Validated for use in the ED setting
Easily learned
Easily administered
Adequate for all relevant patient demographics (e.g. age, socioeconomic status, etc.)
Expeditious
Comprehensive in evaluating most domains of cognitive dysfunction (attention, memory, intellect, judgment, etc.)

The Folstein Mini-Mental Status Examination (MMSE), the Orientation Memory Concentration examination, and the Confusion Assessment Method, have been validated to a limited extent in the ED. Unfortunately, even the briefest of tests takes time in a busy ED.[33] The Clock Drawing Task and the Six-Item Screener are promising alternatives

Table 5.3. Screening instruments for cognitive impairment[34,35]

Six-Item screener

AD8

Mini-Mental Status Examination (MMSE)

Memory impairment screen

Montreal Cognitive Asssement (MoCA)

Mini-cog

7-minute screen

Cognitive assessment screening test

Clock drawing task

Orientation memory concentration

Confusion assessment method (ICU)

Quick confusion scale

Short blessed test

Ottawa 3D/3DY

Table 5.4. The clock drawing test for cognitive impairment[36]

Patient instructions:

Draw a circle.

Draw the face of a clock within the circle (place the numbers of a clock within the circle).

Indicate the time: 11:10.

For the clinician:

Each completely correct action (draws a closed circle, places numbers in correct position, includes all 12 correct numbers, hands in correct position) receives a "1" score. Any sum less than "4" suggests cognitive impairment. Further testing required.

Table 5.5. The short blessed test[37]

(Score 1 point for each error up to maximum per item)

To patient	Maximum error	Score	Weight
The year	1	___ x 4	= ___
The month	1	___ x 3	= ___
Repeat specific phrase			
Time within 1 hour	1	___ x 3	= ___
Count backwards (20 to 1)	2	___ x 2	= ___
Months in reverse order	2	___ x 2	= ___
Repeat prior phrase	5	___ x 2	= ___
		Total score	= ___ /28

A score of 7 or higher requires further evaluation to rule out cognitive dysfunction.

Table 5.6. The six-item screener[34,38]

For the clinician: score 1 point for each correct answer.

To patient:

Remember the following objects:
  Apple
  Table
  Shoe

The year?

The month?

The day of the week?

Repeat the objects
  Apple
  Table
  Shoe

Note: A deduction of two or more points is suspicious for cognitive impairment.

Table 5.7. Key findings on physical exam suggesting medical condition underlying psychosis

Ears: hemotympanum

Eyes: anisocoria, mydriasis, miosis, sclera icterus, nystagmus, papilledema, conjunctival color

Neck: thyromegaly, nuchal rigidity

Chest: subcutaneous emphysema, bruising

Back: crepitus, bruising, CVA tenderness

Skin: needle marks, temperature, moisture, trauma, surgical scars, petechiae, splinter hemorrhages,

Abdomen: Hepatosplenomegaly, trauma (Cullen's sign, Grey-Turner's sign), ascites

Neuro: Cranial nerves, gait, strength, cerebellar functions, reflexes, sensation, abnormal movements (asterixis, myoclonus, tremors[4,5]

pending future studies. They can be administered quickly, validated, easily taught, and have been used in the ED for assessing cognitive impairment specifically in the elderly.[34,36,39] For further discussion, see also the delirium and geriatrics chapters.

While a detailed description of a physical examination is beyond the scope of this chapter, there are specific findings that might indicate a medical basis for a psychosis (Table 5.7).[24]

Ancillary tests

The presumptive diagnosis will depend upon the initial history and the physical evaluation, and then verified, if necessary, by ancillary testing and imaging (Table 5.8). The additional studies should not be protocol-driven, but based on the patient's presentation. Otherwise, the positive yield will be exceedingly low.[3–5,15,22,24]

Table 5.8. Ancillary tests in the acute evaluation of a patient with psychosis

Common	Less common	Uncommon
CBC	<Serum calcium	Folate/B12
Electrolytes/BUN/creatinine	ESR/C-reactive protein	VDRL
Serum troponin	ABGs	HIV screen
Liver function tests	Toxicology panel	Serum cortisol
Serum chemistries	Thyroid studies	FTA-ABS
Myoglobin	CSF analysis	Serum ammonia level
Urinalysis	Lumbar puncture	Heavy metal screen
CXR		EEG
ECG		Neuropsychometric testing
Neuroimaging studies		Evoked potentials (visual, brainstem auditory, somatosensory)

Summary

There are few patient conditions that have the management intricacies that accompany the patient with psychosis. There must be a delicate balance between the care, safety, and civil rights of the patient with those of both staff and others in the vicinity. Every patient with psychosis must be considered a true emergency and a search for a medical cause for the psychosis is warranted in each case, along with close monitoring during the evaluation and treatment course.

Those decisions can be made most competently when the ED personnel come together to review, test, and revise existing policies and procedures on a continual basis.

References

1. Jiang W, Gagliardi JP, Raj YP, et al. Acute psychotic disorder after gastric bypass surgery: differential diagnosis and treatment. *Am J Psychiatry*. 2006;**163**(1):15–19.

2. American Psychiatric Association. *Diagnostic and Statistical Manual of Mental Disorders*. 4th ed. Washington, DC: American Psychiatric Association, 2000.

3. Larkin GL, Beautrais AL. Behavioral disorders: emergency assessment. In Tintinalli JE, Stapczynski JS, Ma OJ, Cline DM, Cydulka RK, Meckler GD (Eds.), *Emergency Medicine: A Comprehensive Study Guide*. 7th ed. http://0-www. accessemergencymedicine.com.carlson. utoledo.edu/content.aspx?aID=6393408. Accessed October 10, 2010.

4. Smith J, Seirafi J. Delirium and dementia. In Marx JA, Hockberger RS, Walls RM (Eds.), *Rosen's Emergency Medicine: Concepts and Clinical Practice*. 6th ed. Philadelphia, PA: Elsevier Health Science, 2005.

5. Sood TR, Mcstay CM. Evaluation of the psychiatric patient. *Emerg Med Clin N Am*. 2009;**27**:669–683.

6. Hockberger RS, Richards JR. Thought disorders. In Marx JA, Hockberger RS, Walls RM (Eds.), *Rosen's Emergency Medicine: Concepts and Clinical Practice*. 6th ed. Philadelphia, PA: Elsevier Health Science, 2005.

7. Zun L. Behavioral disorders: diagnostic criteria. In Tintinalli JE, Stapczynski JS, Ma OJ, Cline DM, Cydulka RK, Meckler GD (Eds.),

Emergency Medicine: A Comprehensive Study Guide. 7th ed. http://0-www.accessemergencymedicine.com.carlson.utoledo.edu/content.aspx?aID=6393408. Accessed October 10, 2010.

8. Wilhelm S, Schacht A, Wagner T. Use of antipsychotics and benzodiazepines in patients with psychiatric emergencies: results of an observational trial. *BMC Psychiatry.* 2008;**8**:61.

9. Fernandez Gallego V, Murcia Perez E, Sinisterra Aquilino J, et al. Management of the agitated patient in the emergency department. *Emergencias.* 2009; **21**:121–132.

10. Rudolph JL. Delirium or dementia. webmm.ahrq.gov/printview.aspx?caseID=200. Accessed September 27, 2010.

11. Wilber ST, Carpenter CR, Hustey FM. The six-item screener to detect cognitive impairment in older emergency department patients. *Acad Emerg Med.* 2008;**15**(7):614–616.

12. Miller MO. Evaluation and management of delirium in hospitalized older patients. *Am Fam Physician.* 2008;**78**(11):1265–1270.

13. Mosholder AD, Gelperin K, Hammad TA, et al. Hallucinations and other psychotic symptoms associated with the use of attention-deficit/hyperactivity disorder drugs in children. *Pediatrics.* 2009;**123**;611–616.

14. Pawsey B, Castle D. Substance abuse and psychosis. *Aus Fam Physician.* 2006;**35**(3).

15. Hughes DH. Acute psychopharmacological management of the aggressive psychotic patient. *Psychiatric Serv.* 1999;**50**(9):1135–1137.

16. Raviprakash T, Mcstay CM. Evaluation of the psychiatric patient. *Emerg Med Clin N Am.* 2009;**27**:669–683.

17. American College of Emergency Physicians Clinical Policies Subcommittee (Writing Committee) on Critical Issues in the Diagnosis and Management of the Adult Psychiatric Patient in the Emergency Department. Clinical policy: critical issues in the diagnosis and management of the adult psychiatric patient in the emergency department. *Ann Emerg Med.* 2006;**47**:79–99.

18. Mattingly BB, Small AD. Chemical restraint. http://emedicine.medscape.com/article/109717-overview. Accessed November 19, 2010.

19. Bell CC. Assessment and management of the violent patient. *J Natl Med Assoc.* 2000;**92**:247–253.

20. Bunney B. The agitated patient in the emergency department. www.uic.edu/com/ferne/pdf/Boston0503/Agitated%20Patient.pdf. Accessed October 25, 2010.

21. Kao LW, Moore GP. The violent patient: clinical management, use of physical and chemical restraints, and medicolegal concerns. *Emerg Med Pract.* 1999;**1**(6):1–24.

22. Piechniczek-Buczek J. Psychiatric emergencies in the elderly population. *Emerg Med Clin N Am.* 2006;**24**: 467–490.

23. Brasic JR, Ainsworth JR. Clinical safety in neurology. http://emedicine.medscape.com/article/1149218-overview. Accessed November 4, 2010.

24. Buckley PF, Noffsinger SG, Smith DA, et al. Treatment of the psychotic patient who is violent. *Psychiatr Clin N Am.* 2003; **26**:231–272.

25. Potash MN, Gordon KA, Conrad LK. Complications after a single ingestion of MDMA (ecstasy) – a case report and review of the literature. *Psychiatry.* 2009;**6** (7):40–44.

26. Powers RE. Physician's guide for management of delirium in adults with mental retardation and developmental disabilities (MR/DD). 2005. http://www.ddmed.org/pdfs/71.pdf. Accessed December 11, 2010.

27. Walsh PG, Currier G, Shah MN, et al. Psychiatric emergency services for the US elderly: 2008 and beyond. *Am J Geriatr Psychiatry.* 2008;**16**(9):706–717.

28. Castagnini A, Berrios GE. Acute and transient psychotic disorders (ICD-10 F23): a review from a European perspective. *Eur Arch*

Psychiatry Clin Neurosci. 2009;**259**: 433–443.

29. Prakash PY, Sughandi RP. Neuropsychiatric manifestation of confusional psychosis due to Cryptococcus neoformans var grubii in an apparently immunocompetent host: a case report. *Cases Journal.* 2009;**2**:9084.

30. Khan MA, Akella S. Cannabis-induced bipolar disorder with psychotic features: a case report. *Psychiatry.* 2009;**6**(12):44–48.

31. Rao NP, Gupta A, Sreejayan K, et al. Toluene associated schizophrenia-like psychosis. *Indian J Psychiatry.* 2009;**51** (4):329–330.

32. Mishra SK, Newton CRJC. Diagnosis and management of the neurological manifestations of falsiparum malaria. *Nat Rev Neurol.* 2009;**5**(4):189–198.

33. Sewell DD, Jeste DV, McAdams LA, et al. Neuroleptic treatment of HIV-associated psychosis. *Neuropsychopharmacology.* 1994;**10**(4):223–229.

34. Zun LS. Medical clearance of the psychiatric patient in the emergency department. http://emedhome.com/ features_archive_detail.cfm. Accessed September 26, 2010.

35. Salen P, Heller M, Oller C, et al. The impact of routine cognitive screening by using the clock drawing task in the evaluation of elderly patients in the emergency department. *J Emerg Med.* 2009;**37**(1):8–12.

36. O'Connor D. Psychotic symptoms in the elderly. *Aust Fam Phys.* 2006;**35**(3):106–108.

37. Carpenter CR, Basset E, Fischer G, Shirshekan J. Four brief screening instruments to identify cognitive dysfunction in older emergency department patients. Poster presentation (#41), Proceedings of the 20th Annual Midwest Regional SAEM Meeting, Wright State University, Dayton, OH; 2010.

38. Carpenter CR. Does this patient have dementia? *Ann Emerg Med.* 2008;**52**:554–556.

39. Keks N, Blashki G. The acutely psychotic patient: assessment and initial management. *Aust Fam Phys.* 2006; **35**(3):90–94.

The delirious patient

Sharon Bord

Background

Delirium is a diagnosis that can be quite elusive to physicians and medical care providers; nearly 75% of cases are missed on initial conventional clinical assessment.[1] Patients with delirium have an in-hospital mortality rate of 22 to 76%,[2] which is on a par with rates associated with acute myocardial infarction and sepsis. Patients with delirium can be difficult to evaluate as the presentation can be confused with a psychiatric disorder. Given the high mortality rates associated with delirium and the multiple conditions that can cause delirium, providers must be careful to consider this diagnosis carefully before other less life-threatening diagnoses are entertained.

The initial discussion must begin by defining what is meant by the term delirium. Defined by both the DSM-IV-TR and the ICD 10 diagnostic criteria, the basic features include impairment of consciousness, thinking, memory, psychomotor behavior, perception, and emotion. Delirium is usually caused by some systemic insult that results in an acute confusional state and is marked by a transient impairment of attention. One key point is that the disturbance of thinking develops over a short period of time and can fluctuate throughout the day, distinguishing the disease from dementia. However, it has been noted that up to two thirds of cases of delirium occur in patients with dementia,[2] making the distinction between the two somewhat challenging. Delirium reflects a state in which there is impaired cognitive functioning generally as a result of an acute or subacute pathological process that needs to be addressed. In all cases, delirium has an organic etiology, and can never be explained by a psychiatric condition itself.

Psychosis (see Chapter 5) is a term that is often used in the context of delirium. Psychosis is a broad term that essentially refers to an impaired reality-testing ability whose hallmarks are delusions and hallucinations. Ultimately psychosis is characterized by false perceptions that may be visual, auditory, tactile, olfactory, or gustatory. Psychosis can be the result of either a psychiatric disorder such as schizophrenia or it can be the result of a transient brain disturbance resulting from trauma, drugs, and/or medical illness – in other words, delirium. A significant challenge for providers occurs when a patient with a psychiatric disease presents with psychosis; the psychosis can either be a manifestation of the psychiatric disease itself, or could be the result of

Emergency Psychiatry, ed. Arjun Chanmugam, Patrick Triplett, and Gabor Kelen. Published by Cambridge University Press. © Cambridge University Press 2013.

Table 6.1. Predisposing factors for delirium

Demographic characteristics
    Age of 65 years or older
    Male sex

Cognitive status
    Dementia
    Cognitive impairment
    History of delirium
    Depression

Functional status
    Functional dependence
    Immobility
    Low level of activity
    History of falls

Sensory impairment
    Visual or hearing impairment

Decreased oral intake
    Dehydration
    Malnutrition

Drugs
    Treatment with multiple psychoactive drugs
    Treatment with many drugs
    Alcohol abuse

Coexisting medical conditions
    Severe illness
    Multiple coexisting conditions
    Chronic renal or hepatic disease
    History of stroke
    Neurologic disease
    Metabolic derangements
    Fracture or trauma
    Terminal illness
    Infection with human immunodeficiency virus

Inyoue S. Delirium in older persons. *N Engl J Med*. 2006;**354**:11.

a delirium (due to some systemic insult such as drugs or medical illness) or a combination of both psychiatric disease and delirium.

The causes of delirium are many and varied and range from adverse medication effects to alcohol withdrawal to sepsis and fever or hypoxemia. Based on multiple studies, the diagnosis of delirium accounts for approximately 10% of emergency department visits. It is imperative to recognize predisposing factors (Table 6.1), as well as precipitating factors (Table 6.2) for the development of delirium. Predisposing factors are those that exist prior to the development of delirium symptoms, while precipitating factors are inciting events that are more proximally related to the development of delirium.

Table 6.2. Precipitating factors that can contribute to delirium

Drugs
  Sedative hypnotics
  Narcotics
  Anticholinergic drugs
  Treatment with multiple drugs
  Alcohol or drug withdrawal

Primary neurologic disease
  Stroke, particularly non-dominant hemispheric
  Intracranial bleeding
  Meningitis or encephalitis

Intercurrent illness
  Infection
  Iatrogenic complaints
  Severe acute illness
  Hypoxia
  Shock
  Fever or hypothermia
  Anemia
  Dehydration
  Poor nutritional status
  Low serum albumin level
  Metabolic derangements: electrolyte, glucose, acid-base

Surgery
  Orthopedic surgery
  Cardiac surgery: prolonged cardiac bypass
  Noncardiac surgery

Environmental
  Admission to an intensive care unit
  Use of physical restraints
  Use of bladder catheter
  Use of multiple procedures
  Pain
  Emotional stress

Prolonged sleep deprivation

Inyoue S. Delirium in older persons. *N Engl J Med.* 2006;**354**:11.

Diagnosing delirium in the emergency department
Conventional history and physical

Evaluation in the acute setting such as an emergency department generally consists of a directed history and physical related to the patient's chief complaint. Elie et al. report that the sensitivity of this conventional clinical assessment to diagnose delirium ranges from 23.5% to 37.5%, resulting in a significant proportion of these patients being misdiagnosed and possibly inappropriately treated or discharged home.[1]

There are many reasons why the diagnosis of delirium is missed. In elderly patients the presence of delirium may be confused with depression because both conditions may have a hypoactive presentation. Complicating the evaluation of patients with delirium is the inability of some patients to provide a clear history. In cases when patients are unable to provide a cogent history, providers are compelled to seek other sources of information. In fact, in apparently stable patients, family and friends may prove the only history suggestive of delirium. One of the most important pieces of information for a diagnosis is a clear understanding of symptom onset, which can be difficult to obtain especially if a family member or caretaker is not readily available.

Providers must also pay close attention to the patient's vital signs. Temperature, if elevated, can indicate an infectious process or hyperthermia; if decreased, then hypothermia may be the underlying cause. Decreased oxygen saturation indicates hypoxia. Tachycardia may point to anemia or an infection. These parameters are clues that a more serious underlying pathology may exist and should not be overlooked.

Physical examination must be performed completely to assess for possible causes of delirium. The patient should be fully disrobed so all components of the physical examination can take place. Many clues as to the cause of delirium can be found on exam; the skin exam might reveal a rash associated with an infectious process, the neurologic exam might reveal a focal deficit. Tremor might suggest alcohol or other substance withdrawal or other central nervous system etiology. All of these findings should help steer the provider to the appropriate diagnosis.

Delirium versus dementia

Delirium can be confused with dementia, which is understandable given that both deal with the cognitively impaired individual. Dementia, on the one hand, indicates a chronic cognitive decline whereas delirium refers only to transient acute-onset cognitive changes that are often associated with a disturbance of consciousness and deficits in attention and perception. To make matters more difficult for the diagnostician, patients with dementia have an increased risk of delirium. A key element in the diagnosis of both entities is the onset of symptoms. Unfortunately, a cogent history may be difficult to elicit from the patient who suffers from either delirium or dementia. Table 6.3 summarizes the differences between the two entities.

One of the more definitive ways to make the diagnosis of delirium is via the electro-encephalogram (EEG), but in the acute setting, obtaining an EEG may not be possible. The use of bedside cognitive tests, the Mini Mental Status Examination (MMSE), as described by Folstein et al. in 1975, and the Confusion Assessment Method are often used. It should be noted that MMSE does not distinguish well between the various confusional states, but it does help to delineate cognitive impairment. Additional limitations to the MMSE are that its questions may be too reliant on the education of the patient. One approach to assess attention and avoid any educational bias is to ask the patient to recite the days of the week or months of the year backward. Another question to help gauge attention, judgment, and insight is to ask a question such as "What would you do if you were in a crowded building and smelled smoke?" A final activity may be to ask the patient to draw a clock face and to set the hands to a specific time to help gauge attention, visuospatial reasoning, and planning. A useful bedside test for delirium is the Confusion Assessment Method (CAM). Both the MMSE and CAM are described below.

Table 6.3. Comparison of delirium and dementia

Feature	Delirium	Dementia
Onset	Abrupt	Usually insidious, abrupt in some strokes/trauma
Course	Fluctuates	Slow decline
Duration	Hours to weeks	Months to years
Attention	Impaired	Intact early; often impaired late
Sleep-wake	Disrupted	Usually normal
Alertness	Impaired	Normal
Orientation	Impaired	Intact early; impaired late
Behavior	Agitated, withdrawn/depressed, or both	Intact early
Speech	Incoherent, rapid/slowed	Word-finding problems
Thoughts	Disorganized, delusions	Impoverished
Perceptions	Hallucinations/illusions	Usually intact early

Data from Butler C, Zeman AZJ. Neurologic syndromes which can be mistaken for psychiatric conditions. *J Neuro Neurosurg Psychiatry.* 2005;**76**:i31–8; Rabinowitz T. Delirium: an important (but often unrecognized) clinical syndrome. *Curr Psychiatry Rep.* 2002;**4**:202–8; and Rabinowitz T, Murphy KM, Nagle KJ, et al. Delirium: pathophysiology, recognition, prevention and treatment. *Expert Rev Neurotherapeutics.* 2003;**3**:89–101.

Mini Mental Status Examination (MMSE), Montreal Cognitive Assessment (MOCA) and Confusion Assessment Method (CAM)

The MMSE and MOCA are tools which have been utilized to assess for cognitive impairment among patients. The MMSE is an easy and reliable test which can be performed at the bedside. It consists of a short series of questions that assess orientation, memory, attention, calculation, language, and recall. A score of 23 or below is considered abnormal and suggests organic brain syndrome or a non-psychiatric cause for the patient's decreased mental status. The MOCA may be more time intensive, but it might also be better at detecting mild cognitive impairment (see Table 6.4).

The CAM is an additional tool to aid in the diagnosis of delirium. It was developed by Inouye et al. to be used by clinicians other than psychiatrists to aid in the diagnosis of delirium. The CAM questionnaire which is seen in Table 6.5 assesses the four features which are present in delirium: (1) acute onset and fluctuating course, (2) inattention, (3) disorganized thinking, and (4) altered level of consciousness. In order to diagnose delirium, the first and second criteria must be present, and either one of the third or fourth criteria. Monette et al. performed a study to validate the CAM in the emergency department and found that it had a sensitivity of 86% and specificity of 100% when compared to the diagnosis made by a geriatrician.[3]

Diagnostic evaluation and ancillary studies

In most delirious patients a complete blood count (CBC), basic metabolic panel (BMP), glucose, calcium, and urinalysis should be obtained. These tests can provide vital

Table 6.4. The Montreal Cognitive Assessment

MONTREAL COGNITIVE ASSESSMENT (MOCA)
Version 7.1 Original Version

NAME :
Education :   Date of birth :
Sex :   DATE :

VISUOSPATIAL / EXECUTIVE		POINTS

Copy cube

Draw CLOCK (Ten past eleven)
(3 points)

[ ]   [ ]   [ ]   [ ]   [ ]   __/5
                                Contour   Numbers   Hands

NAMING

[ ]   [ ]   [ ]   __/3

MEMORY	Read list of words, subject must repeat them. Do 2 trials, even if 1st trial is successful. Do a recall after 5 minutes.		FACE	VELVET	CHURCH	DAISY	RED	No points
		1st trial						
		2nd trial						

ATTENTION	Read list of digits (1 digit/ sec.).	Subject has to repeat them in the forward order	[ ] 2 1 8 5 4	__/2
		Subject has to repeat them in the backward order	[ ] 7 4 2	

Read list of letters. The subject must tap with his hand at each letter A. No points if ≥ 2 errors
[ ] F B A C M N A A J K L B A F A K D E A A A J A M O F A A B   __/1

Serial 7 subtraction starting at 100	[ ] 93	[ ] 86	[ ] 79	[ ] 72	[ ] 65	__/3

4 or 5 correct subtractions: **3 pts**, 2 or 3 correct: **2 pts**, 1 correct: **1 pt**, 0 correct: **0 pt**

LANGUAGE	Repeat : I only know that John is the one to help today. [ ] The cat always hid under the couch when dogs were in the room. [ ]	__/2

Fluency / Name maximum number of words in one minute that begin with the letter F   [ ] _____ (N ≥ 11 words)   __/1

ABSTRACTION	Similarity between e.g. banana - orange = fruit [ ] train – bicycle [ ] watch - ruler	__/2

DELAYED RECALL	Has to recall words WITH NO CUE	FACE [ ]	VELVET [ ]	CHURCH [ ]	DAISY [ ]	RED [ ]	Points for UNCUED recall only	__/5
Optional	Category cue							
	Multiple choice cue							

ORIENTATION	[ ] Date [ ] Month [ ] Year [ ] Day [ ] Place [ ] City	__/6

© Z.Nasreddine MD   **www.mocatest.org**   Normal ≥ 26 / 30   TOTAL   __/30

Administered by: _____   Add 1 point if ≤ 12 yr edu

Table 6.5. The Confusion Assessment Method for the intensive care unit

Delirium is diagnosed when both Features 1 and 2 are positive, along with either Feature 3 or Feature 4.

Feature 1. Acute onset of mental status changes or fluctuating course

– Is there evidence of an acute change in mental status from the baseline?

– Did the (abnormal) behavior fluctuate during the past 24 hrs, that is, tend to come and go or increase and decrease in severity?

Sources of information: Serial Glasgow Coma Scale or sedation score ratings over 24 hours as well as readily available input from the patient's bedside critical care nurse or family.

Feature 2. Inattention

– Did the patient have difficulty focusing attention?

– Is there a reduced ability to maintain and shift attention?

Sources of information: Attention screening examinations by using either picture recognition or Vigilance A random letter test (see Methods and Appendix 2 for description of Attention Screening Examinations). Neither of these tests requires verbal response, and thus they are ideally suited for mechanically ventilated patients.

Feature 3. Disorganized thinking

– Was the patient's thinking disorganized or incoherent, such as rambling or irrelevant conversation, unclear or illogical flow of ideas, or unpredictable switching from subject to subject?

– Was the patient able to follow questions and commands throughout the assessment?

1. "Are you having any unclear thinking?"

2. "Hold up this many fingers" (examiner holds two fingers in front of the patient)

3. "Now, do the same thing with the other hand" (not repeating the number of fingers)

Feature 4. Altered level of consciousness

– Any level of consciousness other than "alert"

– Alert – normal, spontaneously fully aware of environment and interacts appropriately

– Vigilant – hyperalert

– Lethargic – drowsy but easily aroused, unaware of some elements in the environment, or not spontaneously interacting appropriately with the interviewer; becomes fully aware and appropriately interactive when prodded minimally

– Stupor – difficult to arouse, unaware of some or all elements in the environment, or not spontaneously interacting with the interviewer; becomes incompletely aware and inappropriately interactive when prodded strongly

– Coma – unarousable, unaware of all elements in the environment, with no spontaneous interaction or awareness of the interviewer, so that the interview is difficult or impossible even with maximal prodding

Ely EW, Margolin R, Francis J, et al. Evaluation of delirium in critically ill patients: Validation of the Confusion Assessment Method for the intensive care unit. *Crit Care Med.* 2001;**29**:7.

information to the workup. The CBC results can suggest a range of diagnostic considerations. For example, thrombotic thrombocytopenic purpura should be considered in the setting of low platelets, or microangiopathic hemolytic anemia. Acute blood loss should be considered in patients with a low hematocrit. An abnormally high or low white blood cell count (WBC) could indicate an infection. Patients who are febrile should have both a urinalysis and a chest radiograph performed as they are common indicators for infection. The measurement of serum electrolytes can also provide clues as to the etiology of delirium. It is imperative to calculate the anion gap as this may be one of the few indications of a metabolic acidosis. If there is an elevated anion gap, consideration should be given to diabetic or alcoholic ketoacidosis. Other reasons for an increased anion gap include elevated lactate in the setting of sepsis or ingestion of a toxic alcohol (methanol, ethylene glycol), or salicylates. Patients who have a history of cirrhosis or liver failure should have an ammonia level measured. Additionally, if the patient is noted to be hypoxic on vital signs, or have a low respiration rate (elevated pCO_2), an arterial blood gas should be obtained to quantify the acid base abnormality. An electrocardiogram should be obtained, especially in the elderly, to assess for a silent myocardial infarction or arrhythmias. Despite these diagnostic evaluations, Inouye found no identifiable cause for the delirium in up to 16% of patients.[4]

Although frequently sent, the utility of a toxicologic screen is often limited in the evaluation of a patient with delirium. If a patient presents with a specific toxidrome or the cause of delirium is unclear and the patient is not clearing rapidly, a toxicologic screen is appropriate. Additional testing for toxic alcohols should be considered in the appropriate clinical situation. It is important to note that these tests can have a long turnaround time and if the suspicion for one of these ingestions is high, there are other ancillary tests that can provide support for these diagnoses. Serum osmolality will be increased (osmolal gap), and, even in the presence of alcohol, will be higher than expected. Ethylene glycol, used in antifreeze, produces urine (calcium oxalate) crystals in about 50%, and the urine may fluoresce under ultraviolet light. Any further toxicological concerns or questions could be discussed with the regional poison control center.

A lumbar puncture and cerebrospinal fluid (CSF) analysis should be obtained, or considered, in patients who are febrile with cognitive dysfunction, even without meningismus. Patients who are elderly, immunocompromised, or alcoholics might not display the classic signs of meningitis – headache and stiff neck. In any patient in whom there is a concern about elevated intracranial pressure, a head CT scan should be obtained prior to performing a lumbar puncture. The CSF should be sent for cell count, gram stain and culture, protein, glucose and in the proper settings, acid-fast smear, India ink stain, cryptococcal antigen, and VDRL should be sent as well.

Neuroimaging

There is great variability in the emergency department practice of ordering a non-contrast CT scan of the brain in the workup of a confused patient. Patients who have a history of trauma, immunodeficiency, or focal neurologic deficit should have a head CT scan performed to detect a possible structural lesion.[5] Naughton et al. examined the practice of ordering head CT scans in delirious, elderly patients and found two factors associated with an acute abnormality on CT scan; impaired consciousness or a new focal neurologic sign.[6] It is important to note that a normal CT scan does not completely rule out a CNS lesion. Meningitis or encephalitis, early infarctions, and closed head injuries are likely to have a normal head CT. The availability of magnetic resonance imaging (MRI) in the emergency department has been increasing over the last decade; however, its diagnostic utility in delirium has yet to be fully established. The MRI scan has the ability to detect small intracerebral and brainstem lesions, small brain contusions, and certain encephalitides. Perfusion scanning can also help assess for an acute vascular event.

Hyperthermia

Elevated temperature can cause an individual to become confused. Hyperthermia is defined as a rise in body temperature above the hypothalamic set point when heat dissipating mechanisms are overwhelmed by things such as drugs, environmental factors, or internal metabolic heat.[7] Patients who present with severely elevated temperature are frequently unable to provide a history, making the treatment and management challenging.

Heat stroke can be caused either by exposure to environmental heat, which is known as classic heat stroke, or strenuous physical exercise, known as exertional heat stroke. These patients have a temperature > 40 degrees Celsius and can have central nervous system abnormalities such as delirium, coma, or convulsions.[7] Physical exam will also reveal hot and dry skin in addition to the CNS abnormalities. Patients that are at extremes of age, impoverished, or without access to air conditioning are at greatest risk of developing heat stroke. The mainstay of therapy is cooling the patient by applying cold or ice water to the skin which is then fanned. There are no pharmacologic agents which have been found to be effective. Antipyretics have not yet been formally evaluated although theoretically they should be beneficial. When treating heat stroke, seizures can develop and may be treated with benzodiazepines. Central nervous system function should improve in the majority of patients during cooling, however 20% of patients can have residual brain damage and a higher mortality.[7]

In a patient with critically elevated temperature one should also consider other entities including serotonin syndrome and malignant hyperthermia. A large number of medications and poisonings feature hyperthermia/fever. Some endocrine disorders such as hyperthyroidism, particularly thyroid storm and adrenal insufficiency, may present with unexplained fever. Eliciting a precise medication history from family members or any other reliable source in these patients is a valuable strategy.

Hypothermia

Hypothermia is defined as a body temperature of less than 35 degrees Celsius (95 degrees Fahrenheit). Further classification divides hypothermia into mild, 32–35 degrees Celsius (89.6–95 degrees F), moderate, 28–32 degrees Celsius (82.4–89.6 degrees F), and severe, <28 degrees Celsius (< 82.4 degrees F). It is important to note that most conventional thermometers are inaccurate at less than 35 degrees Celsius, therefore a rectal temperature should be obtained and if available a special low-reading thermometer should be utilized. There are many underlying conditions which should be considered that can increase a person's susceptibility to cold, including infancy, old age, alcohol intoxication, and hypothyroidism.[8]

Patients who sustain accidental outdoor cold exposure might be obvious based on their presentation. Alcohol intoxication increases the risk for hypothermia by increasing heat loss via vasodilatation and by impairing behavioral responses to cold.[9] However, there is

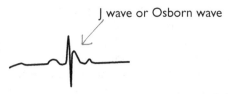

J wave or Osborn wave

Figure 6.1. The J wave (Osborn wave), an EKG finding that occurs in patients with hypothermia.

a subset of individuals who develop hypothermia when indoors either related to excess air conditioning or ice baths. These patients are often elderly and may demonstrate only vague complaints of mental or motor skill deterioration. Additionally, patients with sepsis may present with a low, rather than high, temperature.

When evaluating a hypothermic patient, movement of the patient should be kept to a minimum as significant hypothermia can cause the heart to enter ventricular fibrillation with small jolts or movements of the body.[9] Further evaluation should be pursued including bedside glucose testing, lab analysis to include renal function, coagulation panels and electrolytes and an electrocardiogram (ECG). The classic and well-known hypothermia ECG findings include the presence of J (Osborn) waves (Figure 6.1), which are pathognomonic for hypothermia. Interval prolongation and atrial and ventricular dysrhythmias might also be seen.[10]

Once hypothermia is recognized it is imperative to begin either passive or active rewarming. Passive rewarming, which involves placing the patient in a warm and dry environment, is useful in a patient with mild hypothermia but will increase the body's core temperature slowly. Active external and internal rewarming should be used in cases of moderate or severe hypothermia. Warm lavage of body cavities (bladder, gastric, colonic, or thoracic) can increase the core temperature at a rate of 1 to 2 degrees Celsius per hour.

Substance abuse

Psychiatric diagnoses are often associated with concomitant related substance abuse. Abuse of illicit substances is also an exceedingly common problem with approximately 8 million individuals being dependent on alcohol and 3.5 million dependent on drugs including heroin and stimulants in the United States.[11] Therefore it is necessary to recognize the toxidromes associated with various drug classes when evaluating psychiatric patients. Additionally, some withdrawal states, specifically related to alcohol and benzodiazepine class medications, can be life-threatening especially if not recognized and treated in an appropriate fashion.

Drug-induced delirium in the elderly

When discussing delirium related to drug use, one patient population deserves special consideration, i.e., the elderly. Medications that are commonly prescribed, including anticholinergic medications, benzodiazepines, and narcotics can lead to delirium in a frail elderly individual. Other medications that have been implicated in delirium include the fluoroquinolone class of antibiotics, steroids, theophylline, and antihpertensives (beta-blockers and methyldopa classes). Some studies quote that medications alone may be responsible for

12–29% of all cases of delirium in the elderly.[12] It is imperative for patients presenting with delirium that a complete and thorough list of medications be obtained.

Factors which increase the susceptibility of the elderly to medications include physiological changes, such as a decrease in lean body mass and serum albumin, medical comorbidities, such as hepatic or renal failure, and altered pharmacokinetic parameters, most commonly increased drug half-life.[12] Management of drug-induced delirium in the emergency department consists of stopping the offending agent and the judicious use of antipsychotic medications when needed. Typical antipsychotic medications, such as haloperidol, have been shown to be effective. There is less evidence regarding the effectiveness of the newer atypical antipsychotics. However, Sipahimalani et al. demonstrated that risperidone was effective and reasonably safe for treating agitation related to delirium.[13] Alternative medications should be taken into consideration when prescribing for an elderly patient. For example, a second-generation antihistamine such as loratadine could be recommended as an alternative to diphenhydramine.

Withdrawal from sedatives – alcohol and benzodiazepines

Withdrawal signs and symptoms from alcohol range from minor manifestations such as tremors or tachycardia to more severe complications including seizure and alcohol withdrawal delirium (AWD), more commonly known as delirium tremens. Obtaining an appropriate social history (particularly on alcohol) from the patient or their representatives is necessary in order to make this diagnosis. Current diagnostic criteria in the DSM-IV for AWD include disturbance of consciousness, change in cognition, or perceptual disturbance developing in a short period, and the emergence of symptoms during or shortly after withdrawal from heavy alcohol intake.[14] Clinical presentation includes hyperpyrexia, tachycardia, hypertension, and diaphoresis. Features of alcohol withdrawal can appear within hours of the last drink, but delirium typically does not develop until two or three days after the cessation of drinking.[14] Mortality was initially found to be as high as 15%, but advances in treatment have decreased the mortality to a reported 0–1%.[14]

Studies have found some risk factors that can help predict which patients are at highest risk for developing AWD. A study by Palmistierna found five such risk factors: current infectious disease, tachycardia defined as a heart rate greater than 120 beats per minute at admission, signs of alcohol withdrawal accompanied by an alcohol concentration of more than 1 gram per liter of body fluid, history of epileptic seizures, and a history of previous delirious episodes. Of the 334 alcohol-dependent patients in the study, no patient without these five risk factors developed AWD.[15] Additional studies have found similar risk factors.

Benzodiazepines are noted to be first line agents in the treatment of AWD. Two major reviews of pharmacotherapy for alcohol withdrawal found that benzodiazepines were most effective at decreasing the severity of the alcohol withdrawal syndrome. Benzodiazepines reduced the occurrence of delirium and seizures, and the time to completion of withdrawal. Additionally, they were found to decrease mortality when compared to treatment with neuroleptic agents.[14] Other adjunctive therapies to consider include thiamine (and glucose, especially if Wernicke-Korsakov syndrome is contemplated) and magnesium. Patients at high risk for AWD require close observation and monitoring; those patients with AWD usually require inpatient care and often within an intense care setting.

Cocaine and methamphetamines

Patients who are under the influence of acute cocaine ingestion on presentation will exhibit vasoconstriction, mydriasis, tachycardia, and hyperthermia. These manifestations are related to increased levels of the neurotransmitter norepinephrine and in turn increased sympathetic stimulation.[16] In some patients, cocaine-associated agitated delirium (also known as excited delirium) can occur; these patients are often hyperthermic and grossly psychotic in the early stages, often performing amazing feats of strength, particularly in the setting of being restrained. In a subset of these patients, especially those who have significant exertion, shortly after being restrained, their agitation can cease abruptly. Such patients are at increased risk for sudden death.[17]

Methamphetamine use has become increasingly common over the last 25 years. When this drug class is smoked it leads to an immediate euphoria similar to that seen with cocaine, but lasting much longer. Abuse of high doses of methamphetamines may cause agitation, hallucinations, delirium, excited delirium, seizures, or death. Following use of methamphetamines, the confused patient should also be considered to possibly be post-ictal because of the likelihood of a recent seizure.[18]

Anticholinergic drugs

Emergency medicine physicians often think of medications that possess anticholinergic properties, such as diphenhydramine and promethazine, as relatively benign treatments. However, it is important to note that these medications can cause a quite alarming acute confusional state in patients. Obtaining a medication history is very important, but attention should also be given to over-the-counter medications. As has been previously discussed, elderly patients might be more susceptible to these medication side effects. Agostini et al. found that older patients who had received diphenhydramine during their hospitalization experienced an increased risk for delirium symptoms including inattention, disorganized speech, and altered consciousness.[19] Anticholinergics often produce a classic toxidrome of altered mental status, hyperpyrexia, dry skin and mucous membranes, and flushed appearance.

Metabolic derangements: glucose and electrolytes

The prevalence of diabetes mellitus is on the rise, and correspondingly there are increases in the numbers of emergency department visits related to both hyperglycemia and hypoglycemia. These conditions represent important causes for delirium and mental status changes in the emergency department. Other electrolyte abnormalities such as hypo- and hypernatremia and hypercalcemia might also present with such mental status changes.

Hypoglycemia is often the result of excessive medication use to treat diabetes. However, it may also be precipitated by more ominous underlying issues such as sepsis, hypothyroidism, and worsening renal insufficiency. Patients often become symptomatic when their blood sugar is between 40 and 50 mg/dl, but the symptoms can occur in some patients at levels below 80 mg/dl. Symptoms can range from sweating and nervousness to neurologic symptoms including confusion, seizures, and coma. All patients who present with mental status changes should have blood glucose urgently checked. Patients who have a history of alcohol abuse and those on beta-blockers might have blunted symptoms; therefore increased vigilance is needed in these subgroups. Hypoglycemia should be treated with either oral glucose, via a sugar-containing food, or with one to three ampules of intravenous 50% dextrose in water (D50W). In the setting of alcohol abuse, thiamine should be administered as well to prevent the development of Wernicke-Korsakoff syndrome. If a hypoglycemic patient cannot take anything orally and intravenous access cannot be obtained, 1 to 2 mg of glucagon can be administered intramuscularly or subcutaneously. Depending on the situation in which hypoglycemia developed, patients should either be discharged with close follow-up or admitted to the hospital for further management.

Hyperglycemia can also manifest with mental status changes if diabetic ketoacidosis or hyperglycemic hyperosmolar state are present. Diabetic ketoacidosis (DKA) consists of the triad of hyperglycemia, ketonemia, and acidemia. The annual incidence rate for DKA is estimated to be between 4.6 and 8 per 1000 patients with diabetes.[20,21] The typical patient with DKA has insulin-dependent diabetes and is a lean and thin patient. Patients in DKA can present with a variety of complaints including abdominal pain, nausea, vomiting, polyuria, and polydipsia. On exam Kussmaul respirations and an odor of acetone might be noted. Hyperosmolar hyperglycemic state (HHS), a condition formerly known as hyperosmolar hyperglycemic non-ketotic coma, is more likely to occur in an elderly patient with non-insulin-dependent diabetes. It is imperative in both DKA and HHS to elicit what the precipitating event was. Common precipitating events include infection, with pneumonia and urinary tract infection accounting for 30% to 50% of cases,.[20] myocardial infarction, and medications such as corticosteroids or inadequate or non-compliance with insulin therapy. Therefore, all patients with these diagnoses should have a CBC, CMP, urinalysis, electrocardiogram, and chest radiograph obtained. Additional testing such as a non-contrast head CT, lumbar puncture or cardiac markers should be performed if clinically indicated. The goals of therapy for both DKA and HHS include restoring circulatory volume, decreasing serum glucose and plasma osmolality towards normal levels, clearing the serum and urine of ketones, and correcting electrolyte imbalance.[20]

Infectious disease
Sepsis syndromes

Sepsis is now the 10th most common cause of death in the United States.[22] There exists a spectrum of sepsis syndromes. Systemic Inflammatory Response Syndrome (SIRS) is defined as "a systemic inflammatory response to a variety of clinical insults." In order to make the diagnosis of SIRS, two of the four following criteria must be present in the absence of known causes: tachypnea, hyperthermia or hypothermia, tachycardia, and leukocytosis or bandemia. SIRS can be caused by an infectious process or by a non-infectious process such as pancreatits or trauma. Sepsis is SIRS in the setting of an infection. Severe sepsis is present if the patient demonstrates end-organ damage, hypotension, or hypoperfusion, which in turn can cause acidosis, oliguria, or mental status changes. Septic shock can be defined as a systolic blood pressure of less than 90 despite reasonable fluid resuscitation or that requires a vasopressor or inotropic agents.

Patients with sepsis often display neurologic impairment, specifically altered mental status and lethargy. This condition is commonly referred to as septic encephalopathy. One study demonstrated a correlation between mortality and Glasgow Coma Scale (GCS) score.

A GCS score of 13 to 14 had a mortality rate of 20% while a GCS score of 9 to 12 had a mortality rate of 50%.[23] The pathophysiology behind this condition is likely multifactorial related to direct bacterial invasion, endotoxemia, altered cerebral perfusion or metabolism, and multisystem organ failure. Additionally, impaired renal or hepatic function, without overt heart failure, has been shown to correlate with encephalopathy.

All patients in whom sepsis is considered should have evaluation of the complete blood count including differential, electrolytes and cultures of the blood, sputum, urine, and when appropriate cerebrospinal fluid. A chest radiograph should be obtained to evaluate for pneumonia as well as signs of ARDS. Additional imaging such as head computed tomography, pelvic ultrasound, and an abdominal computed tomography should be obtained based on the patient's clinical picture.

Management of these patients in the emergency department is aimed at decreasing mortality. The initial treatment should consist of managing the patient's ABCs: airway, breathing, and circulation. Rivers et al. developed a protocol that is known as early goal-directed sepsis care. This protocol guides resuscitation by measuring the central venous pressure and continuous mixed venous oxygen level monitoring via central venous access and an arterial line to measure the blood pressure. The goal parameters are maintaining the CVP between 8–12 mmHg in non-mechanically ventilated patients and 12–16 mmHg in ventilated patients, and maintaining the $ScvO_2$ at greater than 70%. In their initial study Rivers et al. found that by following this protocol versus standard emergency department care, there was a 16% mortality reduction in patients with severe sepsis and septic shock.[24] Patients should also be given early and appropriate antibiotic therapy to target the specific infection. If there is no clear identifiable infectious source, broad spectrum antibiotic coverage is recommended.

Meningitis and encephalitides

Diagnosing a patient with a central nervous system (CNS) infection can be a difficult task in the emergency department. Given the high morbidity and mortality associated with CNS infections, it is imperative to maintain a high suspicion for these entities. Meningitis is defined as inflammation of the membranes of the brain or spinal cord, whereas encephalitis indicates inflammation of the brain itself.

When evaluating a patient for a CNS infection, special attention should be paid when performing the neurologic, skin, and ENT portions of the exam. In a prospective study of 696 patients with the diagnosis of bacterial meningitis, Van de Beek et al. found that the classic triad of fever, neck stiffness, and a change in mental status were present in only 44% of patients. It was concluded, however, that 95% of patients had at least two of four symptoms of headache, fever, stiff neck, and altered mental status.[25] Additionally, Kernig's and Brudzinski's signs should be performed on physical exam and, if present, may aid in making the diagnosis of meningitis. Kernig's sign is positive if the examiner is unable to straighten the patient's leg passively when the patient is lying supine and Brudzinski's sign is positive if flexion of the neck leads to flexion of the hips. Each of these signs were found by Thomas et al. to have a sensitivity of only 5%.[26] Patients who are suspected of having meningitis or encephalitis should all undergo a lumbar puncture and cerebrospinal fluid examination. Prior to attempting lumbar puncture, the patient should be evaluated for elevated intracerebral pressure (ICP) and if present, lumbar puncture should be avoided. Elevated ICP can be assessed either via an adequate examination of the

Table 6.6. CSF characteristics

Condition	Pressure (mm H$_2$O)	Cells/ml	Predominant cell type	Glucose (mg/dl)	Protein (mg/dl)
Normal	100–200	0–5	Lymphocyte	50–100	20–45
Bacterial/ purulent	>300	100–10,000	PMNs	<40 >100 (<50% serum glucose)	
Aseptic	N or increased	10–100	Lymphocytes	N	N or Increased
Subacute/ chronic	N or increased	25–200	Lymphocytes	Decreased	Increased

PMN = Polymorphonuclear leukocyte, N= Normal.
It is important to note that values are approximations; exceptions are common. Additionally, CSF pleocytosis may be absent or blunted in immunocompromised patients.
Lavoie FW, Saucier JR. Central nervous system infections. *Rosen's Emergency Medicine*, Sixth Edition. pp. 1714–1718. Mosby, 2006.

posterior fundus of the eye or via a head computed tomogram (CT). Head CT must be considered in all patients with a history of HIV infection, prior surgeries, or known history of brain mass.

Assessing which subset of patients will have the most severe disease course for meningitis and the highest mortality is an integral part of the discussion. The overall mortality rate was found to range from 21% to 27% in two large studies, which further examined prognostic signs.[25,27] Van de Beek et al. found that risk factors for an unfavorable outcome include advanced age, presence of otitis or sinusitis, absence of rash, a low score on the GCS on admission, tachycardia, an elevated erythrocyte sedimentation rate, thrombocytopenia, and a low CSF white count. Additionally the mortality rate was higher among patients with pneumococcal meningitis when compared with meningococcal meningitis.[25] Another study performed by Aronin et al. which examined 269 patients who had been diagnosed with bacterial meningitis found three baseline clinical features that were associated with adverse clinical outcome: hypotension, altered mental status, and seizures.[27]

All cerebrospinal fluid should be analyzed for white and red blood cell count, protein and glucose levels, and gram stain and culture. Additional tests such as cryptococcal antigen, herpes simplex virus, and RPR should be sent in the appropriate clinical situation. The CSF characteristics for bacterial, viral, tubercular, and encephalitis can be found in Table 6.6.

Patients suspected of having a CNS infection should be promptly treated with antibiotics to cover common pathogens. The basic regimen includes Ceftriaxone, Vancomycin, and Acyclovir. It is important to note that these antibiotics can be administered up to two hours prior to performing the lumbar puncture without affecting gram stain or culture results. The benefit of administration of dexamethasone for patients with meningitis was examined by de Gans et al. Treatment with dexamethasone, given either before or with the first dose of antibiotics, was associated with a reduction in the risk of an unfavorable outcome and mortality, with the greatest effects being found in the subset of patients found to have pneumococcal meningitis. Of note, there was no increase in the risk of a gastrointestinal bleed in patients who were administered dexamethasone.[28]

Central nervous system: subarachnoid hemorrhage (SAH) and cerebrovascular accident (CVA)

Strokes are a serious and common problem encountered in the emergency department. They are the third leading cause of death in the United States with an in-hospital mortality of 15% and a 30-day mortality of 20% to 25%. Additionally, patients often experience a dramatic loss in their ability to independently perform their activities of daily living. Stroke is defined as any vascular injury that reduces cerebral blood flow to a specific region of the brain causing neurologic impairment. They can be divided into strokes due to ischemia and strokes due to rupture of a blood vessel. Strokes due to occlusion make up 80% of all strokes, with hemorrhagic stroke due to rupture of a blood vessel making up the remaining 20%.[29]

Patients experiencing a stroke can present with a wide array of symptoms. Focal weakness and sensory deficit contralateral to the lesion is the symptom most commonly considered, but patients may also be found to have aphasia, altered mentation or decreased level of consciousness, gait disturbances, and a gaze preference depending on the location of the stroke. McManus et al. found that of 110 patients presenting with stroke, 23 patients were detected as being delirious with 21 having delirium present on their initial evaluation.[30] On arrival at the emergency department a rapid neurologic examination as well as a brief history should be obtained. The history should focus mainly on the symptom onset, which is defined as the time that the patient was symptom-free or last known to be normal. The neurologic exam should include the patient's score on the National Institutes of Health Stroke Scale (NIHSS). Any patient suspected of suffering from a stroke should promptly have lab tests including CBC, CMP, and coagulation studies sent and an urgent non-contrast head CT should be obtained.

Patients found to have an acute ischemic stroke can be qualified to receive recombinant tissue plasminogen activator (r-TPA). In order to qualify to receive r-TPA, at the time of writing, it must be determined that the patient's symptoms began no more than three hours prior and a rapid assessment should take place to determine if the patient has any contraindications. Based on the NINDS trial and recommendations from the American Heart Association, the decision to administer r-TPA should be made within 60 minutes of arrival in the emergency department as patients who received thrombolysis earlier (90–180 minutes versus 3 hours) were noted to have a better outcome. A blood pressure measured at greater than 185/110 is a contraindication to administering r-TPA. Another contraindication to receiving r-TPA is an elevated prothrombin time (PT) or activated partial thromboplastin time (PTT).[31] While it is appropriate to wait for results of the PT and PTT prior to administration, Gottesman et al. found it unnecessary unless the patient was on warfarin, heparin, had abnormal liver function tests, antiphospholipid syndrome, or end-stage renal disease on hemodialysis.[32]

Subarachnoid hemorrhage (SAH) is a commonly discussed diagnosis in the emergency department given its varying presentation and challenging diagnosis. The classic presentation of SAH is a thunderclap headache that the patient will describe as the worst headache of their life. Reijenveld et al., however, found on retrospective chart analysis that one in 70 patients with SAH present with an acute confusional state that can often mislead the physician in making the appropriate diagnosis.[33] Patients suspected of having an SAH should have a head CT performed. If the CT is negative, but the suspicion of SAH remains high, other diagnostic interventions such as a lumbar puncture (to evaluate for red blood cell count as well as xanthochromia) should be considered.

Summary

Delirium is a serious medical diagnosis that should not be missed as it has a relatively high mortality rate. It can be difficult to diagnose and is often mistaken for psychiatric illness. Often in the initial evaluation the distinction between primary psychiatric illness and delirium cannot be made with certainty. If this is the case, the clinician should err on the side of considering delirium as the diagnosis. Delay in care due to psychiatric referral and evaluation can result in adverse outcomes. Having a systematic method for evaluating patients who present with an acute onset of impairment of consciousness, thinking, memory, psychomotor behavior, perception, and emotion that fluctuates over a day is crucial for managing delirium. A thorough diagnostic evaluation and an understanding of the pathological process that can cause delirium are essential to reducing morbidity and mortality.

References

1. Elie M, Rousseau F, Cole M, et al. Prevalence and detection of delirium in elderly emergency department patients. *CMAJ.* 2000;**163**:8.

2. Inouye SK. Delirium in older persons. *N Engl J Med.* 2006;**354**:11.

3. Monette, J, Galbaud du Fort G, Fung S, et al. Evaluation of the confusion assessment method (CAM) as a screening tool for delirium in the emergency room. *Gen Hosp Psychiatry.* 2001;**23**:20.

4. Inouye SK. The dilemma of delirium: clinical and research controversies regarding diagnosis and evaluation of delirium in hospitalized elderly medical patients. *Am J Med.* 1994;**97**:3.

5. Smith J, Seirafi J. Delirium and dementia. In Marx JA, Hockberger RS, Walls RM (Eds.), *Rosen's Emergency Medicine: Concepts and Clinical Practice.* 7th ed. Philadelphia, PA: Elsevier Health Science, 2006.

6. Naughton BJ, Moran M, Ghaly Y, et al. Computed tomography scanning and delirium in elder patients. *Acad Emerg Med.* 1997;**4**:1107.

7. Bouchama A, Knochel J. Heat stroke. *N Engl J Med.* 2002;**346**:25.

8. Biem J, Koehncke N, Classen D, et al. Out of the cold: management of hypothermia and frostbite. *CMAJ.* 2003;**168**:3.

9. Arora S, McCullough L. Diagnosis and treatment of hypothermia. *Am Fam Physician.* 2004;**12**:70.

10. Mattu A, Brady W, Perron A. Electrocardiographic manifestations of hypothermia. *Am J Emerg Med.* 2002;**20**:4.

11. Kosten TR, O'Connor PG. Management of drug and alcohol withdrawal. *N Engl J Med.* 2003;**248**:18.

12. Alagiakrishnan K, Wiens CA. An approach to drug induced delirium in the elderly. *Postgrad Med.* 2004;**80**:388.

13. Sipahimalani A, Masand PS. Use of risperidone in delirium: case reports. *Ann Clin Psychiatry.* 1997;**9**:105.

14. Mayo-Smith MF, Beecher LH, Fischer TL, et al. Management of alcohol withdrawal delirium. *Arch Intern Med.* 2004;**164**:13.

15. Palmistierna T. A model for predicting alcohol withdrawal delirium. *Psychiatr Serv.* 2001;**52**:820.

16. Warner EA. Cocaine abuse. *Ann Int Med.* 1993;**119**:3.

17. Wetli CV, Mash D, Karch SB. Cocaine-associated agitated delirium and the neuroleptic malignant syndrome. *Am J Emerg Med.* 1996;**14**:425.

18. Albertson TE, Derlet RW, Van Hoozen BE. Methamphetamines and the expanding complications of amphetamines. *West J Med.* 1999;**170**:214.

19. Agostini JV, Leo-Summers LS, Inyoue SK. Cognitive and other adverse effects of diphenhydramine use in hospitalized older patients. *Arch Int Med*. 2001;**161**:2091.

20. Kitabchi AE, Kreisberg RA, Umpierrez GE, et al. Management of hyperglycemic crises in patients with diabetes. *Diabetes Care*. 2001;**24**:1.

21. Chiasson J, Aris-Jilwan N, Belanger R, et al. Diagnosis and treatment of diabetic ketoacidosis and the hyperglycemic hyperosmolar state. *Can Med Assoc J*. 2003;**168**:7.

22. Minino A, Heron M, et al. Deaths final data for 2004. *National Vital Statistics Report*. 2007;**55**:19.

23. Eidelman LA, Putterman D, Putterman C, Sprung CL. The spectrum of septic encephalopathy. Definitions, etiologies, and mortalities. *JAMA*. 1996;**275**(6): 470–473.

24. River E, Nguyen B, Havstad S, et al. Early goal directed therapy in the treatment of severe sepsis and septic shock. *N Engl J Med*. 2001;**345**:19.

25. Van de Beek D, De Gans J, Spanjaard L, et al. Clinical features and prognostic factors in adults with bacterial meningitis. *N Engl J Med*. 2004;**351**:18.

26. Thomas KE, Hasbun R, Jekel J, et al. The diagnostic accuracy of Kernig's sign, Brudzinski's sign and nuchal rigidity in adults with suspected meningitis. *Clin Infect Dis*. 2002;**35**:1.

27. Aronin SI, Peduzzi P, Quagliarello VJ. Community acquired bacterial meningitis: risk stratification for adverse clinical outcome and effect on antibiotic timing. *Ann Intern Med*. 1998;**129**:862.

28. De Gans J, Van de Beek D. Dexamethasone in adults with bacterial meningitis. *N Engl J Med*. 2002;**347**:20.

29. Kothari RU, Crocco TJ, Barsan WG. Stroke. In Marx JA, Hockberger RS, Walls RM (Eds.), *Rosen's Emergency Medicine: Concepts and Clinical Practice*. 7th ed. Philadelphia, PA: Elsevier Health Science, 2006.

30. McManus J, Pathansali R, Hassan H, et al. The course of delirium in acute stroke. *Age Ageing*. 2009;**38**:4.

31. Adams HP, del Zoppo G, Alberts MJ, et al. Guidelines for the early management of adults with ischemic stroke. *Circulation*. 2007;**115**:478.

32. Gottesman RF, Alt J, Wityk R, et al. Predicting abnormal coagulation in ischemic stroke: reducing delay in rt-PA use. *Neurology*. 2006;**67**:9.

33. Reijneveld J, Wermer M, Boonman Z, et al. Acute confusional state as presenting feature in aneurysmal subarachnoid hemorrhage: frequency and characteristics. *J Neurol*. 2000;**247**:112.

The anxious patient

Ashley D. Bone and O. Joseph Bienvenu

Anxiety disorders are among the most common psychiatric conditions worldwide, and persons with anxiety disorders consume a substantial portion of health services, including emergency services. In one study, anxiety disorders constituted 36% of psychiatric diagnoses made in the emergency department (ED), but only a minority of these patients required emergency psychiatric consultation.[1] Patients tended to be referred for emergency psychiatric evaluation only when they had comorbid depression, absence of medical illness, or when a triage nurse elicited psychiatrically relevant information. An understanding of the heterogeneity of disorders that can present with a significant anxiety component is essential to those who practice in acute care environments.

In EDs and many other settings, anxiety-related presentations often receive lower priority than other conditions. Emergency physicians tend not to view anxiety as a condition that is life or limb threatening and thus, are likely to provide only reassurance and small amounts of benzodiazepines or antihistamines to anxious patients who have a comorbid medical illness.[2] However, anxiety sufficient to cause an ED visit is likely to be extremely distressing to the patient. Thus, an understanding of anxiety-related disorders is critical in providing the appropriate treatment, which in some cases, may be to avoid certain medications, including benzodiazepines.

Patients who present acutely with a chief complaint of anxiety, nervousness, or panic attacks may suffer from a range of medical and psychiatric disorders, including anxiety, mood adjustment, and substance-related disorders, in addition to a primary medical condition. If patients are already in treatment for any of the above conditions, they often present to the ED in crisis or for medications.[3] However, it should be noted that requests for benzodiazepines should arouse attention and require careful evaluation. Given the possibility of anxiety presenting as a symptom of a medical illness, when a patient presents to the ED extremely anxious, a medical condition must be ruled out as the cause of the anxiety. Anxiety may assume numerous manifestations, ranging from somatic to behavioral or affective symptoms.

Emergency assessment

Medical stability and safety must be ensured before psychiatric evaluation proceeds. A medical or substance-related cause of anxiety symptoms should be suspected when the following are noted: acute or sudden onset, first presentation (especially after the age of 40), any clouding of consciousness, fluctuation (waxing and waning) in level of consciousness,

Emergency Psychiatry, ed. Arjun Chanmugam, Patrick Triplett, and Gabor Kelen. Published by Cambridge University Press. © Cambridge University Press 2013.

presence of visual, olfactory, or gustatory hallucinations, or autonomic instability.[4] Pollard and Lewis[5] noted that patients suffering from panic attacks typically describe their symptoms in terms of rapid or pounding heartbeat and ill-defined chest pain, as opposed to vice-like, crushing, substernal chest pain. During a panic attack, a patient may feel short of breath but rarely experiences stridor or wheezing. Also, although anxious patients may feel nauseated, they usually do not vomit. Clinical indicators consistent with the presence of panic attacks include: concern about losing control, a positive family history of anxiety disorder, initial onset between 18 and 45 years old, a recent or anticipated major life event, and presence of an agoraphobic pattern of avoidance.

The following signs suggest a primary medical or substance-related condition: pinpoint or dilated pupils, nystagmus, stereotypic movements, facial asymmetry, muscle weakness, or clouded consciousness. In general, patients whose anxiety results from a primary psychiatric illness are alert, clear headed, and are able to articulate a chief complaint and describe the nature of their symptoms. Any change in mental status may indicate a level of disorganization suggestive of a psychiatric condition of a different nature (e.g., psychosis) or may indicate an underlying medical illness. Clinicians should determine whether the symptoms are discrete and circumscribed, such as in panic disorder, or persistent and unremitting, such as in generalized anxiety disorder. Substance use questions should be directed to all patients, and the amount, frequency, and pattern of use should be elicited. Intoxication and withdrawal syndromes may precipitate anxiety symptoms. Family history may be helpful, as anxiety disorders are moderately heritable.

The mental status exam is fairly unremarkable in many patients with a primary anxiety disorder. Patients usually present with somewhat rapid speech, and are typically anxious or restless, but may also be depressed and tearful. Patients may be somewhat distractible, but cognition should be otherwise intact. The physical examination for patients with anxiety is also typically unremarkable. Isolated sinus tachycardia to 120 beats per minute and mild elevation in blood pressure are not uncommon. However, rates of more than 140 beats per minute, a lower than expected blood pressure in the presence of an elevated pulse, an increased respiratory rate in patients with a history of respiratory or cardiac disease, presence of wheezing, or vice-like chest pain suggest the need for further medical workup. Patients over 40 years of age, or those with previous cardiac history or known risk factors, must have a cardiac condition seriously considered as part of the ED evaluation. Risk factors for pulmonary embolism and deep venous thrombosis must also be considered carefully. Perhaps the most important component of any ED evaluation within the realm of anxiety disorders is an assessment of the potential for suicide and homicide.

There are several well-known medical causes of anxiety disorders that will be discussed later in this chapter. First, we will focus on primary anxiety disorders commonly seen in an emergency department.

Primary anxiety disorders
Panic disorder
Definition
The essential feature of panic disorder is recurrent, discrete anxiety or panic attacks. These attacks are characterized by unexpected, extreme anxiety or fear, accompanied by a variety of autonomically mediated symptoms. The latter result from excitation of the sympathetic

nervous system and include heart palpitations, chest tightness or pain, and shortness of breath. Hyperventilation that accompanies this autonomic surge may contribute to additional symptoms, such as dizziness and paresthesias.

The frequency, severity, and duration of these unexpected and recurrent attacks can vary widely. In order to be characterized as panic disorder, the panic attacks must not be due to a substance, general medical condition, or other psychiatric disorder. The relationship of attacks to situational stressors has diagnostic importance; unexpected attacks occur in panic disorder, whereas situational attacks occur in phobias and other anxiety disorders.

Clinical presentation

Typically, symptoms begin suddenly and crescendo rapidly, reaching a peak within 10 minutes. Attacks usually last 10–30 minutes, and rarely do they last as long as an hour. Panic attacks are often accompanied by catastrophic misinterpretations of the danger they represent. Typically patients fear dying, going crazy, or collapsing. In response to palpitations, chest pain, and shortness of breath, patients may believe they are having a "heart attack." With dizziness and depersonalization (a change in an individual's self-awareness such that they feel detached from their own experience, with the self, the body, and mind seeming alien), patients may feel as though they are "going crazy." Similarly, lightheadedness, weakness, and flushing may be interpreted as impending physical collapse.

Patients with panic disorder often present to the emergency department with a primary somatic complaint. For example, Fleet et al.[6] found that approximately 25% (108/441) of chest pain patients that presented to an ED met DSM-III-R criteria for panic disorder. Although almost half of these panic disorder patients had a prior documented history of coronary artery disease, 80% had atypical or non-anginal chest pain, and 75% were discharged with a "non-cardiac pain" diagnosis. Ninety-eight percent of the patients with panic disorder were not recognized as such by attending cardiologists. Non-recognition may lead to mismanagement of a significant group of distressed patients, including those with coronary artery disease.[1] Before chest pain is ascribed to panic or any other psychiatric basis, it is imperative that providers confidently exclude cardiac and other causes of chest pain. Likewise any chest pain patient should have consideration for an anxiety disorder especially when other diagnostic entities have been excluded.

Aside from cardiac manifestations of panic disorder, there is intriguing evidence suggesting pathophysiologic relationships among dyspnea, hyperventilation, and panic symptoms. The symptoms of panic attacks and pulmonary disease overlap, and therefore, dyspnea can reflect an anxiety disorder, and panic symptoms can reflect cardiopulmonary disease. There is reason to believe that the pathogenesis of panic may be related to respiratory physiology by several mechanisms: the anxiogenic effects of hyperventilation, the catastrophic misinterpretation (by the patient) of respiratory symptoms, and/or a neurobiologic sensitivity to CO_2, lactate, or other signals of suffocation.[7] Therefore, in a patient presenting to the ED with dyspnea, with medical causes confidently excluded, panic disorder should be considered and investigated.

Epidemiology

Not only is panic disorder relatively common in the general population, it is especially common in primary care settings. Given that patients typically present with somatic symptoms, panic disorder is particularly relevant to care in EDs and other acute care settings. Panic disorder is roughly twice as common in women as in men,[8] and the incidence of panic disorder is greatest in young persons aged 15–24 years. Also, persons with fewer than 12 years of education are more commonly affected than persons with 16 or more years of schooling.

Comorbidity

Psychiatric comorbidity is extremely common among persons with anxiety disorders. The most common comorbid conditions are other anxiety and depressive disorders, although anxiety disorders are also associated with substance use disorders.[9]

There is reason to believe that pulmonary disease constitutes a risk factor for the development of panic disorder. The connection between the two may be repeated experiences of dyspnea and life-threatening exacerbations of pulmonary dysfunction, as well as repeated episodes of hypercapnia or hyperventilation, the use of anxiogenic medications, and the stress of coping with chronic disease. Panic in pulmonary patients may carry significant morbidity, including phobic avoidance of activity, aggressive treatment with anxiogenic medications, and more prolonged and frequent episodic care visits and hospitalizations. Successful treatment of panic in these patients can improve functional status and quality of life by relieving anxiety and dyspnea.

Cognitive-behavioral approaches and other non-pharmacologic treatments of panic can be useful in patients with concomitant respiratory disease. To avoid respiratory depression, sedating medications such as benzodiazepines should be used with caution. Instead, serotonergic antidepressants may be effective treatments for panic disorder in pulmonary patients because this class of medications has relatively little potential for significant adverse effects on respiration.[7]

Differential diagnosis

Anxiety is often a presenting symptom of other mental disorders, such as mood disorders, delirium, and substance use disorders. Significant anxiety in a patient with no personal or family history of anxiety should heighten suspicion for toxic or medical factors that could be contributing. However, a positive psychiatric history should not blind the clinician to other possible contributing factors, medical or otherwise. Similarly, a previously negative psychiatry history should not blind the clinician to an undiagnosed anxiety disorder; however, first time presentation demands a thorough medical evaluation.

A helpful diagnostic technique is to ask for a description of the patient's first panic attack. Individuals with panic disorder rarely forget the first attack, which is often the single most upsetting experience in his or her life.

Workup

A recent meta-analysis addressed correlates of panic disorder in patients seeking evaluation of chest pain in EDs or outpatient clinics.[10] Five variables were strongly related to panic disorder in these patients: absence of coronary artery disease, atypical quality of chest pain, female sex, younger age, and a high level of self-reported anxiety.

First time presentations have a medical workup dictated by the predominant symptom, past medical history, review of symptoms, and physical exam. First time chest pain presentations will usually require an acute coronary syndrome (ACS) evaluation, but one should also consider the standard ED differential diagnoses for chest pain (i.e., pulmonary embolus, pneumothorax, pericarditis, pneumonia, perforated viscous, and dissection).

Diagnostic tests to consider in the workup of panic symptoms include: a complete blood count (to help rule out infection, anemia, polycythemia, thrombocytopenia, etc.), a comprehensive metabolic panel, cardiac enzymes (if ACS is considered), and urine analysis. Particular attention should be paid to serum values of sodium, calcium, blood urea nitrogen, creatinine, liver transaminases, albumin, magnesium, phosphorus, and thyroid stimulating hormone. Serum and urine toxicology should be performed to screen for the presence of illicit or other substances/medications that may be contributing to the presentation. Even in patients with an established prior history of panic disorder, some of these ancillary tests may be appropriate, as underlying disorders can potentiate anxiety presentations.

Monitoring of the electrocardiogram and cardiac status is essential in patients presenting with chest pain or shortness of breath. Brain imaging studies are dictated by the urgency and uniqueness of the presentation for the patient. As noted before, lateralizing findings and altered sensorium essentially preclude a primary psychiatric diagnosis of anxiety. If a CNS infection is reasonably within the differential diagnoses, then an examination of cerebrospinal fluid is necessary. While an EEG may be helpful in the evaluation of non-convulsive seizures or delirium, presentation of these conditions preclude the ED diagnosis of anxiety.

Treatment

Effective treatments for panic disorder include both pharmacological and psychological therapies. In choosing an approach, the severity of a patient's illness, any coexisting disorders (e.g., major depressive or substance use disorders), and the patient's prior treatment responses should be taken into consideration. Initially, many patients are convinced that they are physically ill and therefore resist psychiatric treatment.

By default, pharmacotherapy has become the standard treatment choice in the ED. Given the high prevalence of substance use disorders in this population, it is often wise to pick non-benzodiazepine medications as a first choice, if possible. Alprazolam, diazepam, and lorazepam have high abuse potential,[11] though patients with addiction histories may also abuse other benzodiazepines. Antihistamines such as diphenhydramine or hydroxyzine have a potential role in helping with panic symptoms by virtue of their sedative properties. Selective serotonin reuptake inhibitors (SSRIs) and tricyclic antidepressants gradually reduce the likelihood and intensity of panic attacks, but the clinical benefit is often not seen for at least 2–3 weeks. SSRIs are not addictive and generally do not cause drowsiness, making them a consideration for the ED setting. However, it is important to keep in mind that patients can become more anxious acutely when starting an antidepressant; this can be minimized by starting patients on lower doses (e.g., half the usual starting dose for the treatment of depression).

Atypical neuroleptics may be useful as adjunctive medications, particularly in patients with comorbid conditions.[12] Olanzapine and quetiapine may be particularly helpful in patients presenting with anxiety who have comorbid bipolar disorder. However, one must balance the risk of weight gain and hyperglycemia associated with these medications. Overall caution should be exercised when prescribing longitudinal medications in the ED, as these patients should have close follow-up with psychiatry, especially if new medications are to be started.

Cognitive-behavioral therapy (CBT) that focuses on relaxation, changes in thinking, and exposure to benign anxiety symptoms and anxiety-provoking situations has been shown to reduce panic. However, CBT expertise is rare in the ED environment. Nevertheless, Swinson et al.[13] have argued for definitive behavioral treatment of panic attacks in the emergency setting. In their study, patients who presented with panic attacks were randomly assigned to receive either reassurance alone, or reassurance coupled with exposure instruction, all of which occurred in the ED or within 48 hours. Those in the exposure group were told that the most effective way to reduce fear was to confront the situation in which the attack occurred. Patients in the exposure group were instructed to return to the situation as soon as possible after the interview and to wait there until the anxiety decreased. In the group of patients that received only reassurance, the frequency of panic attacks increased, and little difference was noted on measures of distress. However, in the exposure group, panic attacks decreased in frequency and measures of distress improved significantly. For many patients with panic attacks, the ED is the first point of contact within the health care system. Interventions, such as CBT, in the emergency setting may reduce the long-term consequences of panic attacks. In the future, other brief cognitive-based interventions may be available to acute care providers in the emergency setting, but more research is needed to establish their effectiveness.

Starting medications or interventions such as CBT in most emergency department settings is just the beginning, and patients should be strongly encouraged to follow up with their primary care physicians or seek the help of a psychiatrist or psychologist if available. In many cases, more frequent visits early in their treatment can be extremely beneficial.

Generalized anxiety disorder
Definition
Generalized anxiety disorder (GAD) is characterized by a prolonged period of excessive worry and anxiety manifesting as restlessness or feeling "keyed up" or "on edge," thereby leading to easy fatigability, difficulty concentrating, irritability, increased muscle tension, or sleep disturbance.

Clinical presentation
GAD has a chronic, fluctuating course; thus, emergency presentation is unlikely unless an acute stressor overwhelms the patient's coping mechanisms. Patients often present with unpleasant overarousal and/or somatic symptoms like muscle aching, fatigue, tension headaches, rapid heart rate, diaphoresis, gastrointestinal distress, or frequent urination.[14]

Epidemiology
GAD is one of the more common anxiety disorders, with a lifetime prevalence of ~6%. Risk factors include female sex, age >24 years, being previously married, being unemployed, and living in the Northeastern United States.[15]

Comorbidity
There are extremely high rates of comorbidity in persons with GAD,[16] and depressive disorders are the most common comorbid diagnoses.

Differential diagnosis
Due to general medical conditions and/or substances, GAD must be distinguished from anxiety disorders. The syndrome is often associated with mood disorders, and it should not

be diagnosed separately if it occurs in the context of these conditions. The diagnosis of an adjustment disorder with anxiety should only be made if the criteria for generalized anxiety disorder are not met. It should also be noted that normal worry, as compared to GAD, is less likely to be accompanied by physical symptoms.

Workup

The workup of generalized anxiety is virtually identical to that for panic.

Treatment

If a patient is presenting to the ED with primary GAD, it is likely severe and usually requires pharmacological treatment. A number of medications, including benzodiazepines, SSRIs, tricyclic antidepressants, azapirones, and sedating antihistamines (e.g., diphenhydramine or hydroxyzine) are helpful in GAD.[17] Benzodiazepines have marked effects on arousal and somatic anxiety, but less pronounced effects on psychic symptoms. The various benzodiazepines are similar in therapeutic properties but differ in pharmacokinetics, as drugs that are rapidly absorbed have greater abuse potential. The greatest drawback to benzodiazepines is their dependence potential, and discontinuation of benzodiazepines may be associated with rebound anxiety that is difficult to distinguish from the primary disorder. Benzodiazepines can also aggravate depression and cause transient amnesia. Alcohol in combination with benzodiazepines can lead to numerous complications, including drug-induced deaths and traffic accidents. In the elderly, the sedative effects can contribute to motor incoordination with a greater potential for falls, as well as cognitive impairment and delirium.

Antidepressants are useful in the long-term treatment of GAD, but their delay in therapeutic action limits their usefulness in the management of acute anxiety. For example, buspirone, the prototypical azapirone, is a partial agonist of the serotonin receptor and, similar to the antidepressants, does not act immediately. Sedating antihistamines are useful in the emergency setting because their anxiolytic effects are rapid, but these medications should be used with caution in elderly patients due to their deliriogenic properties. Patients should also typically be referred for psychotherapy, possibly including CBT.

Obsessive-compulsive disorder

Definition

Obsessive-compulsive disorder (OCD) is characterized by intrusive, distressing thoughts, images, or urges (obsessions) and senseless or excessive, repetitive behaviors (compulsions). A diagnosis of OCD is made if obsessions and/or compulsions are substantially distressing or interfere with functioning.

Clinical presentation

Because the distress of OCD is typically chronic and persistent, patients do not normally present to the ED. Therefore, of all the anxiety disorders, patients with OCD have the lowest rate of treatment through the ED.[18]

Some patients with OCD have excessive concerns that they may have HIV infection or AIDS, even without the presence of any risk factors. The term "FRAIDS" (fear of AIDS) has occasionally been used to describe these patients, as these patients appear repeatedly for HIV testing.

Epidemiology

OCD used to be thought of as being rare but is now recognized as a frequently debilitating anxiety disorder that affects ~2% of the population.[19] OCD affects males and females equally, though onset is generally earlier in males (childhood). Patients occasionally report onset or worsening of symptoms around the time of a stressful event, such as during pregnancy or delivery of their baby. Because many patients are secretive about their symptoms, there is often a delay of 5–10 years after onset before patients seek psychiatric assistance.

Comorbidity

Many patients with OCD struggle with comorbid Axis I conditions (major mental disorders), such as major depression.[20] Skodol et al.[21] found that OCD was two to three times more likely to be diagnosed in combination with a Cluster C personality disorder (the fearful, anxious cluster): dependent personality disorder, obsessive-compulsive personality disorder, or avoidant personality disorder.

Other common comorbid conditions include the "OCD spectrum disorders,"[22] including tic disorders, body dysmorphic disorder, hypochondriasis, and grooming disorders (e.g., trichotillomania). Anxiety is usually not the chief complaint of patients who have these conditions, although they may present with other anxiety-related complaints.

Differential diagnosis

Since a primary diagnosis of OCD is unlikely to be established based on one ED visit, an understanding of the differential diagnosis of conditions that may mimic this condition is of equal importance. Although GAD and OCD have overlapping etiologies, obsessions of OCD should be properly distinguished from the excessive worries seen in GAD. Depressive ruminations are also sometimes confused with obsessions, but the diagnosis of OCD should not be considered unless clear obsessions and/or compulsions are present. In patients with OCD, certain stimuli sometimes provoke anxiety about, and avoidance of, dirt or contamination; however, the co-occurrence of typical obsessions or rituals clarifies the diagnosis of OCD instead of specific phobia. The presence of frank obsessions and ritualistic behaviors also helps to distinguish OCD from obsessive-compulsive personality disorder (OCPD). OCPD is not characterized by anguish, but rather by perfectionism, orderliness, and control. Patients with OCD know that their behaviors are not rational but are nonetheless compelled to do them, thereby causing significant distress.

In some patients with OCD, the symptoms become so severe that the patient seems truly uncertain as to whether his or her concerns are realistic. Such symptoms are termed "overvalued ideas"; for example, a patient may hold the almost unshakable belief that he will contaminate other people unless he washes his hands excessively after urinating. However, the OCD patient can usually acknowledge the possibility that his or her belief may be unfounded. In contrast, the person with a true delusion has a fixed conviction and also is likely to have other psychotic symptoms, such as ideas of reference, paranoia, and/or hallucinations.[23]

Workup

A complete mental status examination should be performed. The patient should be evaluated for disturbances of mood and affect, suicide risk, hallucinations or delusions, orientation, memory, and insight/judgment. All patients with suspected OCD should be evaluated for the presence of tic disorders, as these comorbid diagnoses may influence the treatment strategy. (A tic is an uncontrollable, sudden and repeated movement of a part of the body.) Findings on neurologic and cognitive examinations should otherwise be normal. Focal neurologic signs or evidence of cognitive impairment should prompt evaluation for other diagnoses. Attention should be given to a dermatologic exam, as patients with OCD may have dry, red skin from excessive washing, hair loss from compulsive hair pulling, or lesions from compulsive skin picking. In addition, routine laboratory tests should be performed to rule out medical or substance-induced causes of symptoms.

Treatment

Of the antidepressants, only SSRIs or clomipramine are effective in OCD.[24] Patients with OCD typically require doses in excess of those normally prescribed for the treatment of other anxiety or depressive disorders. Response to treatment is usually quite gradual and may take up to 8–12 weeks. Atypical antipsychotics are often useful augmenting agents.

Though not well-suited in the ED environment, behavioral therapy, specifically exposure and response prevention, is highly efficacious. Meta-analyses and clinical significance analyses indicate that 60%–80% of patients who engage in this treatment improve substantially.[25] Again, starting medications or CBT in most ED settings is just the beginning, as patients should be strongly encouraged to follow up with their primary care physicians or seek the help of a psychiatrist or psychologist. For these patients, more frequent visits early in the treatment course are extremely beneficial, especially given that patients with OCD often have a slower response to treatment.

Acute stress disorder and posttraumatic stress disorder
Definition

Both acute stress disorder (ASD) and posttraumatic stress disorder (PTSD) require exposure to a traumatic event. While there has been debate over the definition of a traumatic event, this definition is the same for both conditions. However, what distinguishes ASD and PTSD is when post-trauma symptoms occur and how long they last. In ASD, symptoms must last at least two days but less than four weeks, whereas in PTSD, the symptoms last for a period of at least a month. Symptoms can include dissociative symptoms (e.g., depersonalization – dissociation is required in ASD) and must include reexperiencing of the trauma, avoidance of associated stimuli, and increased arousal.

With regards to constituting a "traumatic event," DSM-IV requires "an event that involves actual or threatened death or serious injury, or a threat to the physical integrity of self or others." In addition, "the person's response must involve intense fear, helplessness, or horror."

Clinical presentation

Patients present with reexperiencing (e.g., intrusive memories, flashbacks, or nightmares), avoidance of stimuli or numbing, and symptoms of increased arousal. Reexperiencing can occur spontaneously or can be triggered by external sensory stimuli, even though patients typically avoid situations that remind them of the trauma. Numbness refers to a state of detachment, emotional blunting, and relative unresponsiveness to surroundings.

Hyperarousal is indicated by sleep disturbance, difficulty with memory and concentration, hypervigilance, irritability, and an exaggerated startle response.

Patients with this disorder remain trapped by intense past experiences. This interferes with the capacity to maintain involvement in current life activities and relationships. Numbing and decreased responsiveness make it difficult for patients to gain normal rewards from ongoing interactions in social and work environments.

Epidemiology

The lifetime prevalence of PTSD in the United States has been estimated at 7%. However, it is important to note that many people experience traumatic events without developing long-term psychological symptoms or becoming disabled. Kessler et al.[26] found that, in men, the most common traumatic events associated with PTSD were engaging in combat and witnessing death or severe injury, whereas in women, the most common traumatic events associated with PTSD were being raped or sexually molested. Significant sex differences were evident in the types of lifetime traumas experienced: 25% of men had had an accident, in contrast to 14% of women; whereas 9% of women had been raped, in contrast to <1% of men. The association of these events to PTSD varied significantly as well: 48% of female rape victims had PTSD, while 11% of men who witnessed death or serious injury had PTSD.

Since only a fraction of those who are exposed to traumatic events develop either ASD or PTSD, individual vulnerability plays a crucial role in the development of the disorder. Risk factors for ASD include trauma severity, female gender, and avoidant coping style.[27] Potent risk factors for PTSD include trauma severity, female sex, pre-trauma psychiatric illness, and family history of psychiatric illness.[28] A history of psychological treatment can be a better predictor of PTSD than the traumatic event itself.

Comorbidity

PTSD rarely occurs in the absence of other psychopathology. As with all anxiety disorders, comorbidity with other anxiety and depressive disorders is frequent, but substance use disorders are also common comorbid conditions.

Differential diagnosis

Not only are responses to trauma highly variable, but trauma can also precipitate a variety of psychiatric conditions, including generalized anxiety disorder, depression, somatoform disorders, or adjustment disorders. Evidence of an ulterior motive and the absence of distress when a patient believes he or she is unobserved may suggest malingering.

Workup

Patients may present with physical injuries from the traumatic event (e.g., bruises in victims of domestic abuse). The mental status exam may reveal motor agitation, an increased startle response, poor concentration or impulse control, tense mood, suicidal or homicidal thoughts, or evidence of reexperiencing. Routine laboratory tests are important to evaluate for substance-related disorders.

Treatment

Definitive treatment of patients with PTSD is not usually attempted in the acute setting, but management of patients with acute symptomatology may necessitate temporary pharmacologic intervention with a non-benzodiazepine sedative or atypical antipsychotic. Symptoms requiring pharmacologic treatment may include insomnia, poor impulse control, or explosive outbursts. CBT anxiety management techniques, including controlled breathing, muscle relaxation, and guided self-dialogue, are also helpful.

Appropriate treatment of PTSD is essential to reduce symptoms and increase functioning and quality of life for the patient. Early intervention is crucial in order to help prevent the development of secondary chronic comorbidity. There are five treatment goals when treating PTSD: (1) reducing the core symptoms, (2) improving stress resilience, (3) improving quality of life, (4) reducing disability, and (5) reducing comorbidity.[28]

A number of treatment outcome studies for PTSD have focused on CBT, which includes variants of anxiety management, exposure therapy, and cognitive therapy. Successful treatment of PTSD using CBT will involve developing an accepting attitude toward treatment, a capacity to tolerate distress, outside support, and minimization of comorbidities.[29] Exposure therapy has the strongest evidence of efficacy in different populations of trauma victims with PTSD, but a few patients failed to show sufficient gains with this therapy.

PTSD may be successfully treated with CBT alone, but in cases that present to the ED, combined pharmacotherapy and psychotherapy should be considered. The 1999 consensus statement on PTSD[30] recommends starting treatment with an SSRI three weeks after exposure to a traumatic event in those patients with no improvement in their acute stress response. An SSRI should be started at a low dose, and the dose should be gradually titrated upward to the same or higher level than that used to treat depression. An appropriate trial of initial drug therapy is three months, but effective pharmacotherapy should be continued for 12 months or longer, depending on the severity and duration of illness, as well as the presence of any comorbid conditions. In addition, most patients should be referred for CBT.

No studies support the efficacy of benzodiazepines in PTSD, but some evidence does suggest that the clinical condition of patients with PTSD deteriorates when they are treated with benzodiazepines. Even in the setting of sleep disturbance, physicians should typically avoid benzodiazepines. Most recently, atypical antipsychotics have been used off-label for PTSD. They show promise both in their effects on mood and anxiety and in their effects on psychosis. Psychotic-like features may be related to the core PTSD symptoms (i.e., reexperiencing) or reflect comorbid conditions such as major depression.

Recommendations regarding whether medications or CBT should be used as first line treatments depend on local resources. Medication is widely available, whereas CBT is often limited to larger cities with medical schools or universities offering graduate training in clinical psychology. Medication management appointments tend to be shorter than CBT sessions so that, in the short run, fewer human resources are needed to administer medication than to conduct CBT. However, some PTSD sufferers are not willing to take medication, and many would prefer CBT to medication when given a choice.[31] Treatment availability, feasibility, and patient preference should be the primary factors in guiding treatment selection.

Clinical guidelines for primary care management of PTSD include: (1) educating patients regarding the normal stress response and encouraging them to discuss experiences with family and friends in the first few days after exposure to trauma; (2) referring the patient to a mental health professional, especially if there is no clinical improvement within three weeks; (3) ensuring that patients get one or two counseling sessions to deal with distress and create a sense of safety with ongoing monitoring within the first two weeks after the trauma; (4) consider starting a non-benzodiazepine sedative if a patient has had four consecutive nights of sleep disturbance; (5) consider starting a low-dose SSRI and/or (6) continuing effective drug therapy in most patients for 12 months or longer; and (7) referring patients who are refractory to initial drug therapy at three months and those with complicating comorbid conditions to a psychiatrist. In the ED, the most important consideration is to ensure that the patient has close psychiatric follow-up.

Prevention

Given that the ED is often the first line of treatment following traumatic events, the most important role of the ED is to determine if there are preventive measures that can be taken to diminish the progression from acute stress to PTSD. Patients should be educated about the normal stress response and support services should be identified for follow-up counseling.

The terrorist attacks of September 11, 2001 have brought into the forefront the urgent need to prepare for such circumstances. At present, there is little empirical knowledge about effective interventions following terrorism. One potential intervention is aimed at normalizing expected acute stress reactions that are experienced by most people affected by the traumatic event and which are expected to resolve when the situation has been stabilized. This consists mainly of delivering information to the affected community. Psychological debriefing used to be considered the mainstay for community education, as session leaders would ask participants to describe their thoughts, feelings, and behavioral reactions during the event. Leaders would also provide psychoeducation to reassure participants that acute stress reactions are normal responses to horrific events, and not necessarily indicative of mental illness. However, randomized controlled trials investigating the efficacy of psychological debriefing do not support the usefulness of this intervention in preventing chronic stress reactions.

Pitman et al.[32] hypothesized that early administration of propranolol following trauma may decrease the effects of excessive catecholamine release, which was thought to be central in the development and maintenance of PTSD. They administered propranolol or placebo for a period of ten days beginning within six hours after a traumatic event. Rates of PTSD one month following the trauma were 30% in the placebo group and 18% in the propranolol group, a difference that may have had clinical relevance but was not statistically distinct. At three months after the trauma, the corresponding rates were 13% and 11%, respectively. Assessment of skin conductance in response to a tape-recorded description of the trauma three months after the event revealed lower levels of arousal in the propranolol-treated patients. Although results of this small study ($N=41$) are suggestive, replication in a larger sample is warranted before drawing conclusions regarding the efficacy of propranolol as an effective preventative agent for PTSD.

Adjustment disorder with anxious mood

The diagnosis of an adjustment disorder with anxiety is made if a patient becomes anxious in response to an identifiable stressor. Symptoms must develop within three months and resolve within six months. The distress experienced by these individuals is meant to be in excess of what would be expected from the event or result in significant impairment in social or occupational functioning.

Adjustment disorder (AD) is thought to be common, as some studies suggest prevalences as high as 23% in clinical populations. Comorbidity with other psychiatric diagnoses, such as personality disorders, anxiety disorders, affective disorders, and psychoactive substance use disorders, is reported in up to 70% of patients with AD in adult medical settings of general hospitals.[33] Therefore, these comorbidities should be considered when the diagnosis of AD is considered in patients presenting to the ED.

Anxiety symptoms related to medical illnesses or drugs

The number of medical disorders that can directly or indirectly cause anxiety is extensive (see Table 7.1). Clinicians should always consider the possibility that anxiety is caused by a general medical illness or is a side effect of medications, especially when the onset of symptoms is after 35 years of age, when there is no family history of anxiety, and when there is no history of other psychiatric symptoms or recent major stressors.

A variety of drugs are capable of producing anxiety symptoms (see Table 7.2). Information should be obtained routinely about any recent additions of medications (including over-the-counter medications) or changes in dosage.

Table 7.1. Medical conditions associated with prominent anxiety symptoms

General medical illness types/systems	Conditions
Cardiovascular	Angina, arrhythmias, congestive heart failure, hypertension, hyperventilation, hypovolemia, myocardial infarction, shock, syncope, valvular disease
Endocrine	Cushing syndrome, hyperkalemia, hyperthermia, hyperthyroidism, hypothyroidism, hypocalcemia, hypoglycemia, diabetes mellitus, hyponatremia, hypoparathyroidism, menopause
Hematologic	Acute intermittent porphyria, anemias
Immunologic	Anaphylaxis, systemic lupus erythematosus
Infection	Acute or chronic infection
Neoplastic (secreting tumors)	Carcinoid tumor, insulinoma, pheochromocytoma
Neurologic	Cerebral syphilis, cerebrovascular insufficiency, encephalopathies, essential tremor, Huntington's chorea, intracranial mass lesions, migraine headache, multiple sclerosis, postconcussive syndrome, posterolateral sclerosis, polyneuritis, seizure disorders (especially temporal lobe seizures), vertigo, vasculitis, Wilson's disease
Respiratory	Asthma, chronic obstructive pulmonary disease, pneumonia, pneumothorax, pulmonary edema, pulmonary embolism
Other	Beriberi

Table 7.2. Medications associated with anxiety

Anesthetics/analgesics

Antidepressants (tricyclics, SSRIs, bupropion)

Antihistamines

Antihypertensives

Antimicrobials

Bronchodilators

Caffeine preparations

Calcium-blocking agents

Cholinergic-blocking agents

Digitalis

Estrogen

Ethosuximide

Heavy metals and toxins

Herbal remedies: ginseng root, ma huang, guarana (found in herbal diet preparations)

Hydralazine

Insulin

Levodopa

Muscle relaxants

Neuroleptics

Nicotine

Non-steroidal anti-inflammatories

Procaine

Procarbazine

Sedatives

Steroids

Sympathomimetics (often in cold/allergy medicines): epinephrine, norepinephrine, isoproteronol, levodopa, dopamine hydrochloride, dobutamine, terbutaline sulfate, ephedrine, pseudoephedrine, phenylephrine

Theophylline

Thyroid preparations

As noted in the panic disorder section, SSRIs and other antidepressants can induce anxiety symptoms, particularly early in the course of treatment (the first few days) or in combination with other medications. Serotonin syndrome or serotonin toxicity is characterized by neuromuscular excitation (clonus, hyperreflexia, myoclonus, and rigidity), sympathetic hyperactivity (hyperthermia, tachycardia, diaphoresis, tremor, and flushing), and changed mental status (anxiety, agitation, and confusion). There are several drug combinations that cause excess serotonin, the most common being monoamine oxidase inhibitors in combination with SSRIs. Treatment should focus on cessation of one or more offending agent(s) and supportive care. For example, a second-line treatment for methicillin-resistant *Staphylococcus aureus* (MRSA) infections (i.e., after vancomycin) is linezolid, which demonstrates reversible, non-selective inhibition of monoamine oxidase, so clinicians should be mindful of potential serotonin syndrome in patients on a combination of linezolid and SSRIs.[34]

Discontinuation of certain drugs may also be associated with anxiety. If alcohol is abruptly stopped, withdrawal symptoms, including severe anxiety, may appear within the first day. Likewise, benzodiazepines, especially short-acting formulations, can cause similar withdrawal phenomena. Patients dependent on narcotics, whether prescription or illicit, may also experience anxiety as part of a withdrawal syndrome. Many of these patients may be unable or unwilling to accurately report their actual use of these agents. When possible, collateral information from family, friends, and other physicians should be sought, and patients' medication bottles, if available, should be examined closely.

Other drugs that are often overlooked that can generate anxiety include over-the-counter preparations for cold symptoms, weight suppression, or sleep induction.[35] These may include compounds of pseudoephedrine, phenylephrine, and ephedrine. These substances are also found in herbal remedies under a number of pseudonyms such as ma huang.

Anxiety comorbid with a medical disorder

Comorbidity of anxiety disorders and general medical illnesses is common, and anxiety disorders are strongly and independently associated with poor physical health-related quality of life and disability.[36] The disability and related poor physical and economic outcomes associated with anxiety disorders may be as great as with depression. In a sample of 480 primary care patients, the probability of missing time from work in the previous month for persons with an anxiety disorder was as great as for persons with major depression (odds ratio = 2.2).[37] Anxiety disorders are also associated with high rates of medically unexplained symptoms and increased utilization of health care resources.[38]

Special considerations
The acute therapeutic environment

Several hospital-associated factors are associated with anxiety. These include financial burden, intrusive medical procedures, isolation, loss of autonomy, loss of privacy, physical discomfort/pain, possibility of death, and uncertainty regarding cause/prognosis. Often, the environment of the ED can increase anxiety instead of alleviating it.

Since anxious patients are often overstimulated, a properly constructed psychiatric emergency service should offer a quiet environment. In addition, given that anxious patients may be suicidal, it is important to have an environment free of sharp instruments and other hazards. Lastly, anything that might be used for hanging must be tested for load bearing. Given the high level of supervision needed, it is helpful to observe the entire area from a central location. Also, the privacy needs of the patient must be balanced with the need for supervision. Having television or reading materials for distraction is sometimes helpful.[39] Given the number of medical conditions that can present with anxiety, it is important to have the psychiatric emergency service located near a medical ED.

In order to properly reassure anxious patients, appropriate staff availability and space is paramount. The general principles useful in approaching most psychiatric emergencies are equally applicable to the handling of an anxious patient. Early verbal contact is advised because allowing the opportunity to put thoughts and emotions into words invariably helps to reduce initial tension. A private and relaxed setting for the interview is important. However, this can prove challenging when other contributing medical conditions have not yet been excluded. It is important to allow for a delayed final evaluation because many initially overwhelmed anxious people may reconstitute within a matter of hours when allowed to talk, rest, or even sleep. The anxious patient's chief complaint, even if it is somatic, should be taken seriously. A physical examination should be performed routinely in all cases, especially when there is a physical complaint. Within the scope of the ED practice, an "organic" etiology for the anxiety should be ruled out. The emergency physician should be careful to avoid a judgmental or punitive approach, as patients find it most comforting when they experience the feeling of being understood. While in the ED, every attempt should be made to engage the family in caring for the patient. The emergency medicine physician and the acute care team need to assess the degree and adequacy of social support available in the patient's environment, especially since sensible disposition may depend on it.[40]

Suicide

A major priority of any ED is evaluation and disposition of patients who are at risk for self-harm. Among the anxiety disorders, panic disorder may be particularly associated with suicidal behavior. In epidemiological samples, panic disorder was found to be associated with a similar prevalence of lifetime suicidal ideation and attempts as major depression.[41] Uncomplicated panic disorder (i.e., without comorbid conditions) was also associated with an increased suicide risk.[42] Notably, other anxiety disorders (e.g., GAD and social phobia) also appear to be associated with increased suicidal behavior.[43] Some authors report a possible additive effect of major depression and anxiety disorders/agitation, in that patients with both appear at particularly high risk for suicide attempts.[44]

Regardless of the diagnosis, when confronted with an anxious patient in the emergency room, it is important to keep in mind that intense anxious episodes can be antecedents to suicidal behavior. It is best to hospitalize a patient when the clinician is uncertain about the patient's safety and when an adequate plan for follow-up is not available.

Summary

Anxiety disorders are among the most common psychiatric conditions, and the impact of these disorders on patients is substantial. In the acute setting, approach the anxious patient carefully, as anxiety may be a manifestation of a medical disorder as well as a possible comorbid or isolated psychiatric condition. A careful history, including a past medical history and a thorough examination in a safe private setting, is essential. An understanding of the psychiatric conditions that can present with anxiety, along with the judicious use of pharmacotherapy and counseling, will be critical in creating the most appropriate treatment plan.

References

1. Fenichel GS, Murphy JG. Factors that predict consultation in the emergency department. *Med Care*. 1985;23:258–265.

2. Schwartz GM, Braverman BG, Roth B. Anxiety disorders and psychiatric referral in the general medical emergency room. *Gen Hosp Psychiatry*. 1987;9:87–93.

3. Tesar GE. The emergency department. In Rundell RR, Wise MG (Eds.), *Textbook of Consultation-liaison Psychiatry*. Washington, DC: American Psychiatric Press, 1996.

4. Milner K, Florence T, Glick R. Mood and anxiety syndromes in emergency psychiatry. *Psychiatr Clin North Am*. 1999;22:755–777.

5. Pollard CA, Lewis LM. Managing panic attacks in emergency patients. *J Emerg Med*. 1989;7:547–552.

6. Fleet RP, Dupuis G, Marchand A, et al. Panic disorder in emergency department chest pain patients: prevalence, comorbidity, suicidal ideation, and physician recognition. *Am J Med*. 1996;101:371–380.

7. Smoller JW, Pollack MH, Otto MW, et al. Panic anxiety, dyspnea, and respiratory disease: theoretical and clinical considerations. *Am J Respir Crit Care Med*. 1996;154:6–17.

8. Eaton WW, Kessler RC, Wittchen HU, et al. Panic and panic disorder in the United States. *Am J Psychiatry*. 1994;151:413–420.

9. Krueger RF. The structure of common mental disorders. *Arch Gen Psychiatry*. 1999;56:921–926.

10. Huffman JC, Pollack MH. Predicting panic disorder among patients with chest pain: an analysis of the literature. *Psychosomatics*. 2003;44:222–236.

11. Griffiths RR, Wolf B. Relative abuse liability of different benzodiazepines in drug abusers. *J Clin Psychopharmacol*. 1990;10:237–243.

12. Gao K, Muzina D, Gajwani P, et al. Efficacy of typical and atypical antipsychotics for primary and comorbid anxiety symptoms or disorders: a review. *J Clin Psychiatry*. 2006;67: 1327–1340.

13. Swinson RP, Soulios CS, Cox BJ, et al. Brief treatment of emergency room patients with panic attacks. *Am J Psychiatry*. 1992;149:944–946.

14. Noyes R, Hoehn-Saric R. *The Anxiety Disorders*. New York, NY: Cambridge University Press, 1998.

15. Wittchen HU, Zhao S, Kessler RC, et al. DSM-III-R generalized anxiety disorder in the National Comorbidity Survey. *Arch Gen Psychiatry*. 1994;51:355–364.

16. Brawman-Mintzer O, Lydiard RB. Generalized anxiety disorder: issues in epidemiology. *J Clin Psychiatry*. 1996;57:3–8.

17. Hoehn-Saric R, Borkovec TD, Belzer K. Generalized anxiety disorder. In Gabbard GO (Ed.), *Treatments of DSM-IV-TR Psychiatric Disorders*. Washington, DC: American Psychiatric Press, 2007.

18. Deacon B, Lickel J, Abramowitz JS. Medical utilization across the anxiety disorders. *J Anx Disord*. 2008;22:344–350.

19. Björgvinsson T, Hart J, Heffelfinger S. Obsessive-compulsive disorder: update on assessment and treatment. *J Psychiatr Pract*. 2007;13:362–372.

20. Antony MM, Downie F, Swinson RP. Diagnostic issues and epidemiology in obsessive-compulsive disorder. In Swinson RP, Antony MM, Rachman S, Richter MA (Eds.), *Obsessive-Compulsive Disorder: Theory, Research, and Treatment*. New York, NY: Guilford, 1998.

21. Skodol AE, Oldham JM, Hyler SE, et al. Patterns of anxiety and personality disorder comorbidity. *J Psychiatr Res*. 1995;29:361–374.

22. Bienvenu OJ, Samuels JF, Riddle MA, et al. The relationship of obsessive-compulsive disorder to possible spectrum disorders: results from a family study. *Biol Psychiatry*. 2000;48:287–293.

23. Jenike MA. An update on obsessive-compulsive disorder. *Bull Menninger Clin*. 2001;65:4–25.

24. Koran LM, Hanna GL, Hollander E, et al. American Psychiatric Association. Practice guideline for the treatment of patients with obsessive-compulsive disorder. *Am J Psychiatry*. 2007;**164**(Suppl 7):5–53.

25. Fisher PL, Wells A. How effective are cognitive and behavioral treatments for obsessive-compulsive disorder? A clinical significance analysis. *Behav Res Ther*. 2005;**43**:1543–1558.

26. Kessler RC, Sonnega A, Bromet E, et al. Posttraumatic stress disorder in the National Comorbidity Survey. *Arch Gen Psychiatry*. 1995;**52**:1048–1060.

27. Harvey AG, Bryant RA. Acute stress disorder after mild traumatic brain injury. *J Nerv Ment Dis*. 1998;**186**:333–337.

28. Davidson JRT, Stein DJ, Shalev AY, et al. Posttraumatic stress disorder: acquisition, recognition, course, and treatment. *J Neuropsychiatry Clin Neurosci*. 2004;**16**:135–147.

29 Foa EB. Psychosocial treatment of posttraumatic stress disorder. *J Clin Psychiatry*. 2000;**61**(Suppl 5):43–51.

30. Ballenger JC, Davidson JR, Lecrubier Y, et al. Consensus statement on posttraumatic stress disorder from the International Consensus Group on Depression and Anxiety. *J Clin Psychiatry*. 2000;**61**(Suppl 5):60–66.

31. Zoellner LA, Feeny NC, Cochran B, et al. Treatment choice for PTSD. *Behav Res Ther*. 2003;**41**:879–886.

32. Pitman RK, Sanders KM, Zusman RM, et al. Pilot study of secondary prevention of posttraumatic stress disorder with propranolol. *Biol Psychiatry*. 2002; **51**:183–188.

33. Strain JJ, Smith GC, Hammer JS, et al. Adjustment disorder: a multisite study of its utilization and interventions in the consultation-liaison psychiatry setting. *Gen Hosp Psychiatry*. 1998;**20**:139–149.

34. Sternberg M, Morin AK. Mild serotonin syndrome associated with concurrent linezolid and fluoxetine. *Am J Health Syst Pharm*. 2007;**64**:59–62.

35. Goldberg RJ. Anxiety in the medically ill. In Stoudemire A, Fogel BS (Eds.), *Principles of Medical Psychiatry*. Orlando, FL: Grune & Stratton, 1987.

36. Kroenke K, Spitzer RL, Williams JB, et al. Anxiety disorders in primary care: prevalence, impairment, comorbidity, and detection. *Ann Intern Med*. 2007;**146**:317–325.

37. Stein MB, Roy-Byrne PP, Craske MG, et al. Functional impact and health utility of anxiety disorders in primary care outpatients. *Med Care*. 2005;**43**: 1164–1170.

38. McLaughlin TP, Khandker RK, Kruzikas DT, et al. Overlap of anxiety and depression in a managed care population: prevalence and association with resource utilization. *J Clin Psychiatry*. 2006;**67**:1187–1193.

39. Allen MH. Level 1 psychiatric emergency services. *Psychiatr Clin North Am*. 1999;**22**:713–734.

40. Kercher EE. Anxiety. *Emerg Med Clin North Am*. 1991;**9**:161–187.

41. Weissman MM, Klerman GL, Markowitz JS, et al. Suicidal ideation and attempts in panic disorder. *N Engl J Med*. 1989;**321**:1209–1214.

42. Johnson J, Weissman MM, Klerman GL. Panic disorder comorbidity and suicide attempts. *Arch Gen Psychiatry*. 1990;**47**:805–808.

43. Cox BJ, Direnfeld DM, Swinson RP, et al. Suicidal ideation and suicide attempts in panic disorder and social phobia. *Am J Psychiatry*. 1994;**151**(Suppl 6);882–887.

44. Busch KA, Fawcett J, Jacobs DG. Clinical correlates of inpatient suicide. *J Clin Psychiatry*. 2003;**64**:14–19.

Mood disorders

Eric L. Anderson

Introduction

Mood disorders are a complex set of diagnoses. Patients suffering from mood disorders present in a variety of ways – happy, sad, despondent, elated, suicidal, or dysphoric to name a few. In the emergency setting, it is often hard to distinguish mood disorders from other medical and psychiatric disorders. Mood disorders include the *Diagnostic and Statistical Manual of Mental Disorders, 4th Edition, Text Revision* (DSM-IV-TR) diagnoses of major depressive disorder and bipolar affective disorder.[1]

Mood *disorders* are comprised of mood *episodes*. Specific disorders can be described according to the mood episodes experienced by the patient (see Table 8.1).

In the acute and urgent care setting, making a definitive psychiatric diagnosis is not as important as recognizing the type of mood episode the patient is experiencing and assessing the implications of that mood episode in terms of danger to themselves or others and their ability to function. Acute care providers must be vigilant about mood episodes as they are often underrecognized. On the other hand, when a mood disorder is suspected, a thorough search for a medical cause must occur before attributing symptoms solely to the mood episode. This chapter will examine the three most common mood episodes (depressive, manic/hypomanic, and mixed states) in an effort to guide management efforts.

Depression

Major depressive disorder (MDD), also known as depression, is one of the most common psychiatric disorders worldwide.[2–5] In the United States alone, 5–12% of men and 10–25% of women will experience MDD in their lifetime.[6–9] In pregnant women, 7–26% will meet criteria for depression during pregnancy and 10–15% will suffer post-partum depression.[9] Over one million psychiatric-related emergency department (ED) visits in 2000 were due to complaints of depressive symptoms, with an estimated 30% prevalence amongst ED patients regardless of the chief complaint.[10,11] It tends to first strike patients when they are younger and, as a result, significantly impedes their opportunities to flourish.[12,13] Major depression is not restricted to the young, however: 30% of older patients who present to the ED may in fact be depressed.[14,15]

Emergency Psychiatry, ed. Arjun Chanmugam, Patrick Triplett, and Gabor Kelen. Published by Cambridge University Press. © Cambridge University Press 2013.

Table 8.1. The mood disorders

Diagnosis	Depressive	Manic	Hypomanic
Major depressive disorder	Yes	No	No
Bipolar affective disorder, type I	Maybe	Yes	Maybe
Bipolar affective disorder, type II	Yes	No	Yes

Depression is a remitting-relapsing disease. Patients may experience depressive episodes only rarely or several times per year. For some patients, symptoms are mild, and they can continue to function relatively normally. For other patients symptoms are severe to the point that they suffer psychotic features, with as many as 19% of depressed patients experiencing psychoses.[16] Many patients contemplate taking their own life. Suicide is very common in depression, with self-inflicted injuries accounting for over 12% of ED visits.[17] The rate of suicide in the United States is estimated to be 11 per 100,000 individuals and is comprised in large part of patients suffering from mood disorders such as major depression.[18]

Diagnostics

The presenting signs and symptoms in depression can vary from patient to patient, but in general they consist of changes in the patient's *mood*, *vital sense*, and *self-attitude*. In this triad, "mood" is the patient's pervasive state of mental and emotional existence. Depressed patients may experience sadness and not be depressed (just as manic patients may experience happiness and not be manic), but when a patient is depressed their mood is predominantly sad or lackluster. Even though sadness is the most common (and easily recognized) mood state, apathy, anxiety, and anhedonia (inability to experience pleasure) are also possible in patients who are clinically depressed. If anxiety is the predominant mood state, the presence of an independent or comorbid anxiety disorder must be suspected as well.

Some patients experience anger attacks, which are intense periods of anger that resemble panic attacks but lack the elements of fear and anxiety.[19] Somatic complaints, such as headache or chest pain, are also common as an initial complaint, especially in adolescents.[20–22]

The second part of the triad is a patient's vital sense, which can be thought of as their level of energy – their "pick-up-and-go." In a depressive episode, a patient's vital sense is disrupted. As part of that constellation, sleep is disrupted. The quantity of sleep may be normal, but the quality of sleep is often described as fitful, non-restorative, and interrupted. Early awakening is common. Concentration is impaired. This may include memory and attention problems, slowed speed of thought, and disordered thought. Appetite changes occur: patients may refuse to eat; others find they have an unusually voracious appetite. Food often loses its taste, becoming bland. Activity levels also change. Most depressed patients have a decreased level of activity as compared to their pre-depressed state. As one patient described it: "If I were to be seated on a chair on one side of the room, and the cure to my depression lay upon the mantel on the other side of the room, I would not have the ability to rise up and retrieve it."

Self-attitude is the third component in the triad. Patients may think they deserve to feel poorly. Others believe they have no hope of ever feeling well, and that they would not deserve it even if they could feel better. They do not engage in pleasurable activities as before. In part, this is due to their poor vital sense. In other respects, it is because they do not feel they deserve to experience pleasure.

Patients who experience depression may contemplate death. Assessments for these thoughts are critical in the evaluation of a depressed patient. It is also very important to distinguish what a patient means when they say they wish to die. Do they wish that they want to go to sleep and never wake up, or are they actively thinking about taking their own life? If the latter, do they have a plan for doing so? Do they have access to means, making it even more likely they can carry out their plans for suicide?

In the emergency setting, evaluation of the mood, vital sense, self-attitude, and desires for death can best be quickly performed using the following mnemonic: "SIGECAMPS." It stands for:

Sleep disturbances

Interest decline, including a drop in sexual interest or impotence

Guilt or feelings of worthlessness or hopelessness

Energy loss

Concentration impairment

Appetite changes

Mood changes

Psychomotor changes

Suicidal ideations or passive death wishes

According to the DSM-IV-TR, the presence of low mood or anhedonia plus five or more of the above symptoms for two or more weeks constitutes a major depressive episode (see http://www.mental-health-today.com/dep/dsm.htm).

Other elements of the history that can help the clinician decide if depression is present include family, personal, and substance use histories. A family history of a mood disorder could suggest a genetic predisposition. Developmentally, did the patient have any childhood difficulties such as poor school attendance or performance due to depression? A brief employment history could be useful to help understand how well the patient has been able to cope with symptoms and may be a clue to how long the symptoms have been present. It is important to ascertain if the patient currently is employed. If they have been unemployed for a long time, reasons should be sought. A thorough substance use or abuse history is also critical, since mood disorders and substance use disorders have a very high concordance rate.[12,23–25] For example, 60% of all patients who chronically abuse alcohol have depressive symptoms.[26] Intoxication and withdrawal syndromes (such as withdrawal from opioids or intoxication with alcohol) can mimic depressive episodes.

The issue of substance use also raises an important diagnostic question. Most experts agree, and even the DSM-IV-TR stipulates, that for a mood disorder diagnosis the patient's mood symptoms cannot be due to the influences of a medication or illicit drug.[1] Definitive diagnosis is best made by serial observations of the patient, the kind of observations which are *not* usually conducted or necessary in the emergency setting. However, it is important to try to assess whether an organic cause such as medication is the root or a major contributor to the observed behavior, as the approach to treating an organic cause of mood disorder is different than if one can be confident the observed behavior is psychiatric in origin.

The past medical history is also important, as there are multiple medical problems that can mimic, incite, or are coincident with depression. These diagnoses include chronic pain, hypothyroidism, hyperthyroidism, epilepsy, dementia, stroke, cancer (especially

Table 8.2. Medical conditions that may mimic or precipitate depression (Based on information supplied in[27–37])

Anemia

Cancer (especially pancreatic, oropharyngeal, and breast)

Cardiovascular disease

Chronic pain

Congestive heart failure

Coronary artery disease

Cranial neoplasms

Dementia (especially Alzheimer's)

Diabetes mellitus

Epilepsy

HIV/AIDS

Hyperthyroidism

Hypothyroidism

Hypoxemia

Migraines

Mononucleosis

Multiple sclerosis

Myasthenia gravis

Obesity

Parkinson's disease

Post-cerebral vascular accident/stroke

Shock

Subdural hematoma

Substance intoxication (such as alcohol or opioids)

Traumatic brain injury

pancreatic), and HIV/AIDS (Table 8.2). Medications should be considered because there are many medications, both iatrogenic and over-the-counter, which can cause a depression-like presentation (Table 8.3). This part of the evaluation should complement efforts made to assess the medical status of the patient, including vital signs, physical examination, laboratory testing, and toxicology screens (including urine drug screening) to rule out medical etiologies to the patient's presentation.

A brief review of the patient's psychiatric history, if any, is helpful. The following are useful in the evaluation: date of first time encounter with a mental health professional, previous psychiatric admissions (number, duration, and reasons), past and current psychiatric treatments (therapy, medication, electroconvulsive therapy, etc.), number and

Table 8.3. Medications that may mimic or precipitate depression (based on information supplied in[32,36–38])

Amantadine

Ampicillin

Anticholinergic agents (cimetidine, metoclopramide)

Anticonvulsant agents (carbamazapine, phenytoin)

Antihypertensive agents (clonidine, digitalis, beta-blockers, procainamide, reserpine)

Antineoplastic agents (vincristine, C-asparaginase, bleomycin)

Antipsychotics (especially butyrophenones and phenothiazines)

Baclofen

Barbiturates

Benzodiazepines

Bromocriptine

Corticosteroids

Disulfuram

Ephedra

Ibuprofen

Indomethacin

Levodopa

Metronidazole

Ranitidine

Trimethoprim

Table 8.4. ED-DSI

1.	Do you often feel sad or depressed?	Yes	No
2.	Do you often feel helpless?	Yes	No
3.	Do you often feel downhearted and blue?	Yes	No

description of self-injurious behaviors, and psychiatric diagnoses that may be contributing to their current symptoms. Specific psychiatric diagnoses to be aware of include anxiety disorders and impulse control disorders. These have high comorbidity with depression.[12] Understanding the extent of the disease and the presence of comorbid conditions is essential to crafting an effective management plan.

Multiple screening tools exist to aid in the diagnosis of MDD. These include the Beck Depression Inventory (BDI), Montgomery-Asberg Scale (MA Scale), and Zung Self-Assessment Depression Scale. The recently developed Emergency Department Depression Screening Instrument (ED-DSI) was developed for use in elderly patients. It consists of three questions and has demonstrated validity in early studies.[39] See Table 8.4.

Interventions

The most critical initial intervention to make for depressed patients is to ensure their safety. Any patient presenting for depression, sadness, suicidal thoughts, or the like should be kept under constant observation. If specific facilities are available for these patients, they should be utilized. If not, then placement in a quiet, secluded area with an observer is best. These patients should never be left alone. A tactful and compassionate search of the patient and their belongings is also necessary; many patients will bring pills, sharp objects, or something worse with them. These items must be removed for the safety of the patient and all other persons present. Until such a search has been conducted, it is advised that patients presenting for depression are not allowed to be alone, which includes unattended use of restroom facilities.

As part of this safety evaluation, the risk for harm to self or others needs to be assessed. A focused mental status examination should be conducted and at a minimum include questions about thoughts of suicide, plans to act on the thoughts if present, and access to means. This assessment should also include thoughts of harm or violence to other people. Tools exist which can help clinicians in the acute setting, such as the Beck Scale for Suicide Ideation, but these tools do not replace a face-to-face evaluation of the patient.[18]

Assessment of the patient's safety should be followed by the decision about whether or not the patient requires hospitalization for treatment of their depressive symptoms. The presence of suicidal thoughts, psychoses, or active substance withdrawal (especially alcohol) should prompt the clinician to seek admission. In the ideal case, the patient will willingly be admitted. However, clinicians should be aware of the legal, medical, and emergency options available to them should they have a patient who requires admission but refuses to be admitted. For outpatient clinic settings, some states allow clinicians to obtain an emergency petition which authorizes law enforcement personnel to take the patient to the nearest ED – even against their wishes. For hospital settings, including the ED, involuntary admission based upon certification may be an option. Laws vary from state to state, thus careful review of the law in one's state of practice is necessary.

In either the clinic setting or the ED, if the decision not to admit is made, then prompt referral to outpatient mental health services should be performed. Ideally, clinic or ED staff should make contact and arrange for a confirmed follow-up appointment that the patient can take with them. Involvement of social work may also be of use in connecting the patient with available community support resources.

Whether to initiate antidepressant treatment in the ED is a matter of debate. Before the advent of newer agents, such as the selective serotonin reuptake inhibitors (SSRIs), long-term treatment was not started because most antidepressant agents had a narrow therapeutic margin and high lethality risk in overdose. SSRIs and the other new antidepressant medications generally have lower risk. Nonetheless, some caution should be exercised in starting these agents in the ED. For example, there is some risk of paradoxical exacerbation of agitation or anxiety, even of inciting a manic or hypomanic episode in vulnerable patients. Patients started on antidepressants or other psychotropics in the ED who are not being hospitalized would need to be monitored closely after leaving the ED for adverse reactions and require close follow-up. It would be important to know the supports in place to help monitor for clinical worsening and respond appropriately, ensure adherence to medication regimen, and confirm follow-up with a prescribing care provider in the very near future. More severe forms of depression, such as those marked by suicidal thoughts, psychosis, and/or agitation, will more likely merit inpatient admission. For patients already in a treatment relationship with a psychiatrist or other provider, any changes in psychotropics contemplated in the ED should be discussed with the outpatient provider and the same safety considerations weighed.

Depression summary

- Depression is extremely common and likely to be routinely seen in acute care settings.
- Use the "SIGECAMPS" mnemonic to remember the diagnostic criteria for a depressive episode.
- Patients presenting with the chief complaint of feeling depressed and/or suicidal should be kept safe. Use an observer as needed.
- After safety, determine if the patient requires inpatient admission.
- Initiation of treatment may be considered with caution, only if careful monitoring and close and timely follow-up can be assured.

Mania

Another mood disorder commonly seen in the ED is bipolar affective disorder (BPAD), which is also known as manic-depressive disorder. Less severe cases, "hypomania," differ from the more severe cases, "mania," by the duration and severity of symptoms. Bipolar disorder occurs in roughly 1–6% of the US population and affects men and women equally.[7,8,40,41] Symptom onset occurs typically around the late teens or early twenties, although evidence for the disorder is usually present many years before then.[41] It has an episodic course, with the prognosis being poorer for patients who suffer from multiple mood disturbance episodes.[42] Bipolar disorders also have a high comorbidity with alcohol and illicit drug abuse or dependence, with as many as 61% of bipolar patients suffering from comorbid substance use.[23,24,26,41] BPAD seriously impairs patients in all facets of their life: work, school, leisure, and interpersonal activities.[4,43] Psychosis is very common in mania and contributes significantly to overall impairment.[44]

Depressive episodes are very common in bipolar illnesses. As such, patients suffering from BPAD can also experience thoughts of suicide, especially in a depressed or mixed state. In the manic state patients may die from self-inflicted injuries or poor behavioral choices, such as speeding down the wrong side of an interstate.[45]

Diagnostics

The manic patient is relatively easy to identify. Truly manic patients are usually bursting with energy. They are a veritable fountain of motion, and their thought patterns often mirror their physical actions. Mania is a state of hyperactivity, both in body and mind, and it is usually (although not always) accompanied by a feeling of euphoria, extreme happiness, grandiosity, or joy. Unlike someone who is just "happy," the manic patient feels an over-the-top sense of elation.

Three broad areas of observation can be used to evaluate the manic patient: *vital sense, self-attitude,* and *mood.* For patients who are manic, their vital sense is on overdrive. They describe an excessive amount of energy, unlike their usual state of energy. For example, patients might relate how, after working 36 hours straight, they still had enough energy to go another 36 hours. Alternatively, they might find they engage in numerous activities they normally would not do.

One patient described how she ironed her clothes and vacuumed her house for hours on end. The clinical significance of this became clear once she admitted that she absolutely loathed ironing and vacuuming when in her normal mood state. Manic patients may also engage in more risky or impulsive behaviors as part of the increased activity level.[46] Such behaviors can include criminal activities, sexual indiscretions, or sports they would not normally engage in (like skydiving or bungee jumping). Related to the activity increase, manic patients often have little or no need for sleep. They can do things for days and not sleep, yet they still feel they have plenty of energy to stay awake and active for long periods of time.

With respect to self-attitude, manic patients have an inflated sense of self. In extreme cases, their grandiosity may take on a note of the bizarre or nonsensical. For example, one patient related that he was *the real* Donald Trump and seemed quite upset that he was not believed. Such grandiosity is universally delusional during a manic episode because the patient's judgment is fixed, false, and idiosyncratic. For other patients, their grandiosity may be more subtle. For example, they might feel that others, including complete strangers, are watching them. At first glance, this may seem like paranoia. But on closer questioning, the manic patient will usually relate that they are being constantly observed because they are special or possess unique qualities somehow. Other patients relate a heightened sense of purpose, special meaning, or connectedness that they usually do not feel. The key to evaluating for grandiosity is to ascertain how the patient *usually* views him/herself. As in depression, collateral information from friends and family can be very helpful in such cases.

Manic patients often have rapid speech. Their ideas and thoughts are moving so rapidly that they have to speak at the same pace that their minds are going. These speech patterns are usually loud and fast. Clinicians find it difficult or impossible to interrupt manic patients. The speech also often has a "pressured" quality to it, as if the patient will explode if they do not get the words out. These speech patterns directly reflect the racing thoughts they are experiencing.

Racing thoughts are not unique to mania, however. They can also be found in anxiety and even depressive disorders. What is unique to manic patients is that the racing thoughts have a grandiose or "good" quality to them, unlike the worried nature of racing thoughts in anxiety or despondent ruminations in depression. These "flights of ideas" are difficult for the patient to keep up with, but they are not usually bothered too much by it because more wonderful ideas are coming along every minute (or even every second). Because they are having so many thoughts coming at them at once, and because these thoughts are usually quite pleasant in nature, manic patients are also easily distracted.

The mood in manic patients is usually elated, euphoric, or in some patients irritable. Manic patients describe their mood as incredibly high. As one patient who also suffered from cocaine abuse put it, "When I'm manic, I'm higher than I can ever get with coke." Manic patients smile at and start conversations with strangers as if they had been best friends for many years. They feel good about life – *very* good. However, some manic patients do not experience elation. Rather, their manic periods consist mainly of feelings of irritability. Such irritability is out of character for them, and they may find themselves snapping at friends, family, or strangers for no clear reason.

The DSM-IV-TR describes a manic episode as the presence of unusually elated or grandiose mood, or irritable mood, for at least one week (see http://www.mental-health-today.com/bp/man.htm). There must also be at least three of the following symptoms present (four if the primary mood is irritability). These symptoms can be remembered by using the mnemonic, "DIG-FAST":

Table 8.5. Medical conditions that may mimic or incite mania or hypomania (based on information supplied in[29,32,36,37,47])

Cancer (CNS involvement)

Collagen vascular disease (CNS involvement)

Complex partial seizures

Cushing's disease or exogenous steroid excess

Endocrine disturbances (especially hyperthyroidism)

Epilepsy (right temporal lobe)

Traumatic brain injury

Hemodialysis (electrolyte disturbance)

Hyperthyroidism (hyperdynamic state)

Infection (e.g., influenza, Q fever, encephalitis)

Multiple sclerosis

Sleep deprivation

Substance intoxication (especially stimulants)

Substance withdrawal (especially sedatives or alcohol)

Wilson's disease

Distractibility
Indiscretions (risky behavior)
Grandiosity
Flight of ideas
Activity increase
Sleep deficits
Talking more

In addition, the patient must suffer psychoses, severe impairment in social or occupational functioning, and/or require hospitalization.

Hypomanic episodes are similar to manic episodes, with a few subtle distinctions. For one, the length of the episode need be only four days instead of a week. Also, the patient does not experience the severity of symptoms that manic patients do, such as psychoses or serious impairment of social or occupational functioning. That being said, if a patient presents in the acute care setting with symptoms consistent with mania, the discrimination between mania and hypomania becomes academic, losing its importance to the overall treatment needs of the patient (see http://www.mental-health-today.com/bp/hypo.htm).

The family, personal, and substance use history is helpful in the evaluation of these patients. Given the evidence for a genetic link, it is reasonable to look for a family history of a mood disorder such as bipolar affective disorder. School or work attendance problems may be a clue. A thorough substance use history is critical because certain drugs can mimic manic states during intoxication (see Table 8.5). For example, a past or current history of use of amphetamines, cocaine, or ecstasy is important since the use of these substances can

Table 8.6. Medications that may mimic or incite mania or hypomania (based on information supplied in[32,36–38,47–49])

ACTH

Alcohol (withdrawal from)

Antidepressants (withdrawal from)

Antiretroviral antibiotics

Baclofen

Bromide

Bromocriptine

Corticosteroids

DHEA

Ephedra

Ginseng

Isoniazid

Levodopa

Levothyroxine

Phenylpropanolamine (especially when combined with caffeine)

Sedatives (withdrawal from)

Stimulants (amphetamines, cocaine, PCP)

Testosterone

Yohimbine

mimic manic symptoms. As with acute depression, according to the DSM-IV-TR, patients cannot be diagnosed as suffering from mania if the effects of drugs, medications, or medical conditions are the root cause of their symptoms.[1]

In the absence of strong collateral information, it is sometimes difficult to determine if the patient's symptoms are indicative of an underlying bipolar disorder or are secondary to some other medical or pharmacologic etiology. Patients who present and appear to be in a manic state but also have other possible causes to explain their symptoms are no less at risk from behavioral sequelae than patients suffering from idiopathic mania. In either case, the initial approach to management (see below) is the same.

Medical problems should be explored, as there are several conditions, such as delirium, that can mimic or exacerbate mania. Delirium can be caused by a variety of medical conditions including hyperthyroidism, cancer, infections, and sleep deprivation (Table 8.5). Medications should also be considered, as several prescription or over-the-counter medications can present with manic-like symptoms. Examples include corticosteroids, antiretroviral antibiotics, antidepressants, and ginseng (Table 8.6). This part of the evaluation should complement efforts made to assess the medical status of the patient, including vital signs, physical examination, laboratory testing, and toxicology screens to rule out medical etiologies to the patient's presentation.

The patient's psychiatric history is also important, including previous hospitalizations, treatments, psychiatric medications prescribed (whether compliant), and family and friends' behavioral observations.

Interventions

As with patients who are depressed, patients who are manic need to be kept safe as the first priority. Many manic patients do not come to the acute care setting of their own accord; often, it is a friend, loved one, or law enforcement personnel who bring the patient to be seen. Such being the case, these patients also require safety evaluations. Manic patients may not feel suicidal during their mania, but they can engage in risky behaviors which may bring harm to themselves or others. A risk assessment for suicide as well as potential harm to themselves and others is mandatory in these patients.

Manic patients should also be discreetly searched for any items which may cause them or others harm. It is not unusual for manic patients to feel invincible or above the law, and so the risk of them acting in an unsafe manner is great. A manic patient should never be left alone while in the acute care setting. If possible, they should be located in a quiet, secluded area with as minimal stimulation as possible. Confrontation with the patient should be avoided, as this will invariably cause symptom escalation. The counterbalance to confrontation is firm and direct communication with clear setting of limits.

After assuring safety, the next two steps are to determine whether or not the patient requires hospitalization for the treatment of their mania, and to make a decision about pharmacological interventions. Should the patient be suffering from thoughts of self-harm or harm to others, psychoses, medical instability, or withdrawal from substances, they should be admitted for their safety. Patients with organic causes of their mania will likely require a "medical" admission. In addition, if the patient lacks a support network and is unable to care for him/herself, consideration for admission should be strongly entertained. Patients for whom admission is not felt to be warranted should be given prompt mental health follow-up. Additionally, clinicians are advised to strongly consider medication in these patients in order to prevent their symptoms from worsening.

The question of treatment is, for manic patients, more straightforward than for depressed patients. Medications which attenuate hyperdynamic manic symptoms should be considered. These treatments should ideally be rapid in action, minimal in sedation, and quick to control or minimize agitation.[51] There are three major classes of medications which are used in the emergency setting: mood stabilizers, neuroleptics (also known as antipsychotics), and benzodiazepines. Each have their own merits and drawbacks. When possible, it is preferable to administer the medications in a liquid or quick dissolve form as this formulation usually has a more rapid onset of action. Injectable versions of these medications can be used if the patient is agitated to the point that they pose a danger to themselves or others.

"Mood stabilizer" is a bit misleading, as many different agents on the market today have been advertised as having mood stabilizing qualities. Classically, a mood stabilizer is either lithium or an antiepileptic drug which has demonstrated efficacy in the treatment of bipolar disorder. Mood stabilizers such as lithium and valproic acid are the standard of care when it comes to acute and maintenance treatment of bipolar affective disorder. Even though evidence exists that response is more rapid with intravenous (in the case of valproic acid) or oral loading (in the case of lithium) of certain mood stabilizers, their full effect will

Table 8.7. Commonly used emergency drugs and their doses (based on information supplied in[32,36,55])

Antipsychotics

Drug	Oral dose (mg)	Intramuscular dose (mg)	Interval between doses (minutes)
Haloperidol (Haldol®)	2.5–10	2.5–10	60
Risperidone (Risperdal)	1–3	N/A	75
Olanzapine (Zyprexa®)	5–20	5–10	90
Ziprasidone (Geodon®)	N/R	10–20	90
Quetiapine (Seroquel®)	50–200	N/A	75
Aripiprazole (Abilify®)	2–15	5.25–9.75	120

Benzodiazepines

Drug	Oral dose (mg)	Intramuscular dose (mg)	Interval between doses (minutes)
Lorazepam (Ativan®)	1–3	0.5–3	60
Diazepam (Valium®)	5–15	N/A	75

N/A: Not available in this form
N/R: Not recommended for this setting

require days to weeks.[45,51,52] Thus, these medications are generally impractical in the acute care setting for the management of agitation. Additionally, these medications require monitoring (including serum laboratory tests such as liver enzymes, renal function, electrolytes, and complete blood counts) initially and throughout treatment. Depending on the medication, it will be necessary to monitor serum levels of the drug as well.

Neuroleptics are one of the chief pharmacologic interventions for agitated manic patients in the acute setting. High-potency neuroleptic agents such as haloperidol have been studied extensively in the acute care setting.[53] Generally, neuroleptics have both sedating and antipsychotic properties which benefit the patient in the following ways. Sedation helps them sleep, the lack of which contributes to their mania. The antipsychotic properties help dampen the delusions and hallucinations which are common in mania. These pharmacologic effects often have a modest stabilizing effect on the patient. It is not unusual to have a floridly manic patient become more cooperative and insightful after a single dose of neuroleptic. However, these medications can have distressing acute and chronic side effects whose onset is not very predictable. In the acute setting, extrapyramidal symptoms and tardive dyskinesia are not as common as the sedation, possible orthostatic hypotension, QTc prolongation, akathisia, restlessness, acute dystonic reactions, and, in rare cases, neuroleptic malignant syndrome. For detailed discussions of these effects the reader is referred elsewhere.[36,54] Commonly used neuroleptics and their recommended dose ranges are listed in Table 8.7. Another point that is especially important in neuroleptic-naïve patients, but true for almost all patients requiring these medications, is to strongly consider co-administering an anticholinergic medication such as diphenhydramine. In addition to benefits in preventing some of the acute side effects of neuroleptics, anticholinergic medications also tend to be sedating, a desired side effect in the manic patient.

Benzodiazepines, like neuroleptics, have the benefit of sedation, but they tend to lower the inhibition level of patients who are manic.[56] Thus, until the sedative effects of the medications begin, it is quite possible the manic patient will actually escalate in behavior before calming. If benzodiazepines are used, shorter-acting agents such as lorazepam are recommended over longer-acting agents such as diazepam and clonazepam, or ultra-short agents such as alprazolam. Dosing guidelines are also provided in Table 8.7.

There is strong evidence for a better response with the co-administration of a benzodiazepine with specific neuroleptics. By doing so, the overall dose of both medications necessary to achieve symptom relief is reduced.[56] Examples include oral or intramuscular benzodiazepine administration with oral or intramuscular haloperidol, risperidone, or ziprasidone.[53,55]

Bipolar summary

- Bipolar disorders are extremely common. They consist of at least one manic episode (bipolar disorder, Type I) or one hypomanic episode (bipolar disorder, Type II). In bipolar, Type II, evidence for a history of depression must also be present.
- Manic and hypomanic patients have elated, irritable, or grandiose mood, and an abnormally elevated vital sense and self-attitude.
- Clinicians who suspect mania or hypomania can diagnose it based upon the patient's symptoms. Three or more of the following (four if the predominant mood is irritability) raise suspicion for mania or hypomania. The symptoms of mania are recalled using the mnemonic, "DIGFAST."
- The manic or hypomanic patient must first and foremost be kept safe and closely monitored. Patients who are suffering from psychoses, are feeling or expressing suicidal or homicidal thoughts, are withdrawing from substances, are medically unstable, or are unable to function (care for themselves) should be admitted.
- After safety and the question of admission are addressed, clinicians should strongly consider instituting medications for the patient who presents with mania. The recommended medications in the acute care setting are neuroleptics, benzodiazepines, and mood stabilizers.

Mixed states

The DSM-IV-TR defines a mixed state as the presence of both depression and mania during the same period of time, the symptoms of which are present for at least a week.[1] Mixed states are relatively common and are dangerous because they are both difficult to treat and have a higher risk of suicide.[57] Patients have the energy and disordered thought processes that occur in mania, but they have an irritable, poor, or despondent mood such as occurs in depression. The risk of suicide in a mixed state is very high. Contrary to popular belief, mixed states are not merely the transitioning of one predominant mood to the next; they appear to be their own discrete clinical entity.[58] Because of the severity of symptoms and danger to the patient, prompt recognition and intervention by clinicians is necessary to prevent further deterioration of the patient's condition.

Diagnostics

Mixed states, as noted above, contain both elements of mania and of depression simultaneously.[59] This maelstrom of emotions and energy creates for the patient a quite unpleasant experience. The patient's condition can be understood by examining their *mood, vital sense,* and *self-attitude.* Their predominant mood is rarely consistently happy or euphoric. It tends, rather, often to be dysphoric or irritable. Dysphoria is a subjective sense of internal tension that is expressed externally as irritability, hostility, or suspiciousness.[57] In a mixed state, the patient's mood does not remain fixed, but shifts quickly, sometimes from second to second: at one moment they seem happy, the next they seem infinitely miserable.

The patient's vital sense is also skewed. They have energy, but it seems misplaced, uncontrolled, and haphazard, coming and going as it pleases with no predictability. Their sleep is disrupted, and at other times they sleep to excess. Their appetite is voracious at one moment, but completely anorexic at the next. As one patient described his vital sense, "It is like a hundred bombs went off in me, but I kept all the force inside. I'm imploding but I want to explode."

The patient's self-attitude also varies. In some moments they are extremely self-confident, and they feel like nothing is wrong, but that can quickly change to hopelessness, the sense that all is lost. This rapid shifting of feelings and self-perception is part of what makes a mixed state so dreadful for patients: the mismatch between vital sense and self attitude.

Given that mixed states represent both manic and depressive states, in order to diagnose a mixed episode the patient must fulfill criteria for a depressive episode (see http://www.mental-health-today.com/dep/dsm.htm) and a manic episode (see http://www.mental-health-today.com/bp/man.htm) during a minimum one week period. As with other mood episodes, the mixed state cannot be due to the influences of a medical disorder, substance intoxication or withdrawal, or the effects of medication (see http://www.mental-health-today.com/bp/mix.htm).

Interestingly, it is very difficult to find patients who fit the DSM criteria completely.[57] This may be resolved in the upcoming edition of the DSM (DSM-V), but for the time being if elements of both mania and depression are observed, a preliminary diagnosis of a mixed episode may be given. Even if the patient is only in an irritable form of depression or mania instead, defaulting to a mixed episode will ensure the most conservative path of treatment for the patient. In this case the name given to the clinical presentation is not as important as the interventions which follow.

The same exploration of the patient's past family, personal, substance use, and psychiatric history as mentioned above for patients in depressive or manic episodes needs to be conducted for patients suspected of being in a mixed state. An evaluation for medical conditions, medications (illicit, prescribed, and over-the-counter), a physical examination, and laboratory studies (including urine toxicology) should be performed to rule out medical or chemical causes for the patient's symptoms.

Interventions

The interventions outlined for depressive and manic episodes also apply to mixed episodes. The first priority is the safety of the patient. This includes a thorough risk assessment, both for harm to self and harm to others. Following this assessment, the next issue is whether or not the patient requires emergent treatment (pharmacological intervention) and inpatient admission. Patients in a mixed state tend to be labile, agitated, and thought-disordered. As such, they are unpredictable. Clinicians should have a very low threshold for offering medications to alleviate the patient's distress. If the patient is judged non-competent to make such a decision, clinicians should err on the side of active treatment with pharmacologic agents. Neuroleptics are the initial treatment of choice, both for their antipsychotic and sedative effects (see Table 8.7). Anticholinergic treatment, such as with diphenhydramine, should also strongly be considered to mitigate potential side effects of the neuroleptic and also to provide some sedation. Benzodiazepines may also be used with caution. Again, by themselves, they may disinhibit an already unstable patient, making them more uncontrolled. However, coupled with neuroleptics, benzodiazepines add a calming effect to the patient, which is desirable in mixed states. Mood stabilizers may be initiated, but their effects will not be seen for many days, even weeks. Evidence exists for a better response to valproic acid (loaded at 20 mg/kg/day) than to lithium.[45]

Most patients who present in a mixed state are very distressed. They are suffering from disordered thought, an inability to function in society or care for themselves. Frequently, thoughts of violence towards themselves or others are in accompaniment. Patients should be placed in an area with as little stimulation as possible. Firm setting of limits is desirable, but direct confrontation is not. Given the great risk of self-harm or harm to others, strong consideration for psychiatric admission should be given to these patients. In the acute setting, the patient should be in continuous observation.

Mixed summary

- Mixed episodes are not felt to be as common as manic, hypomanic, or depressive episodes, but they are still encountered in mood-disordered patients.
- Patients in a mixed state have features of both depression and mania at the same time.
- Patients in a mixed state are at a high risk of harm to self or others.
- Critical interventions include a safety evaluation, pharmacological interventions, and strong consideration for inpatient hospitalization.
- Medications of choice include neuroleptics, benzodiazepines (along with neuroleptics), and mood stabilizers.

Acknowledgements

The author wishes to thank Roberta Boyd-Anderson, BSN, MSN, and Dennis Anderson, DO, for their review of this chapter.

References

1. American Psychiatric Association. *Diagnostic and Statistical Manual of Mental Disorders, 4th Edition, Text Revision.* Washington, DC: American Psychiatric Association, 1994.

2. Nandi A, Beard JR, Galea S. Epidemiologic heterogeneity of common mood and anxiety disorders over the lifecourse in the general population: a systematic review. *BMC Psychiatry.* 2009;9:31.

3. Ohayon MM. Epidemiology of depression and its treatment in the general population. *J Psychiatric Res.* 2007;41:207–213.

4. World Health Organization. *The Global Burden of Disease: 2004 update.* Geneva: World Health Organization Press, 2004.

5. WHO World Mental Health Survey Consortium. Prevalence, severity, and unmet need for treatment of mental disorders in the World Health Organization world mental health surveys. *JAMA.* 2004;**291**:2581–2590.

6. Flynn HA, Davis M, Marcus SM, et al. Rates of maternal depression in pediatric emergency department and relationship to child service utilization. *Gen Hosp Psychiatry.* 2004; **26**:316–322.

7. Kessler RC, McGonagle KA, Zhao S, et al. Lifetime and 12-month prevalence of DSM-III-R psychiatric disorders in the United States. *Arch Gen Psychiatry*. 1994;**51**:8–19.

8. Kessler RC, Berglund P, Demler O, et al. Lifetime prevalence and age-of-onset distributions of DSM-IV disorders in the national comorbidity survey replication. *Arch Gen Psychiatry*. 2005;**62**:593–602.

9. Moses-Kolko EL, Roth EK. Antepartum and postpartum depression: healthy mom, healthy baby. *JAMA*. 2004;**59**:181–191.

10. Hazlett SB, McCarthy ML, Londner MS, et al. Epidemiology of adult psychiatric visits to US emergency departments. *Acad Emer Med*. 2004;**11**:193–195.

11. Kumar A, Clark S, Boudreaux ED, et al. A multicenter study of depression among emergency department patients. *Acad Emer Med*. 2004;**11**:1284–1289.

12. Kessler RC, Berglund P, Demler O, et al. The epidemiology of major depressive disorder: results from the national comorbidity survey replication (NCS-R). *JAMA*. 2003;**289**:3095–3105.

13. Kessler RC, Angermeyer M, Anthony JC, et al. Lifetime prevalence and age-of-onset distributions of mental disorders in the World Health Organization's world mental health survey initiative. *World Psychiatry*. 2007;**6**:168–176.

14. Kowalenko T, Khare RK. Should we screen for depression in the emergency department? *Acad Emer Med*. 2004;**11**:177–178.

15. Meldon SW, Emerman CL, Schubert DSP, et al. Depression in geriatric emergency department patients: prevalence and recognition. *Ann Emerg Med*. 1997;**30**:141–145.

16. Ohayon MM, Schatzberg AF. Prevalence of depressive episodes with psychotic features in the general population. *AJP*. 2002;**159**:1855–1861.

17. Harman JS, Scholle SH, Edlund MJ. Emergency department visits for depression in the United States. *Psychiatric Services*. 2004:**55**:937–939.

18. Healy DJ, Barry K, Blow F, et al. Routine use of the Beck scale for suicide ideation in a psychiatric emergency department. *General Hospital Psychiatry*. 2006:**28**: 323–329.

19. Fava M, Rosenbaum JF. Anger attacks in patients with depression. *J Clin Psychiatry*. 1999;**60**:21–24.

20. Porter SC, Fein JA, Ginsburg KR. Depression screening in adolescents with somatic complaints presenting to the emergency department. *Ann Emerg Med*. 1997;**29**:141–145.

21. Scott EG, Luxmore B, Alexander H, et al. Screening for adolescent depression in a pediatric emergency department. *Acad Emer Med*. 2006;**13**:537–542.

22. Srinivasan K, Joseph W. A study of lifetime prevalence of anxiety and depressive disorders in patients presenting with chest pain to emergency medicine. *General Hospital Psychiatry*. 2004;**26**:470–474.

23. Brown ES. Bipolar disorder and substance abuse. *Psych Clin North Am*. 2005;**28**:415–425.

24. Kessler RC. Impact of substance abuse on the diagnosis, course, and treatment of mood disorders: the epidemiology of dual diagnosis. *Biol Psychiatry*. 2004:**56**:730–737.

25. Glantz MD, Anthony JC, Berglund PA, et al. Mental disorders as risk factors for later substance dependence: estimates of optimal prevention and treatment benefits. *Psychol Med*. 2009;**39**: 1365–1377.

26. Quello SB, Brady KT, Sonne SC. Mood disorder and substance use disorder: a complex comorbidity. *Research Review – Mood and Substance Use Disorders*. 2005;13–24.

27. Benedetti F, Bernasconi A, Pontiggia A. Depression and neurological disorders. *Curr Opin Psychiatry*. 2006;**19**:14–18.

28. Campbell LC, Clauw DJ, Keefe FJ. Persistent pain and depression: a biopsychosocial perspective. *Biol Psychiatry*. 2003;**54**:399–409.

29. Demet MM, Ozmen B, Deveci A, et al. Depression and anxiety in hyperthyroidism. *Archives Med Res.* 2002;**33**:552–556.

30. Evans DL, Charney DS, Lewis L, et al. Mood disorders in the medically ill: scientific review and recommendations. *Biol Psychiatry.* 2005;**58**:175–189.

31. Fenton WS, Stover ES. Mood disorders: cardiovascular and diabetes comorbidity. *Curr Opin Psychiatry.* 2006;**19**:421–427.

32. Glick RL, Berlin JS, Fishkind AB, et al. *Emergency Psychiatry: Principles and Practice.* Philadelphia, PA: Lippincott Williams & Wilkins, 2008.

33. Kanner AM. Depression in epilepsy: a complex relation with unexpected consequences. *Curr Opin Neurol.* 2008;**21**:190–194.

34. McDonald WM, Richard IH, DeLong MR. Prevalence, etiology, and treatment of depression in Parkinson's disease. *Biol Psychiatry.* 2003;**54**:363–375.

35. Riggio S, Wong M. Neurobehavioral sequelae of traumatic brain injury. *Mt Sinai J Med.* 2009;**76**:163–172.

36. Sadock BJ, Sadock VA. *Kaplan & Sadock's Synopsis of Psychiatry.* 10th ed. Philadelphia, PA: Lippincott Williams & Wilkins, 2007.

37. Stern TA, Fricchione GL, Cassem NH, et al. *Massachusetts General Hospital Handbook of General Hospital Psychiatry.* 5th ed. Philadelphia, PA: Mosby, 2004.

38. Maglione M, Miotto K, Iguchi M, et al. Psychiatric effects of ephedra use: an analysis of Food and Drug Administration reports of adverse events. *AJP.* 2005;**162**:189–191.

39. Fabacher DA, Raccio-Robak N, McErlean MA, et al. Validation of a brief screening tool to detect depression in elderly ED patients. *Am J Emerg Med.* 2002;**20**:99–102.

40. Judd LL, Akiskal HS. The prevalence and disability of bipolar spectrum disorders in the U.S. population: re-analysis of the ECA database taking into account subthreshold cases. *J Aff Dis.* 2003;**73**:123–131.

41. Merikangas KR, Akiskal HS, Angst J, et al. Lifetime and 12-month prevalence of bipolar spectrum disorder in the national comorbidity survey replication. *Arch Gen Psychiatry.* 2007;**64**:543–552.

42. Turvey CL, Coryell WH, Solomon DA, et al. Long-term prognosis of bipolar I disorder. *Acta Psychiatr Scand.* 1999;**99**:110–119.

43. Calabrese JR, Hirschfeld RMA, Reed M, et al. Impact of bipolar disorder on a U.S. community sample. *J Clin Psychiatry.* 2003;**64**:425–432.

44. Swann AC, Daniel DG, Kochan LD, et al. Psychosis in mania: specificity of its role in severity and treatment response. *J Clin Psychiatry.* 2004;**65**:825–829.

45. Dilsaver SC, Swann AC, Shoaib AM, et al. Depressive mania associated with nonresponse to antimanic agents. *AJP.* 1993;**150**:1548–1551.

46. Swann AC, Dougherty DM, Pazzaglia PJ, et al. Increased impulsivity associated with severity of suicide attempt history in patients with bipolar disorder. *AJP.* 2005;**162**:1680–1687.

47. Krauthammer C, Klerman GL. Secondary mania: manic syndromes associated with antecedent physical illness or drugs. *Arch Gen Psychiatry.* 1978;**35**:1333–1339.

48. Brown ES, Suppes T, Khan DA, et al. Mood changes during prednisone bursts in outpatients with asthma. *J Clin Psychopharmacol.* 2002;**22**:55–61.

49. Lake CR. Manic psychosis after coffee and phenylpropanolamine. *Biol Psychiatry.* 1991;**30**:401–404.

50. Currier GW, Allen MH, Bunney B, et al. Intramuscular antipsychotics: clinical experience review. *J Emerg Med.* 2004;**27**:S3–S4.

51. Grunze H, Erfurth A, Amann B, et al. Intravenous valproate loading in acutely manic and depressed bipolar I patients. *J Clin Psychopharmacol.* 1999;**19**:303–309.

52. McElroy SL, Keck PE, Stanton SP, et al. A randomized comparison of divalproex oral loading versus haloperidol in the initial treatment of acute psychotic mania. *J Clin Psychiatry*. 1996;**57**:142–146.

53. Garza-Trevino ES, Hollister LE, Overall JE, et al. Efficacy of combinations of intramuscular antipsychotics and sedative-hypnotics for control of psychotic agitation. *AJP*. 1989;**146**:1598–1601.

54. Labbate LA, Fava M, Rosenbaum JF, et al. *Handbook of Psychiatric Drug Therapy*. 6th ed. Philadelphia, PA: Lippincott Williams & Wilkins, 2009.

55. Allen MH, Currier GW, Carpenter D, et al. Expert consensus guidelines on the treatment of behavioral emergencies. *J Psychiatr Pract*. 2005;**11**:S1–S108.

56. Swann AC. Treatment of aggression in patients with bipolar disorder. *J Clin Psychiatry*. 1990;**60**:S25–S28.

57. Dayer A, Aubry JM, Roth L, et al. A theoretical reappraisal of mixed states: dysphoria as a third dimension. *Bipolar Disorders*. 2000;**2**:316–324.

58. Akiskal HS, Benazzi F, Perugi G, et al. Agitated "unipolar" depression re-conceptualized as a depressive mixed state: implications for the antidepressant-suicide controversy. *J Aff Dis*. 2005;**85**:245–258.

59. Swann AC, Secunda SK, Katz MM, et al. Specificity of mixed affective states: clinical comparison of dysphoric mania and agitated depression. *J Aff Dis*. 1993;**28**:81–89.

Personality disorders

Frederick Houts and Glenn Treisman

Personality disorders are among the most poorly understood conditions in psychiatry. Current "lore" includes numerous faulty assumptions and stigmatizing descriptions of patients with these conditions. In the emergency department (ED) setting, the use of the term "personality disorder" is usually reserved for those patients with behaviors that sabotage the physician's efforts to help them. The appellation of "difficult" patient is rarely used for patients with a difficult to diagnose, treatment resistant, or medically complex disease. The term "difficult" usually describes a patient who provokes frustration in his or her treating clinicians. In the ED setting, these patients often have time and resource consuming interactions with the staff and often have a less than satisfactory outcome for the clinician, the patient, or both. These patients include but are not limited to: individuals with chronic pain, addiction, personality disorders, unexplained symptoms, or those who have poor interpersonal boundaries or acceptance of set limits. Despite multiple interventions, these patients will be dissatisfied or will display excessive emotion, and many of these patients will have either undiagnosed or well-established personality disorders. This chapter will review some useful strategies to manage personality disorders in the acute care setting.

Personality or character is the set of behaviors that the patient "characteristically" exhibits in response to a given stimulus. Personality emerges out of the interaction between temperament (nature – the natural affectively driven response to the stimulus) and learning or through shaping by the environment (nurture). Our experience has led us to focus on describing the temperament of patients with personality disorders as a way of understanding them. Despite a long debate about which is more important, temperament is a measurable human endowment or dimension. While different psychologists have measured temperament in different ways, we will focus here on the description of temperament discussed in the book *Perspectives of Psychiatry*, which summarizes ideas from several sources. This model focuses on two dimensions of temperament, the introversion-extraversion axis (summarized in Figure 9.1) and the stability-instability axis (see Figure 9.2). The first figure shows the population measured on an axis of introversion at one end and extraversion on the other. As it is shown, introverts are consequence avoiding, future focused and function oriented, while extraverts are reward seeking, now focused and feeling oriented. Most people are shown as being in the middle of the curve, with the average temperament having a balance of traits. People with extreme endowments fall at the wings of the curve and are highly

Emergency Psychiatry, ed. Arjun Chanmugam, Patrick Triplett, and Gabor Kelen. Published by Cambridge University Press. © Cambridge University Press 2013.

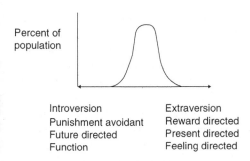

Figure 9.1. Simplified model of disposition

Percent of
population

Introversion	Extraversion
Punishment avoidant	Reward directed
Future directed	Present directed
Function	Feeling directed

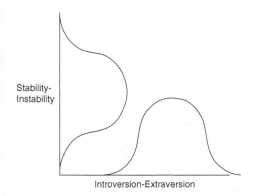

Figure 9.2. Population disposition

Stability-
Instability

Introversion-Extraversion

specialized; they do well in environments where their endowments work for them but poorly in others. For example, many physicians are introverted, and do well with studying for a test to avoid failing, working on preparing for the future, and getting things done. Extraverts make good politicians, actors, and CEOs, and have a "get it done" attitude that is based on feelings, now, and rewards. In general, intensely extraverted patients have strong feelings that drive their choices, often to the exclusion of considering the consequences that will occur later.

The second axis shown vertically in Figure 9.2 is orthogonal to the first. Stability and instability (instability is often referred to as neuroticism) describe how much emotion is generated by a stimulus, how intensely emotions occur, and how predictably they occur. People with prominent instability have large emotional responses to stimuli, have strong emotions, and have unpredictable emotional responses. As expected, unstable, extraverted people are the patients that present with the most problematic personality styles in the ED.

The concept of unstable extraversion allows for an understanding of why the patient sees their feelings as an emergency, and is not a pejorative description. The more commonly used terms are somewhat stigmatizing and often carry a pejorative label. The DSM IV-TR uses the term Cluster B (borderline, narcissistic, histrionic, or antisocial) personality disorders for those patients with heavy endowments of extraversion and instability. The subgroups overlap considerably, and thus the term "Cluster B personality" is usually sufficient to describe these patients. It is useful to think of Cluster B patients as unstable extraverts. This quantitative, dimensional approach allows for "lumping" Cluster B patients together, as they all tend to be focused on getting what they want in the now and have an unstable personality structure prone to labile emotions.

Patients with other personality disorders do present to the ED. Persons with instability (intense reactive emotions) who are introverted (more consequence avoidant) have obsessive-compulsive, passive-aggressive, dependent, or avoidant behaviors (the DSM Cluster C category) that can also be problematic. They have trouble making decisions and may ruminate endlessly over every issue in their care due to their obsessional and ambivalent styles. These patients may end up in the ED because they have been too ambivalent to act on problems until they become a crisis. Patients labeled as Cluster A schizoid, schizotypal, or paranoid personalities may also present late because they may avoid medical care, but when they do present to an acute care setting their reticence to accept care can be problematic.

Unstable extraverts (Cluster B patients) are driven by feelings, and may place unreasonable demands on their doctors and other members of the health care team. In some situations, their behavior may be appropriate; for instance, if a Cluster B patient were experiencing a myocardial infarction, there may be some tolerance and understanding for their outspoken requests for immediate attention and treatment of chest pain. When a potentially serious medical condition is present, clinicians tend to be empathetic about the patient's condition, even in cases where the patient is demanding to be seen without delay. Unfortunately, unstable extraverts often exhibit the same behavior whether they are in a serious medical crisis or are uncomfortable from symptoms such as withdrawal symptoms, cravings, or even a viral syndrome. Clinicians are less sympathetic with patients demanding specific treatments such as lorazepam, promethazine, or hydromorphone for their condition. These patients do not distinguish between a medical crisis and a circumstance where they have an urgent desire or discomfort. In the first example, the patient is presenting with a potentially life-threatening condition, whereas in the second example the patient is demanding specific treatments involving controlled substances and is always in crisis, but has no life-threatening condition. Although the doctor sees the difference, the patient does not.

In the ED, problematic patients soon realize that their ability to get what they want varies between different shifts, staff members, and hospitals. Unfortunately, intermittent positive reinforcement increases problematic behavior. These patients are relatively insensitive to consequences and failure but are highly motivated to obtain their goal. Like a car salesman who is rebuffed again and again, each new opportunity is a new challenge. Car salesmen (indeed any salesperson) are intermittently reinforced, and while introverts do poorly because they have difficulty with the repeated failures, extraverts thrive on the intermittent but large rewards. Positively reinforcing elements of emergency care, such as vigorous pain management, promotion of comfort, relief from distress, and intense attention can be a trap for the patient with a personality disorder. Although they will learn to avoid certain doctors and settings, their remarkable drive to obtain rewards motivates them to continue. Opiates and benzodiazepines cause intense positive reinforcement, and can condition patients to overuse EDs. In a busy emergency setting, the fastest and easiest way to respond to patients may be to give them what they say they need. For a dose of intravenous opioid, a patient may visit multiple EDs or pit staff against each other until someone finally provides a dose of medication. Although the providing team may try to talk to the patient about his/her inappropriate behavior, the behavioral learning message is clear to the patient: increasingly problematic behavior will eventually bring about a reward.

The correct management of these patients is straightforward but difficult. An assessment of the real danger to the patient, an explanation of what the diagnosis and treatment plan will be, and a description of the requirements for the patient behaviorally to access the treatment should be offered. In a situation where the patient is in danger, their excessive focus on their feelings may impair their decision-making capacity and thus limit their autonomy, but when the danger is limited, the patient can decline the treatment. Limit setting can take the form of: "This is what I think is wrong with you, do you agree? If so, this is the most appropriate treatment." If the patient rejects your diagnosis and they are not in any significant danger, they should get a second opinion (probably elsewhere). If the patient accepts the diagnostic formulation but rejects the treatment plan, then they are refusing treatment. Physicians are not obligated to provide treatment recommended by the patient, another doctor, or what the patient says works for them.

Setting limits can be done on an institutional level. Many EDs have specific care plans for frequent visitors (see Chapter 1), or may have a policy forbidding the dispensing of certain drugs in specific situations, such as methadone to patients who are receiving the drug from elsewhere, as is illustrated in the case below:

A 28-year-old female with a history of opioid and cocaine dependence presents with suicidal ideation, having recently cut her wrist to the point of requiring several stitches. On initial questioning, she complained that, "I was feeling real bad and missed my methadone appointment and then I wanted to kill myself. I'm okay now and I want to go home." On further questioning, she revealed that she missed her scheduled methadone appointment because she went out to use cocaine. Once she got to the ED and received her methadone and care for her superficial injuries, she felt better and requested to be discharged.

In cases like the one described above, the simplest course would be to discharge the patient without further intervention. For many EDs, this may be the most pragmatic disposition depending on current constraints of the department. It is clear that this patient has no hesitation in doing something very drastic to obtain what she wants. It can be difficult for many physicians to comprehend how such dangerous behavior can develop solely as a means to manipulate clinicians.

If the emergency staff had decided against providing the patient with methadone, she may have left the ED to seek alternative mechanisms, such as illegal methadone. The issue here is choosing the course of action that is most likely to help this patient. A systematic approach that requires patients to engage in healthy behaviors in order to get what they want can provide benefit and change behavior over time. For example, requiring the patient to watch an educational video about substance abuse treatment and meeting with an addictions counselor prior to providing methadone is helpful. Requiring that the patient enter an ED-linked addictions unit to get opiates in the context of treatment would be even more beneficial. In many cases, EDs are not well suited to provide on-site adjunctive interventions, and making use of existing community-based or hospital programs should be an option as well.

Physicians must constantly struggle with pressure to provide medications that may harm patients, including those medications that have led to or enabled addictions. In particular, physicians in the ED are under time constraints and have a little time to go above and beyond their primary responsibility of solving the immediate problem to actually managing the big picture of the whole patient.

Consider the case of Mr. Jones, a 53-year-old homeless male with a left below-the-knee amputation who presents with lower extremity pain. Prior to the doctor's entering the examination room, nursing staff report that Mr. Jones was chatting amiably with peers in the waiting room and had politely asked for food. However, when the doctor goes in to see the patient, he looks ill and behaves as if he has intolerable pain. Before entering the room, the physician notes that the patient appeared comfortable and at ease and seemed to enjoy the attention of the staff.

As the interview continues, Mr. Jones confesses to the ED physician that he is using illegally obtained opiate medication. However, he repeats that his pain is intolerable and demands a prescription and opiates for immediate pain relief. Although some patients can tolerate pain and "put a good face on things" until they see the doctor, the judgment of the clinician is essential. In this case, as Mr. Jones has an opioid abuse or dependence problem complicated by prior experiences with outpatient providers, Mr. Jones believes he is in crisis, and the only remedy in his mind is the continued opioids. As a result, Mr. Jones engages with his outpatient providers only to gain what he wants.

For a physician working in a busy ED, more opioids would placate Mr. Jones and could result in a short ED length of stay, which in turn has a positive impact on all the patients waiting to be seen. However, if the physician really wants to help the patient, he must engage in a difficult conversation with Mr. Jones; the physician must be prepared to share his goals for treatment, which in all likelihood will have little in common with the patient's goals. This conflict is not new to the patient, and it can be helpful to point this out to him. However, confrontations are most effective when they are pleasant and are without accusation, frustration, or anger on behalf of the physician. Manipulative patients will try to provoke an antagonistic interaction, but smiling and insisting that we are there to help usually diffuses this. The profound emphasis on the present without regard for the past or future is common among problematic patients, and it drives solutions that provide increased immediate comfort at the cost of future function.

The best intervention for this circumstance is a review of the doctor's goals for treatment of their patients. A clear and detailed discussion of beneficial health and treatment options is the best alternative, but is often rejected by the patient. Patients may say, "You have no idea what I'm going through," or "How can you sit there and tell me that you can't help me?" This problem is exacerbated by the patient's off-putting nature and is further complicated by a taxed or overburdened clinical staff. Problematic patients have difficulty taking responsibility for their behavior and often see themselves as victims of their environment; seldom do they say, "I am addicted to opioids and have no more long-term goals. Please help me obtain detoxification and physical therapy." Instead, they believe that they feel bad, and thus, only opioids and people who can prescribe them opioids can help them. Despite the fact that the patient's treatment plan has been tried in the past and has failed repeatedly, these patients reject the doctor's prescription in favor of their own. A clear description and discussion of this will usually result in the patient either leaving the ED or accepting the treatment plan.

Patients with personality disorders can complicate management possibilities by making statements that require action on behalf of acute care personnel. As an example, Mr. Smith is a 47-year-old opioid-dependent man who presents to the ED requesting detoxification. He has undergone detoxification with buprenorphine four times in the last three months at various short-stay programs and has relapsed immediately upon discharge from each one.

MR. SMITH: You have to help me. I want to get better.

ED PHYSICIAN: Mr. Smith, I see you've had several attempts at detoxification and sobriety in the past few months. What would be different this time around?

MR. SMITH: I really need to get on track, doc. I'll do anything.

ED PHYSICIAN: That's great! Tell me, what usually happens when you're discharged from detox?

MR. SMITH: I go back to using because I don't always change people, places, and things.

ED PHYSICIAN: What's your experience in 12-step been like? I'm not saying that it's the answer, but I wonder if you've found any support there.

MR. SMITH: I did a second step.

ED PHYSICIAN: It sounds like your sobriety falls apart because you don't have any community support. Since you said that you'd do anything to get better, I'm going to ask you to do something difficult. I want you to go to ten 12-step meetings and bring in a form to our outpatient clinic that documents your attendance. That way, we will know you have some support in the community when you leave detox, and that you are serious about taking the important steps to help yourself.

MR. SMITH: But if I leave now, I'm going to kill myself.

ED PHYSICIAN: Mr. Smith, I cannot let you leave the hospital if you tell me that. Because I don't have an appropriate bed for you and will have to search to find one, you will need to stay in this safe environment for now.

MR. SMITH: I don't feel suicidal. I want to leave.

ED PHYSICIAN: Mr. Smith, I can't let you go if you've just told me you're going to kill yourself. I'll be back in an hour or so, and we can talk again.

This patient was eventually discharged, but returned to the outpatient clinic two weeks later with a Narcotics Anonymous slip indicating attendance at ten meetings. He subsequently completed detoxification without any issues. The transformation of a patient from a crisis mindset to a rehabilitation mindset has seldom been achieved in one visit, but the goal should still be the same, eventual successful recovery. By moving the onus of recovery from the physician to the patient, both the physician and the patient were able to do their jobs. However, it is remarkable to see how often threatened suicide is utilized as a coping skill in problematic patients during the crises preceding such a transformation. Although threatened suicide is used as a manipulation tool in many cases by patients with personality disorders, a number of them do impulsively seriously injure or kill themselves. The patient must be carefully evaluated as someone who is at risk for self-injury, and the appropriate precautions must be taken. In many cases like the one described above, the statement may have reflected a temporary sentiment or was an indication of the patient's frustration with the situation. Allowing the patient to think more on that sentiment, or giving them the opportunity to talk about their level of frustration, can result in the patient feeling more secure to the point where both provider and patient feel that the patient is safe for outpatient management.

In the next case, a 27-year-old homeless patient with HIV who has had three days of night sweats and two weeks of non-productive cough says that she would like to leave against medical advice. While she exhibits signs of opioid withdrawal, she denies that she is leaving to use drugs. She can clearly describe the reasons as to why the ED physician wants her admitted to the hospital, one of them being the possibility of tuberculosis. She can also reliably say that she could die from untreated tuberculosis, but regardless of that possibility, she would like to leave so that she can ensure receipt of her disability check.

The ethical arguments about autonomy and beneficence in cases like this are shaped by both economic factors and traditional medical ethics. The first question is whether or not the patient is acting autonomously, as patients with addictions, personality disorders, and chronic mental illness may appear to superficially describe the risks and benefits of a decision, but often have a fundamental impairment in their ability to act in their best interests. States vary with regards to the requirements for involuntary hospitalization, but in general, they require documentation that the patient has a mental illness, a treatable disorder, suffers from a serious or mortal heath risk, and that there is no safer or less restrictive course of action other than involuntary hospitalization. The best course of action is to make decisions clinically rather than based on one's interpretation of legal issues. In this case, while one could probably make a case for involuntary admission, it is better and easier to persuade the patient to stay. Patients with personality disorders seem to respond best when given a choice to do the best thing medically because it is the most comfortable choice. In addition, it is important have a fine balance between making it clear to the patient that leaving the ED is not possible in a life-threatening situation and allowing the patient to "save face" and have some level of autonomy. In the case described above, the patient agreed to admission once the availability of opioid agonist treatments was explained and social work helped her arrange for her mother to get her check; thus ensuring that involuntary admission for this patient was unnecessary.

Summary

Personality disorders are chronic aberrations in patterns of behavior. Patients with personality disorders often are emotionally labile and often resort to inappropriate language or raised voices in the ED. Managing the threats of suicide and the wanton wasting of resources that are associated with the behavioral repertoire of these patients is beyond the training of most doctors. While comorbid mental illness is a frequent complication in patients with unreasonable behavior in the ED, the usual goal is to manage the behavior of the patient and direct them towards more effective health care. The goal for emergency practitioners is improved health, longevity, function and quality of life, while **for these patients, their goal is usually feeling better *now*, even if it is at the cost of poorer health later**. With patients experiencing personality problems, allowing them to dictate the outcome of health care interactions may result in shorter ED stays, but can also result in poor long-term outcomes, frustration on behalf of the providers, and patients habitually misusing the medical system including the ED. Effective interventions that are prescribed by doctors rather than patients are usually directed by the goals of function, longevity, and quality of life. In many cases, these interventions take longer, require more effort, and can result in longer ED stays, but lead to better outcomes as well as greater clinician satisfaction. Although this method may impede ED patient flow in the short term, uniform ED management of these patients should result in a more effective health care system overall. It must be stated that reaching these goals for patients with personality disorders can be difficult and may not always lead to the ideal disposition. Also, it should be noted that having conversations with patients might not always be as peaceful as illustrated above. However, approaching patients with honesty, sincerity, and a sense of empathy and understanding, will minimize the patient's anger and frustration and can help to bring about a more efficient and reasonable disposition.

(The Personality and Personality Disorders Work Group has proposed a new diagnostic criteria for personality disorders that is likely to be reflected in the DSM V. It includes six specific personality disorder types which are as follows: Antisocial, Avoidant, Borderline, Narcissistic, Obsessive-Compulsive, and Schizotypal. Each criteria is characterized by specific impairments in functioning and has pathological personality traits.)

Legal issues in the care of psychiatric patients in the emergency department

Cynthia Major-Lewis, Dennis Barton, Patrick Triplett, and Darren Mareiniss

Care for patients with active psychiatric problems in the emergency department (ED) requires an understanding of the complex intersection of emergency medicine, psychiatry, and law. The ED is frequently a site of concentrated risk and sometimes without the commensurate resources to address the complexity of patient presentations. Decisions must be made in an expeditious manner often without complete information, adequate time, or access to legal counsel. Although the old adage, "Think like a doctor first and like a lawyer second" is appropriate in emergency psychiatry, the well-informed clinician should have a working knowledge of the potential legal issues that are involved in providing care in this setting. A review of some the key issues is below.

Presentation to EDs

Although some patients present themselves voluntarily to the ED to seek treatment, others may be brought to the ED involuntarily. The process by which patients may be brought involuntarily for emergency psychiatric evaluations varies from state to state and is most usually codified in state law.[1] Because state laws vary, clinicians should be familiar with the legal requirements in the local jurisdiction in which they are practicing. Particular attention should be paid to ensure that the correct procedures (including transport) are followed when a patient is brought to the ED and that the timelines for evaluation and decisions regarding admission or release are followed.

Some states allow citizens to petition a court to authorize police to detain and bring persons with potentially dangerous behaviors to an ED for emergency evaluation. Most states use the "probable cause" standard when determining if a patient poses a sufficient danger to self or others or whether the patient demonstrates grave disability. States also vary with regard to who may file a petition or who may issue a temporary hold allowing for psychiatric evaluations. Some states have statutes that assume an evaluation will be done in an ED before release or voluntary or involuntary admission to a psychiatric unit. Other states allow a short period of time (typically less than 72 hours) during which a patient may be evaluated on an involuntary admission basis before determining the necessity of subsequent steps in the civil commitment process.

In Maryland, for example, emergency petitions (EPs) constitute the means by which an emergency evaluation is started. EPs may be initiated and executed by law enforcement officers (peace officers) if the officers document that an individual's behavior "present[s] a

---

Emergency Psychiatry, ed. Arjun Chanmugam, Patrick Triplett, and Gabor Kelen. Published by Cambridge University Press. © Cambridge University Press 2013.

danger to the life or safety of themselves or others." Licensed physicians, psychologists, social workers, or nurse practitioners who have examined the patient may endorse an EP for a peace officer to act upon without a judge's order.[2]

Other citizens, including family members or loved ones, have the right to petition that an individual be psychiatrically evaluated on an emergency basis. Although states vary in the methods by which this is accomplished, most require that a judge or commissioner authorize such an evaluation. Many states provide access for the authorization of these kinds of evaluations on a 24 hours a day, seven days a week basis. Typically, a judicial overseer uses a probable cause standard to determine whether an individual requires an emergency evaluation.

In Maryland, the statute authorizing emergency petitions requires that the petitioner or "lay person" have "reason to believe" that the individual presents a danger to the life or safety of themselves or others.[3] This includes endangering oneself by not eating or drinking, not recognizing actions that could lead to dangerous consequences, and neglecting serious or life-threatening medical conditions. If the judge approves the petition, a law enforcement officer will be authorized to pick up the evaluee and transport them to the nearest ED for evaluation. If the judge does not sign the petition, it is denied, and no further action may be taken.[4]

Admission to an inpatient psychiatric unit

Following assessment and possible treatment in the ED, patients will be either released or admitted to an inpatient unit. When admission is to an inpatient psychiatric unit, it may be on a voluntary or involuntary basis.

When the determination is made by an evaluating clinician that a patient is in need of inpatient psychiatric hospitalization, the patient will be offered admission as a voluntary patient. Most jurisdictions require that a voluntarily-admitted patient sign a voluntary admission agreement, which may also be signed by the physician seeking the patient's admission. The majority of states require that a patient give an acknowledgement or assent to their voluntary admission.

In Maryland, for example, an individual may request voluntary admission through either an informal (not requiring a signed application by the individual) or formal proced-ure.[5] Under either procedure, the individual must meet the following criteria: (1) the individual has a mental disorder; (2) the mental disorder is susceptible to care or treatment; (3) the individual understands the nature of the request for admission; (4) the individual is able to give continuous *assent* to retention by the facility; and (5) the individual is able to ask for release (emphasis added).[6]

A minority of states require that a patient give informed consent to a voluntary admission. A pivotal landmark case in this area is *Zinermon v Burch*.[7] Under Florida law at the time, voluntary admission required "application by express and informed consent."[8] Zinermon alleged that his procedural due process rights had been violated when he was admitted voluntarily to a Florida psychiatric hospital because, he argued, he was unable to provide informed consent for his admission. Although not directly answering the question of whether voluntarily admitted patients must provide informed consent for admission, the US Supreme Court did find that Florida should have procedures in place to exclude those not able to give informed consent. States have adopted various methods to screen for incompetent patients following the *Zinermon* decision.

Decision-making capacity and informed consent

Competent patients, as a pre-requisite, must have decision-making capacity. Competence is a legal determination whereas capacity is a medical determination that may be made in the ED. A patient must have capacity in order to give informed consent.[9] As alluded to above, an assessment of capacity may be prudent before a patient is voluntarily admitted to a psychiatric unit. Further, a capacity assessment is even more important before a patient can be allowed to leave against medical advice or refuse care. This may be an issue for psychiatric patients who are not candidates for involuntary admission, but still require medical evaluation and treatment. Before such a patient or any other patient may be allowed to leave against medical advice, decision-making capacity must be assessed by a provider. Once decision-making capacity is verified, the patient can then be informed about the risks and benefits of leaving against medical advice and opt to leave AMA.

The informed consent standard has its roots in the common law of both England and the United States. Treatment of patients without such consent was and is considered a battery. In 1914, Justice Cardozo, in the oft-cited case of *Schloendorff v. Soc'y of New York Hospital*, stated that, "Every human being of adult years and sound mind has a right to determine what shall be done with his own body: and a surgeon who performs an operation without his patient's consent commits an assault for which he is liable."[10] This rule governing consent remains in the American and English common law today.

Similar to the law, modern bioethics supports the concept of informed consent. Respect for autonomy can be traced back to the Nuremberg Code, the Belmont report, and principlism.[11] Autonomous decisions require three basic elements: (1) disclosure of information; (2) comprehension; and (3) voluntariness.[11] A patient must be informed of the risks, benefits, and alternatives of a procedure and a clinician must ensure that the patient understands this information.[9] Further, a patient's decision must be voluntary. Only decisions that are substantially informed and free of duress are considered autonomous.[12]

Decision-making capacity

A pre-requisite to informed consent is a patient's intact capacity to make decisions. Evaluation of such capacity is a decision-specific determination that focuses on the patient's ability to understand and communicate a rational decision.[13] The key considerations in an assessment of decision-making capacity are:

1. **Ability to express a choice:** The person must be able to express his or her choice and communicate that choice.
2. **Ability to understand relevant information:** The person must be able to understand information about the purpose of treatment, remember the information, and show that he or she can be part of the decision-making process.
3. **Ability to appreciate the significance of the information and its consequences:** The person must understand the consequences of treatment refusal and the risks and benefits of accepting or refusing treatment.
4. **Ability to manipulate information:** The person must be able to engage in reasoning as it applies to making treatment decisions (e.g., use logical processes, weigh treatment decisions, and manipulate information about treatment decisions).[14]

It is usually inappropriate to assume that a patient with mental pathology, sedation, or cognitive deficit lacks decision-making capacity. Instead, a formal evaluation is necessary. As noted above, capacity is different from competence. Competence is determined by a court of law and uses issues of capacity in evaluating the legal ability to contract, write wills, or conduct one's affairs.[14] As the standard of competence varies by jurisdiction, an exhaustive discussion of competence is beyond the scope of this chapter.

Involuntary admissions

Emergent psychiatric assessment may be the first in a series of events that leads to an involuntary hospitalization and potential civil commitment. Involuntary commitment is the act of placing an individual in a psychiatric ward or hospital against his or her will. This commitment is usually time-limited and requires periodic re-evaluation. Certain statutory mandates regarding criteria, which vary from state to state, must be met in order for an individual to be involuntarily committed. Licensed physicians, psychiatrists, and some mental health professionals have the ability to initiate the involuntary commitment of a patient. While procedures vary from state to state, the informed clinician will be familiar with the legal parameters around such involuntary admission so as not to have the patient released from a civil commitment hearing because procedural issues were not followed according to law. Ultimately, the commitment decision is made by a court or by a mental health commission.[15]

State statutes differ in the exact wording of civil commitment laws. Nonetheless, there are three general criteria that are usually considered around the civil commitment process:

(1) The individual must be mentally ill, which loosely defined means they must be suffering from a mental illness which substantially impairs their mental health;

(2) They must be deemed a danger to themselves or others; and/or

(3) They must be unable to provide for their basic needs because of their impaired mental state.[15]

In addition to the main criteria above, other factors may be considered in determining that an individual is in need of an involuntary psychiatric hospitalization. Grave disability rendering persons unable to care for themselves to the point of probable self-harm may allow for civil commitment in some jurisdictions. Still others may allow persons who are in need of hospitalization but who refuse it to be considered for civil commitment. Individuals displaying a danger to property, individuals who lack capacity (see above) to make rational treatment decisions, and individuals for whom hospitalization represents the least restrictive environment may meet criteria for involuntary admission.[15]

Once individuals are involuntarily admitted to a psychiatric hospital, they will be afforded legal representation to appear before a judge or other designated representative to determine whether procedures have been followed appropriately and whether they meet the civil commitment criteria for further hospitalizations and treatment. At that time, clinicians may present information related to the need for ongoing involuntary admission and treatment. A judge will determine whether the facility/treatment team has met the "minimum standard of proof" constitutionally required for continued long-term commitment of the individual.[15] In *Addington v. Texas*, the US Supreme Court held that the standard of proof required in a civil commitment proceeding was "clear and convincing evidence."[16] This standard of proof is less than the standard of "beyond a reasonable doubt" required in criminal proceedings but more than the required "preponderance of the evidence" standard used in most civil cases.

When an individual continues to meet criteria for involuntary commitment, the case is generally reviewed by the court or judicial body that conducted the initial hearing every 3, 6, or 12 months, according to the specific state statute. Psychiatrists also have the ability to release patients when they believe the patient no longer meets commitment criteria.

Psychiatric hospitalization of minors

As with other topics discussed in this chapter, states differ in their statutes outlining the guidelines for the psychiatric hospitalization of minor children. Generally, children are considered to be those 18 years and younger. The American Psychiatric Association's Task Force on the Commitment of Minors published guidelines to ensure that children in need of mental health care would be protected against needless hospitalization and deprivations of liberty.[17] In these guidelines, the Task Force recognized the importance of parents' authority to make medical decisions for their children and the need for "medical decisions to be made in response to clinical needs and in accordance with sound psychiatric judgment."[17]

Under these guidelines, children under the age of 16 can be admitted without their consent to a psychiatric hospital but with the consent of their parents, if a treating or admitting physician determines that the child is in need of psychiatric hospitalization. Children aged 16 and over have the right to contest the admission. States vary on the exact mechanisms put in place for a child over the age of 16 to contest the admission. The treating physician has the ability to move forward with involuntary commitment of a child aged 16 and over who refuses psychiatric hospitalization but meets involuntary commitment criteria. Also, children age 16 and over have the ability to admit themselves, without the consent of their parent or guardian, if the treating or admitting physician agrees that psychiatric hospitalization is indicated. Parents do have the right to be notified immediately in the event that their child age 16 and over is self-admitted to a psychiatric hospital.

Tarasoff issues

The concepts of duty to warn and duty to protect arose in the context of two court decisions from the Supreme Court of California in the 1970s.[18,19] Both decisions sprang from the same set of facts and legal case. *Tarasoff v. Regents of the University of California* was a civil suit filed by the surviving parents of a college-age woman who had been killed by a student being treated by the university psychologist.

In this case, a University of California student (Prosenjit Poddar) disclosed to his student health center psychologist that he planned on harming his former girlfriend, Tatiana Tarasoff. The psychologist notified campus police, who questioned Poddar, found him to be rational, and made him promise to stay away from Tarasoff. Two months later, Poddar killed Tarasoff, which led to a suit brought by the parents of Tatiana Tarasoff against the University of California, the university health center, and the police. At trial, the case was dismissed on the grounds that, because of confidentiality between a doctor and patient, the physician has a duty only to the patient and not to third parties.

The family appealed to the Supreme Court of California. They asserted that the defendants had a duty to warn Tatiana or her family of Poddar's threat and that steps should have been taken to ensure his confinement.[18] The Supreme Court of California reversed the trial court's decision and stated that a "therapist bears a duty to use reasonable care to give threatened persons warnings as are essential to avert forseeable danger." (*Tarasoff I*). Following the *Tarasoff I* ruling, there was discontent among the mental health and police communities, and the court took the unusual step of hearing the case again.

In 1976 (*Tarasoff II*), the Supreme Court of California held: "When a therapist determines, or pursuant to the standards of his profession should determine, that his patient presents a serious danger of violence to another, he incurs an obligation to use reasonable care to protect the intended victim against such danger. The discharge of this duty may require the therapist to take one or more of various steps. Thus, it may call for him to warn the intended victim, to notify the police, or to take whatever steps are reasonably necessary under the circumstances."[19]

This case illustrates that confidentiality no longer takes precedence when there is a direct threat of imminent danger or harm toward a third party. States differ in their interpretation of *Tarasoff*, and clinicians should consult their state's laws as they pertain to the duty to warn.

EMTALA

EMTALA was passed in 1986 as part of the Consolidated Omnibus Budget and Reconciliatory Act (COBRA).[20] The term EMTALA now commonly refers both to the statute and the regulations enacted and amended to enforce the statute. Sometimes referred to as an "anti-dumping law," EMTALA requires hospitals with an ED to provide an appropriate medical screening examination "within the capability of the hospital's emergency department, including ancillary services routinely available to the emergency department, to determine whether or not an emergency medical condition exists."[21]

The US government defines an "emergency department" as a "specially equipped and staffed area of the hospital used a significant portion of the time for initial evaluation and treatment of outpatients for emergency medical conditions."[4] An "emergency medical condition" is defined as "a condition manifesting itself by acute symptoms of sufficient severity such that absence of immediate medical attention could reasonably be expected to result in placing the individual's health (or health of an unborn child) in serious jeopardy, serious impairment to bodily functions, or serious dysfunction of bodily organs."[5]

EMTALA applies to "participating hospitals," which are those that accept payment from the Department of Health and Human Services, Centers for Medicare and Medicaid Services (CMS) under the Medicare program. However, EMTALA's provisions apply to all patients and not just Medicare patients.

Hospitals have three main obligations under EMTALA. First, a hospital must determine whether an emergency medical condition exists for any individual who comes and requests a medical screening. Second, treatment must be provided until the medical condition is resolved or stabilized or the hospital must transfer the patient to another hospital that can appropriately treat the patient. Lastly, hospitals with specialized capabilities must accept transfers from other hospitals and may not discharge a patient until the condition is resolved and the patient is able to provide self-care or is transferred to another facility.[22]

There are penalties for violating EMTALA, which is enforced by CMS and the Office of the Inspector General (OIG). The most severe of these penalties can include termination of the hospital or physician's Medicare provider agreement. Hospitals can be fined up to $25,000 if they have less than 100 beds and up to $50,000 if they have more than 100 beds.

Physicians, including "on call" physicians, can be fined up to $50,000. Patients may bring personal injury suits against hospitals, and a receiving hospital or facility can file a suit to recover damages if it suffered a financial loss as a result of another hospital's EMTALA violation.

There are myriad issues that can come up when trying to apply EMTALA to psychiatric patients or patients who are suspected of having a mental illness. An "emergency medical condition" as it pertains to psychiatric patients requires the patient to be determined "dangerous to self or others." Guidelines to the federal regulations make it clear that simply expressing the intent to harm oneself or others by itself is not necessarily sufficient to create an emergency medical condition for the purpose of EMTALA.[22] The expressed intent would require the examining physician to assess the dangerousness and seriousness of the threat. Once the individual is assessed as being "dangerous to self or others," EMTALA would apply, and it would be the duty of the treating physician or mental health professional to stabilize and treat the condition or to transfer to a facility that has the capabilities of treating the patient.

EMTALA does not require forcible detention or treatment. EMTALA does not preempt state statutes or regulations requiring that informed consent be obtained before treatment is provided, nor does it preempt state emergency commitment statutes.[22]

HIPAA

The Health Insurance Portability and Accountability Act (HIPAA) is a federal law passed in 1996 by Congress.[23] There are several provisions and titles under HIPAA that address different issues including: protecting health insurance coverage for workers and their families when they change or lose their jobs; the Administrative Simplification Provision that requires the establishment of national standards for electronic health care transactions; and national identifiers for providers, health insurance plans, and employers. There is also a federal privacy rule that is a component of HIPAA, which is aimed at protecting a patient's health care information.

The component of HIPAA aimed at protecting a patient's health care information can have significant impact on the treatment of psychiatrically ill individuals in an emergency setting. The federal privacy rule of HIPAA attempts to help patients maintain their medical history and retain control of how that information will be used and disseminated. The privacy rule allows for patients to see and make corrections in their medical record and requires that patients authorize the release of their medical information.

The concept of confidentiality requires that information given in confidence to a physician will be kept secret and revealed to others only with permission. In psychiatric emergency settings, other interests may take priority and lead to a permissible breach of confidentiality. In these situations where confidentiality must be breached, the clinician should be careful to consider what information will be disclosed and documentation should support why confidentiality is being broken. An emergency situation is usually sufficient grounds to reveal health information without a patient's consent if the information obtained will help with emergency treatment. Another situation where a patient's confidentiality can be breached is when there may be risk to a third party. Clinicians may also have to breach confidentiality when they are concerned about potential child or elder abuse.

Patients who believe their rights have been violated under HIPAA can file a complaint with the Secretary of Health and Human Services (HHS) within 180 days of the date of the violation. HHS can then refer complaints to the Department of Justice for criminal prosecution and penalties.[22]

Seclusion and restraint

Although there has been a national focus on reducing the use of seclusion and restraint, in the emergency setting such use may be necessary at times. In the United States, the Centers for Medicare & Medicaid Services (CMS) and the Joint Commission on Accreditation of Healthcare Organizations (JCAHO) set standards and regulate the use of seclusion and restraints. Providers should be familiar with specific state laws or regulations that impact providing care for patients requiring seclusion or restraint.

Summary

Patients with psychiatric disorders who need emergency treatment pose a number of unique challenges. The assurance of safety and provision of appropriate care must be the primary goal. Knowledge of applicable federal, state, and local regulations is critical as care is delivered in the ED and a plan of care is created. The intersection of psychiatry, emergency medicine, and law commonly involves the process of involuntary referral and assessment, informed consent, involuntary commitment, decision-making capacity, duty to warn, HIPAA, EMTALA, and seclusion and restraints. Familiarity with these issues in advance of actual patient presentations can help providers create a more efficient and effective treatment system of care.

References

1. Rubin WV, Snapp MB, Panzano PC, et al. Variation in civil commitment process across jurisdictions: an approach for managing and monitoring change in mental health systems. *J Ment Health Admin*. 1996;**23**:375–388.

2. Maryland Health-General Article, §10–620 et seq.

3. Maryland Health-General Article, §10–622 (a)(2).

4. Janofsky JS, Tamburello AC. Diversion to the mental health system: emergency psychiatric evaluations. *J Am Acad Psychiatry Law*. 2006;**34**:283–291.

5. Maryland Health-General Article, §10–609.

6. Maryland Health-General Article, §10–609(c).

7. *Zinermon v. Burch*, 494 U.S. 113 (1990).

8. Florida Statutes, Sections 394.465(1)(a), 394.455(22)(1981).

9. Morgan H, Mayo TW. Ethical aspects of neurosurgical practice. In *Textbook of Neurological Surgery, Principles and Practice*. Philadelphia, PA: Lippincott Williams & Wilkins, 2003.

10. *Schloendorff v. Soc' of New York Hospital*, 105 N.E 92 (N.Y. 1914).

11. Shapiro MH, Spece RG, Dresser R, Clayton EW (Eds.), *Bioethics and Law*. 2nd ed. St. Paul, MN: West Publishing Co., 2003.

12. Beauchamp TL, Childress JF. *Principles of Biomedical Ethics*. 4th ed. New York, NY: Oxford University Press, 1994.

13. Kapp MB. Ethical and legal issues. In Duthie EH (Ed.), *Practice of Geriatrics*. 3rd ed. Philadelphia, PA: Saunders, 1998.

14. Mufson M. Evaluation of competence in the medical setting. In Samuels MA (Ed.), *Office Practice of Neurology*. 2nd ed. Edinburgh: Churchill Livingston, 2003.

15. Riba MB, Ravindranath D. *Clinical Manual of Emergency Psychiatry*. Washington, DC: American Psychiatric Publishing, 2010.

16. *Addington v. Texas*, 441 U.S. 418 (1979).

17. http://www.psych.org/lib_archives/ archives/198101.pdf. Accessed September 11, 2011.

18. *Tarasoff v. Regents of the University of California*, 529 P.2d 533 (Cal. 1974).

19. *Tarasoff v. Regents of the University of California*, 551 P.2d 334 (Cal. 1976).

20. 42 USC 1395dd.

21. 42 USC 1395dd(a).

22. Stefan S. *Emergency Department Treatment of the Psychiatric Patient: Policy Issues and Legal Requirements*. Oxford: Oxford University Press, 2006.

23. Health Insurance Portability and Accountability Act (HIPAA) of 1996 (P.L.104–191).

Geriatric psychiatry

Crystal Watkins and Patrick Triplett

Introduction

With the expanding geriatric population in the US and an estimated 71 million people over the age of 65 by 2030, the number of older patients that use the hospital emergency department (ED) for evaluation and treatment will increase accordingly.[1] Patients aged 65 or older, defined as "geriatric," represent about 13% of the population and currently use an estimated 5–6% of all services in emergency psychiatry.[2] There is high overall prevalence of mental illness in the geriatric population.[3,4]

The most common neuropsychiatric affliction in this group is cognitive impairment. On average 10–15% of the population over 65 report some degree of memory deficit. Over 69% of patients with significant intellectual decline live in skilled nursing facilities or similar institutions.[3,4] However, many older adults with some degree of cognitive impairment continue to live in the community. As the "baby boomers" mature, and older patients are increasingly remaining in the community with relatives or in assisted living, more geriatric patients are anticipated to present to the ED for management of related psychiatric complaints.[5] A review of the literature suggests that many of the studies examining utilization of psychiatric emergency services in the geriatric population are decades old, though the trend has been for geriatric patients to present to the ED when they are at their most vulnerable, most disruptive behaviorally, the most medically complex, or at the severest point in their illness.

Special considerations for this group of patients

Geriatric patients embody a special demographic group whose presenting complaints may be more somatically focused than psychiatrically oriented. The elderly are often on a fixed income and sometimes have little social support. Delirium, depression, dementia, suicidal thoughts, and failure to thrive are not, however, characteristics of the majority of geriatric patients.[6] Nonetheless, these conditions are more common in older adults and thus geriatric patients are more susceptible to present acutely with a psychiatric emergency.[2] Presentations in this age group often pose a diagnostic and management dilemma since psychiatric symptoms can be atypical, non-specific, or masked by physical impairments. Classic psychiatric presentations in this age group are also more likely to be due to an acute underlying medical condition. As examples, an acute urinary tract infection can present as a change in mental status; shortness of breath can manifest as aggressive behavior in a demented patient; and metabolic disturbances can be related to symptoms of fatigue and anorexia. See Table 11.1.

Emergency Psychiatry, ed. Arjun Chanmugam, Patrick Triplett, and Gabor Kelen. Published by Cambridge University Press. © Cambridge University Press 2013.

Table 11.1. Geriatric medical conditions associated with psychiatric symptoms

	Medical diagnosis	Psychiatric symptoms	Related illnesses
Cardiovascular	Congestive heart failure, coronary artery disease	Depression, anxiety	Recent MI
	Mitral valve prolapse	Panic	
Pulmonary	COPD, asthma	Depression, anxiety, panic	Smoking history, pneumonia
Metabolic	Hyponatremia	Delirium, irritability, lethargy, psychosis, seizures	SIADH from carbamazepine and SSRIs; psychogenic polydypsia
	Hypokalemia	Depression	Failure to thrive, malnutrition from laxatives and diuretic abuse
	Hypophosphotemia	Delirium, anxiety, hyperventilation, weakness, seizures	Alcoholism, malnutrition
	Hypomagnesemia	Agitation, irritability, seizures	Alcoholism, malnutrition hypocalcemia
	Hypocalcemia	Depression, delirium	Hypoparathyroidism
	Hypercalcemia	Depression, psychosis	Primary or metastatic cancer Hyperparathyroidism Vit. D intoxication
Endocrine	Hypothyroidism	Depression, psychosis	
	Hyperthyroidism	Hypomania, anxiety, depression	Myxedema
	Hyperparathyroidism	Depression, personality change	
	Testosterone deficiency	Low energy, decreased libido	
Renal	Renal insufficiency – end stage	Depression, anxiety, delirium	
Rheumatologic	Rheumatoid arthritis	Chronic pain syndrome, depression, anxiety	
Trauma	Subdural hematoma/ traumatic brain injury	Personality change, delirium, cognitive disorder, focal neurological deficits	
	Burns	PTSD, adjustment disorder, delirium	
Oncologic	Any type of cancer	Depression, fatigue, delirium	
	Brain metastases	Focal neurologic deficits, delirium, depression	Breast, lung

Table 11.1. (cont.)

	Medical diagnosis	Psychiatric symptoms	Related illnesses
Infectious	Urinary tract infection	Delirium, agitation, depression	Sepsis
	Syphilis	Tertiary- encephalopathy, personality changes, memory impairment, depression, delirium	
	HIV	Delirium, dementia, memory impairment, depression	
Vitamin deficiencies	B-12	Dementia, personality and mood changes, delirium, neurological deficits	
	Folate	Cognitive impairment, depression	
	Thiamine	Confabulation, delirium, depression	Wernicke-Korsakoff syndrome, alcoholism
	Niacin	Dementia	

Adapted from Ferrando, S. Psychiatry in Review

On the other hand, serious psychiatric problems may only yield non-specific diagnostic clues, such as weight loss, headache, fatigue, weakness, or insomnia. Even when the diagnosis is major depressive disorder (MDD), geriatric patients may not report feeling "sad," but may endorse feelings of guilt, anhedonia, loss of concentration, and decreased attention.[6,7]

Chronic and acute medical conditions often add to the diagnostic challenge. As patients age, certain organs are directly affected, including the kidneys, lungs, and the immune system. These organ systems lose their reserve capacity to manage physiologic stress and also have a decline in basal physiologic function.[8] This decrease in reserve and function makes older patients more vulnerable to infections and acute illnesses. This change in functional capacity also contributes to the delay in recovery that is often observed when the elderly become ill. Furthermore, because of the comorbid physical and neurological symptoms, geriatric psychiatry patients[9] often will have more than one acute process that requires attention when they present to the ED. This may lead to longer ED stays and possibly complex disposition decisions.

Depression and mild cognitive impairment are commonly associated with acute and chronic cerebrovascular diseases[10–13] and cardiovascular conditions.[14–17] Patients recovering from a stroke, a recent myocardial infarction (MI), or congestive heart failure (CHF) may report low mood, poor sleep, decreased energy, and loss of interest. Studies demonstrate that these symptoms are directly related to changes in chemokines and cytokines in the immune system.[18,19] As a result of these changes, post-stroke and post-MI patients are now considered a group at high risk for recurrence of MDD as well as a first episode of MDD, late in life.[20] Many providers and patients mistakenly believe that these symptoms are the result of the underlying medical problem (e.g., stroke or CHF), and thus, recognition and treatment for MDD is not considered.

Given the multiple, co-existing medical problems, geriatric patients are more susceptible to developing polypharmacy-related problems that can also become evaluation and management issues in the emergency department. The normal pharmacokinetics (the study of the mechanisms of absorption and distribution of an administered drug) and pharmacodynamics (biochemical and physiological effects of drugs on the body) are known to change with age. Older patients take longer to metabolize and clear medications from their bodies compared to younger patients. Although a particular drug may have serum levels that are in the normal target range for a younger person, geriatric patients can sometimes become toxic if the medication is not reduced to account for age-related decreases in renal and hepatic function. In addition, geriatric patients tend to take more medications because of comorbid illnesses, leading to higher risks for drug-drug interactions and adverse side effects. According to the 2003 report released by Families USA, a Washington-based consumer health organization, seniors represent 13% of the total population and yet they account for about 34% of all prescriptions dispensed and 42% of all prescription drug spending.[21]

Polypharmacy is inherently difficult to manage. A significant effort is required to keep track of the number of medications, as well as the times to take the medications. Furthermore, medications may be managed by different physicians, who may not be well acquainted with drugs prescribed by other specialists. In addition, the exorbitant costs of the medication regimens can contribute to poor adherence to medication regimens in the elderly or result in patients taking reduced doses to save money.

Suicide risk is an important factor to assess in the geriatric psychiatric patient. Bereavement, social isolation, and clinical depression may all contribute to the markedly elevated risk of suicide among older patients. MDD is the primary factor related to suicide in the elderly, with 85% of completed suicides among patients 65 or older having this diagnosis.[22–24] While attempted suicides are less frequent in older patients, completed suicide occurs at a higher proportion in this population. According to the Centers for Disease Control (CDC) and the National Institute of Mental Health (NIMH), an estimated 14.3 of every 100,000 people aged 65 and older died by suicide in 2007, compared to the national average of 11.3 suicides in the general population. White males aged 85 or older have an alarming rate of 47 suicide deaths per 100,000.[25] For these reasons, geriatric patients, perhaps more than other groups, need an integrated approach to psychiatric diagnosis and coordinated management of medical and social issues in the ED setting. Whether a clinician is comfortable or feels challenged at times during the assessment of an elderly patient, this chapter is designed to address the evaluation, diagnosis, and management of conditions commonly seen in geriatric emergency medicine and geriatric psychiatry. We outline a practical approach to assessment and management of older patients when they present to the ED.

CASE: Mr. J is a 75-year-old white male with a history of MI two years ago and CVA one year ago, resulting in mild cognitive impairment and right-sided residual deficits, and chronic pain from osteoarthritis. He is currently housed in a skilled nursing facility (SNF) for subacute rehabilitation. Since residing at the SNF for the past four weeks, he has complained of headaches and become more withdrawn, with difficulty sleeping and decreased interests. Over the past two days, he has been angry, verbally aggressive to staff, refusing to take his medications, and not participating in physical therapy. Today, the situation escalated and he struck a staff member. He was bought to the ED for a psychiatric evaluation.

Diagnostics

As with any patient population seen in the ED, the immediate goals are patient safety, appropriate triage, evaluation, and appropriate management. The first step begins with a thorough medical evaluation followed by a psychiatric examination.

Important elements in the geriatric psychiatric history	
1	Background
2	Initial risk assessment
3	Collateral information
4	Medical and psychiatric factors
5	Cognitive impairment and capacity assessment
6	Medication use and/or substance abuse
7	Disposition

Background

Most elderly patients are brought to medical and psychiatric treatment by family members or caregivers; rarely do they refer themselves.[26] Presentations often occur after caregivers have been struggling with subacute or chronic issues for some time.[2,26,27] A survey by the National Alliance of Caregiving found that at least 22 million households in the US involve family caregivers. Providing care for an aging parent or another elderly family member can be physically exhausting, emotionally taxing, and often a financial strain.[28] With 7.4% of individuals over 75 living in SNFs, facilities are another major primary source of referral for emergency psychiatric evaluation and treatment.[2,26,27] As with any 24-hour operation, nursing facilities and private homes are vulnerable to having periods of time when staff and other resources are limited. These tend to be during evenings and weekends. Not only are staffing levels decreased, but the outpatient psychiatrist or primary care physician may not be available during these low-resource times. Care providers become more concerned and perhaps less tolerant of a resident who may be disruptive to the milieu. An agitated, cognitively impaired, combative, and/or assaultive patient is just as difficult to manage in an SNF as in a family care setting. Although it can feel as if the responsibility for the patients is being passed on to the ED staff, these patients are often more appropriate for the ED because they may require more intensive monitoring, and at times aggressive pharmacological management and even use of restraints. Ultimately they need a comprehensive medical and psychiatric evaluation in a safe controlled environment, which, in most cases, can only be accomplished by emergency services and acute care hospitals at times of crisis.

Initial risk assessment

The immediate concern in the ED is whether the patient is a danger to him/herself or others. Among geriatric patients, compared with other age groups, suicidal action is highly correlated with lethal outcomes. Mood disorders are common among older psychiatric patients, and the presenting affect, even in a manic state, is more often dysphoric compared with that of younger patients. Other risk factors for suicide, such as being unmarried and having a chronic medical illness, are also common in this population.[20] Screening tools such as the self-rated Geriatric Depression Scale can be used to assess symptoms (see Appendix). **The most effective risk assessment uses direct questions and follow-up questions.** Clinicians should specifically ask about suicidal thoughts, intentions, specific plans, access to guns, and other means. While suicide assessment tools like the Chronological

Assessment of Suicide Events scale and Suicide Ideation scale exist, clinical recognition, immediate safety precautions, and prompt treatment of MDD are the most effective strategies to manage elderly people at risk for suicide.[29]

Collateral information

Family members, caregivers, and treating physicians can provide valuable information, such as the patient's baseline level of functioning and past and current history of mood and behavioral changes, that can help formulate a diagnosis in the geriatric patient. These collateral sources of information can provide the longitudinal history that is needed to make an appropriate assessment. Particularly when dealing with disorganized, delirious, or demented patients, caregivers and family members help to establish the patient's baseline mental status. Additional informants may also identify the acute event precipitating the need for evaluation, such as a physical or verbal altercation or an acute change in the patient's ability to perform necessary activities of daily living. Information should be obtained from at least one caregiver, family member, facility nurse, or other physician. Geriatric patients may not be able to identify or may deny environmental or other variables that are antecedents to the emergency evaluation.[27] A great deal of objectivity must be maintained by the emergency providers when obtaining collateral information from informants; providers must be aware of any potential bias, the informant's agenda, and have a clear understanding of the informant's relationship to the patient. Signs of neglect or other indications of potential elder abuse must be explored in full.

A full review of the past written or electronic medical record can be instructive, especially if a patient has a past psychiatric history. When a previous psychiatric history is identified, a call to the treating psychiatrist or therapist can provide information about psychotropic medicines and any recent changes noted in the patient, including any recent changes in the patient's management. For ED physicians who do not routinely care for older patients with mental illness in the ED, it may be appropriate to consult other colleagues with experience in geriatrics to help manage the patient's medical and psychiatric issues,[2] though access to such specialists may be hard to come by in many settings, particularly at off-hours.

Medical and psychiatric factors

Although episodes of depression and other psychiatric conditions do occur later in life, new-onset conditions require thorough evaluation[2] (see Table 11.2). Delirium, characterized by waxing and waning levels of consciousness and problems with attention and cognition, is one of the most frequent emergencies and reasons for ED evaluation (see Chapter 6). Delirium can be related to infection, trauma, myocardial infarction, hypoxemia, fever, overmedication, and other medical causes, but may be further influenced or complicated by other chronic or subacute conditions such as dehydration, visual and hearing impairment, deconditioning, anemia, and lack of sleep.

Hallucinations or delusions in a person with no history of psychotic symptoms should lead to an evaluation of cognitive function to determine whether underlying delirium or other conditions exist. At a minimum, a urinalysis and culture, complete blood count, metabolic profile, ECG, and chest x-ray should be obtained to rule out reversible causes of delirium. Other laboratory testing, such as thyroid stimulating hormone, B12 level, and rapid plasma reagin are not part of the routine work-up in most ED settings due to the delay

Table 11.2. Suggested elements of a geriatric psychiatry evaluation

- Complete medical and psychiatric history

- Physical exam

- Neurological and mental status exams

- Laboratory tests:

  o Comprehensive metabolic panel (CMP) to evaluate electrolytes, including a magnesium level

  o BUN, Creatinine (renal function), liver function, albumin for nutrition status,

  o Complete blood count (CBC) for acute and/or chronic anemia and white blood cell count for infection

  o Urinalysis, urine toxicology, and urine cultures

  o Electrocardiogram (ECG) for baseline before treatment and to consider acute cardiac pathology

  o Optional considerations: B-12, folate, RPR, thyroid function tests,

  o HIV, ammonia level, ABG, lumbar puncture and CSF fluid examination

- Imaging

  o Chest radiograph

  o CT or MRI of the brain if trauma, space occupying lesion, stroke, or encephalopathy are suspected

  o Electroencephalogram (EEG) if delirium highly suspected; Delirium will show diffuse slowing; Alcohol withdrawal will have a normal or overexcitable pattern (may be difficult to obtain in the ED setting)

- Cognitive assessment

  o Folstein Mini-Mental State Examination for all able patients (for severe impairment due to dementia, consider the Severe Impairment Rating Scale (SIRS))

  o Montreal Cognitive Assessment

  o OPTIONAL: Confusion Assessment Method; Trail-Making Test; Clock Drawing (executive function); Memorial Delirium Assessment Scale; Delirium Rating Scale; CAM-ED

- Differential diagnosis

in obtaining results, though may be of utility for the individual admitted to an inpatient service or in a subacute facility. Decisions about obtaining a lumbar puncture, MRI, or CT scanning are usually determined by the details of the patient's presentation and examination. Brain imaging should be considered in the workup of older patients presenting with acute changes in cognition, but may be particularly instructive in the workup of some patients, for example with histories of cancer (i.e., metastases) or recent falls (subdural hematoma presenting as clouded sensorium).

Cognitive function

Routine screening of cognitive function by emergency physicians and psychiatrists is another important part of the geriatric assessment. In contrast to the acute change in cognition that may be seen in delirium, conditions such as Alzheimer's disease and other forms of dementia are usually marked by a progressive decline over a period of months or years. There may also be symptoms of MDD that affect cognitive domains such as attention, concentration, memory, and others. There are times when patients with depression may be hyper-attentive to any memory problems, even seemingly mild ones, whereas patients with dementia may minimize or even attempt to refute or camouflage memory deficits. One study suggests that cognitively impaired patients are at high risk for misunderstanding their treatment plan and follow-up instructions from the emergency setting.[30] This raises clear safety concerns for these patients and, at a minimum, jeopardizes their ability to obtain needed care.

The rapid pace and changing acuity of patients in the ED can create a challenging atmosphere in which to assess a patient's cognitive status. Although several research groups are trying to establish assessment tools to screen for delirium and dementia in the emergency setting, these tools have not been validated for the geriatric population. A reliable and efficient screening tool for cognitive function is the Folstein Mini-Mental State Examination[31] (also, see Table 6.5). The Montreal Cognitive Assessment tool (MoCA; see mocatest.org) is also a brief cognitive screening tool with high sensitivity and specificity for detecting mild cognitive impairment (MCI).[32] It is best suited for patients performing in the normal range on the MMSE but with symptoms suggestive of MCI. A patient's agitation and threatening or aggressive behavior may be related to their cognitive impairment, which is often driven by their impaired ability to interpret stimuli and the associated miscommunication that can result from these situations. An objective cognitive evaluation for all patients over 65 should be considered, especially in high-risk individuals, to help determine the appropriate intervention.

Capacity

Determination of cognitive capacity should be a part of the initial evaluation. The terms capacity and competency are sometimes used interchangeably, but have distinctly different meanings in the psychiatric assessment. Capacity is the ability to understand information relevant to a treatment decision and to appreciate the reasonably foreseeable consequences of an affirmative or passive decision or refusal of care.[33] Competency is a legal determination, made by a court, which addresses whether the person can be held accountable for the consequences of his or her decisions and actions. In an emergency, the treating team does not require informed consent for interventions that are meant to mitigate "life or limb" threats. However, if there is not an immediate risk, the patient must be able to communicate a reasoned choice for informed consent to be valid. Psychiatrists and neurologists are often sought as medical experts in preliminary determination of capacity, but any physician can judge the decision-making capability of a patient and an official consult often is not needed. Patients lacking the ability to make an informed decision should have detailed documentation regarding that capability as well as the reasons for any interventions performed without informed consent. In some cases where interventions or admission to a facility is deemed warranted, patients may require involuntary commitment. This may be due to lack of decision-making capacity on behalf of the patient or may be the result of formally declared lack of competency (by a judge), including guardianship of person. The details regarding involuntary commitment are beyond the scope of this chapter and there is some variability from state to state. In addition to state law, hospital and department policies regarding informed consent should be followed when managing patients who do not have capacity. Advice from the hospital legal department should be considered before implementing any non-emergency intervention.

Medications and substance abuse

Drug-drug interactions are relevant to the geriatric evaluation in the ED because medications have the capacity to mimic psychiatric symptoms including low mood, insomnia, anxiety, loss of appetite, and lethargy. Polypharmacy can be defined as using five or more chronic medications and is the most prevalent explanation for delirium seen in the ED.[2,34] Psychiatric medications are managed increasingly more often by a primary care physician (PCP) than a psychiatrist. The most common medications prescribed for the geriatric population are for the cardiovascular system or the central nervous system.[35] Overall, antidepressants have become the most prescribed class of drugs in the United States and now exceed prescriptions for antihypertensives.[34,35] Elderly patients with a history of depression are at the highest risk for potential drug interactions and require an audit of all of the drugs in their medication regimen. Direct pharmacy contact, review of medication charts from the SNF, or an examination of all pill bottles and over-the counter medicines, is the first step in investigating potential drug interactions related to the symptoms.

Vitamins and herbal remedies are popular supplements in the geriatric population and should be included in the medication evaluation, since they also have potential drug-interactions and CNS side effects. For example, St. John's wort is commonly used by many for depression, despite evidence (including a randomized controlled study) that the herb is no better than placebo.[36] Other research studies suggest that St. John's wort inhibits the proper functioning of antihypertensives, antidepressants, antiepileptic medications, chemotherapy agents, contraceptives, and antiretroviral treatments.

Substance abuse, particularly alcohol intoxication and withdrawal, are recognized as common problems treated in the ED that may alter mental status. A substance use history, including alcohol, tobacco, illicit drugs, and intentionally misused pharmaceuticals, should be included in the emergency evaluation of all older patients. Surveys estimate that 17% of adults over age 65 have an alcohol abuse problem, compared to about 10% of the population in the United States.[37] Caregivers and family members may minimize an older patient's substance abuse or be hesitant to entertain that there may be a problem. Substance abuse history is often not documented in the elderly during medical evaluations[37] so an ED evaluation that includes a substance abuse history may capture critical information for evaluation and management. Repetitive falls, unexplained bruises, memory loss, low or labile mood, chronic diarrhea, weight loss, and worsening legal trouble may be signs and symptoms of a medication and/or substance abuse problem.

Disposition

Elderly patients with a diagnosis of delirium or another condition causing an imminent danger of harming themselves or others are usually admitted to the hospital. Determining whether the elderly patient should be admitted is the central decision of the emergency providers, but deciding where the patient is to be admitted is just as important. The decision for a medical admission can sometimes be made by the physician during the initial evaluation or triage stage, based on the chief complaint or the gravity of symptoms and findings. New or first time behavioral presentations usually require a comprehensive medical evaluation which usually cannot be accomplished in the ED setting. On the other hand, with the exception of the above caveat, aggressive behavior in the SNF and suicidal and homicidal actions often lead to 24-hour observation and voluntary or involuntary psychiatric admissions. In the elderly in particular, all suicidal thoughts, intentions, and plans should be taken seriously and warrant an in-depth risk assessment.

Other factors for consideration in a decision for or against hospitalization may involve psychosocial issues. Axis IV on the DSM-IV-TR axes of psychiatric diagnoses recognizes environmental and psychosocial variables that may influence the patient's mental state. Caregiver fatigue is a recognized entity in psychiatry.[38] A compelling book on this topic is *The 36-Hour Day: A Family Guide to Caring for Persons with Alzheimer Disease, Related Dementing Illnesses, and Memory Loss in Later Life* by Mace and Rabins. The family dynamic and home environment can accelerate the need for psychiatric management that is beyond the standard PMD or outpatient psychiatrist visit.

Geriatric patients with memory impairment can be vulnerable to elder abuse. Recent falls, social isolation, and low mood can be the result of elder abuse, but mistaken for depression. A portion of the patient's history should be obtained separately from caregivers, in order to evaluate for patient intimidation and abuse. If abuse is suspected or confirmed, formal reporting standards (e.g., police, adult protective services) must be followed. Admission or extended observation may be needed until the safety of the patient can be assured and outreach and other services arranged prior to discharge.[2]

Once it is clear a patient needs admission, determining where the patient should be admitted can be a complex task. Where the patient should be admitted depends on a number of factors including the availability of beds, willingness of admitting providers to accommodate patients with multiple problems, admitting service capabilities, and existing policies. The emergency provider must often negotiate with several services before a final disposition can be made to ensure the patient's safety. In cases where the patient needs admission, a discussion in which all the potential admitting services participate can help to improve the efficiency of decision-making and reduce potential miscommunication.

Interventions and treatment

The delirious patient

As discussed above and in Chapter 6, delirium is a fairly common condition, occurring in an estimated 1–2% of the general population and 14–24% of patients in the general hospital setting.[39] Given the high morbidity and mortality associated with delirium, the initial challenge is early detection. Demented patients are particularly vulnerable to delirium. In many geriatric patients, delirium can be superimposed on dementia. An important clue can be sudden changes in cognition from baseline. Hypoactive and hyperactive delirium are both described in the literature.[39] Hypoactive delirium is more common in the elderly and is marked by slowed cognition, decreased responsiveness, and/or apathy. The hyperactive, delirious patient may have hallucinations, delusions, aggressive behavior, and restlessness. Patients in the ED may also have a "mixed" presentation with features of both delirium subtypes. Even when the history of confusion is not entirely clear, because in many cases the findings of delirium can be subtle, the workup for delirium should take precedence.

Several assessment tools exist to help distinguish delirium from depression, dementia, and psychosis. Few have been shown valid or reliable in older adults in the emergency setting. The Memorial Delirium Assessment Scale and the Confusion Assessment Methods (CAM; see Table 6.4) are two diagnostic instruments that may help to diagnose delirium in geriatric patients.[39] Once a diagnosis of delirium is suspected, the patient must undergo a careful and thorough medical evaluation. Brain imaging should be considered if a focal lesion is suspected in the brain from a stroke, mass, or infection.

Research shows the best management for delirium is to implement measures to prevent it.[39] Since prevention is not an option in an emergency presentation, acute management should begin with a comprehensive medical evaluation while treating the patient with non-pharmacological approaches (to the degree that the patient's condition allows) and behavioral interventions.[39] Although few clinical trials have examined these supportive measures in the emergency setting, non-pharmacological interventions appear to be effective in managing the behavioral aspects of delirium.[39,40] For example, the clinician should attempt to orient the patient and provide simple instructions using understandable terms and brief sentences. Sentences should be as simple as possible and phrased in the form of questions that can be answered with a simple yes or no. Eye contact with the patient is important. Patients should be provided with their glasses to help their visual perception. Hearing aids should be turned on and tested to see if they are working to minimize problems with communication. Though it may be difficult to achieve in a busy ED, attempts should be made to make the patient feel comfortable by providing an environment with minimal noise. Patient handoffs should be minimized as much as possible, maintaining the same treatment team during the duration of the evaluation.[17] Physical restraints can worsen agitation and exacerbate delirium. They should not be used, except as a last resort.

Clinicians may have to resort to the use of pharmacological approaches, if the behavioral interventions do not succeed or the patient's behavior threatens the patient's safety or the safety of others. The majority of the medications used for aggressive and agitated patients in an emergency can also worsen the patient's cognitive status and delay resolution of the delirium. Medications should be administered at the lowest dose possible, with preference for medications with short half-lives.[41] The three main classes of medications commonly used are neuroleptics (antipsychotics including "typical" (older) and newer, atypical antipsychotics), anticholinergics (used both to counter the side effects of neuroleptics and for their sedating effects), and benzodiazepines.

Randomized controlled trials in geriatric patients with delirium have shown that haloperidol reduces symptom severity and duration of delirium.[42] Side effects of neuroleptics to monitor include Parkinsonian symptoms including stiffness, bradykinesia, tremor, gait difficulties (with attendant increased risk of falls), and dystonias. Anticholinergics are often given at the same time to reduce these side effects, but must be used sparingly, given their risk of worsening delirium and falls. The new class of "atypical" antipsychotics has fewer side effects than older antipsychotics and has been shown to be equally efficacious to haloperidol for delirium.[43] Haloperidol, fluphenazine, olanzapine, aripiprazole, and ziprasidone are available in injectable forms, which make them an efficient choice for emergency situations. It should be remembered that both the atypicals and haloperidol can prolong the QT interval and should be used cautiously, if at all, with at-risk patients. Atypical antipsychotic medications have also been shown to increase the risk of stroke and all-cause mortality in patients with dementia, leading to a black box warning in 2005 for their use in elderly patients with behavioral disturbances.[29,44–46]

Benzodiazepines do not appear to improve delirium. Studies have shown a potential paradoxical or "rebound" effect of over-excitation, followed by worsening confusion, respiratory depression, and sedation in some patients.[42] Benzodiazepines are an effective treatment for substance abuse withdrawal (i.e. alcohol or benzodiazepine dependence), diffuse Lewy Body Dementia (a not uncommon form of dementia marked by psychotic and Parkinsonian symptoms and cognitive decline as well as poor tolerance of neuroleptic medications), or when the first line antipsychotics are not effective.[39] Clinicians must also be mindful of the increased fall risk that use of these sedating medications can induce.

Patients with delirium, even with an identifiable precipitating factor, generally require inpatient medical management. If the delirium can be readily corrected in the ED, the clinician must be careful not to simply return the patient to the environment where, for lack of resources or for inadequate care, the delirium was precipitated, without some thought to addressing the underlying precipitating factors.

The demented elderly patient

Unlike delirium, the demented patient is usually alert and consciousness is preserved (see Table 11.3). Dementia is the deterioration of higher cortical processes, including memory, cognitive processing, language, judgment, and the ability to learn new tasks. Dementia is more prevalent in the elderly, but can occur at any age. In the emergency setting, these patients may appear to neglect their personal hygiene, have anxiety or paranoia about the clinician or environment, lack impulse control, and become irritable and aggressive.[2,26] "Pseudo-dementia" (an imprecise term to describe the reversible dementia syndrome that may be seen in severely depressed persons) should be suspected in a patient with a history of a mood disorder, recent life stressors, and loss of short and long-term memory. Amnestic disorder is a condition limited to memory impairment with no other cognitive dysfunction and no impairment in activities of daily living. This disorder can be related to Wernike-Korsakoff encephalopathy, a recent traumatic event, an extended course of electroconvulsive therapy, or severe psychological stress.[41] Common *medical* conditions in the elderly associated with memory loss include subdural hematoma, Parkinson's disease, meningitis, normal-pressure hydrocephalus, and recovery from hypoglycemic or anoxic metabolic states.[27]

In assessing patients for dementia, the history should focus on the specific mental status change and the acute reason for emergency evaluation. It is important to know and understand the patient's baseline in the past six months to better understand the immediate mental status change. For example, determining whether the patient has a history of mental status changes following a diurnal pattern, worsening in the late afternoon into evening and night (sundowning), or previous treatment for similar symptoms, can influence the clinician's next step in management. Understanding the pattern of confusion and relating that to any associated shortness of breath, chest pain, or weakness may point to an emergency medical situation, such as a myocardial infarction, pulmonary embolism, or stroke. Similar to the delirious patient, the clinician should focus on a detailed review of medications including dosages, recent changes, and who administers the medication. Elevated temperature, blood pressure, heart rate, or respirations should be followed and investigated. If there is the possibility of an organic cause involvement, a standard ED approach to the physical and neurological exam is necessary.

Continuous observation should be provided for patients with dementia that are at risk for harming themselves or others.[41] In the ED setting this usually implies a "sitter," someone who has appropriate training and is assigned the task of continuously watching over the patient and intervening or alerting others as needed. Creating an environment that feels safe to the patient may be necessary before proceeding with additional laboratory tests or evaluations, depending on the degree of confusion and agitation the patient has. Further management is similar to the delirious patient, including identifying any

Table 11.3. Differential diagnosis of the geriatric patient in the ED setting

	Delirium	Dementia	Depression	Withdrawal/ Intoxication
Onset	Acute	Insidious or step-wise change	Cyclical	Acute
Course	Variable	Progressive	Diurnal variation	Rapid (24–72 hours)
Consciousness	Impaired	Clear until later stages	Generally unimpaired	Continuum of unimpaired to impaired
Attention	Poor	Generally good	Poor	Poor
Memory	Poor	Poor short and long-term	Intact	Intact
Mood	Variable	Neutral	Low	Elevated, neutral, or depressed
Hallucinations	Visual more than auditory; can be tactile, gustatory, or olfactory	Auditory or visual	Usually pseudo-auditory	Visual and tactile; Can be auditory
Delusions	Transient, usually persecutory	Fixed and often paranoid	Mood congruent and complex	Fleeting but often paranoid
Behavior			Psychomotor retarded	

Adapted from Levenson JL. *Textbook of Psychosomatic Medicine*. Arlington, VA: American Psychiatric Publishing, 2010.

underlying medical illness. Assessment tools like the MMSE can be employed to monitor the patient's progress.

With demented, elderly patients, using fewer pharmacological interventions is better for preservation of cognition. Behavioral interventions, although less practical in the emergency setting, should be the first line management for the demented patient. As in delirium, benzodiazepines, anticholinergic medications, and specifically diphenhydramine should be reserved only for severe agitation and true emergency situations. Haloperidol at a low dose (0.5 to 1.0 mg twice per day) is usually well tolerated by demented patients with agitation.[41,43] Atypical antipsychotics such as quetiapine, ziprasidone, and risperidone can be effective in the acute setting because of fewer extrapyramidal side effects.[46] However, atypical antipsychotic long-term use in the demented patient has been associated with higher mortality rates and carries an FDA black box warning.[43,46]

The aggressive and/or agitated elderly patient

The words aggression and agitation are used interchangeably, but often mean different things to the clinician evaluating the patient. Describing the behavior in detail is often more telling to other clinicians than just naming the behavior. For our purposes, aggression is defined as a hostile act toward self, objects, or others. These behaviors can be verbal, vocal, physical, or sexual.[43,46] In contrast, agitation is defined as observable, situation-inappropriate behavior that is characterized by excessive motor or verbal activity.[47,48] As with delirium, which may contribute to both agitation and aggression, the best initial intervention is to identify an underlying cause. Obtaining history about the quality and duration of the agitation may help to pinpoint the source.[40,47] Factors that can contribute to agitation include inability to communicate needs, unfamiliar environment, reinforced inappropriate behavior, and biological changes in the brain. A longitudinal study of patients with vascular dementia, Alzheimer's disease, and mixed dementia (both vascular and Alzheimer's) revealed that 96% of them displayed ongoing and sometimes severe aggressive behavior at some point of their dementia illness.[29,43,46]

Agitation should also be distinguished from anxiety, which is associated with a "fight or flight" response, distress, and fear. Akathisia, the personal feeling of restlessness, which may be related to use of antipsychotic medications and sometimes selective serotonin reuptake inhibitors (SSRIs), is also often misdiagnosed as agitation or anxiety.

Management of the agitated patient is discussed in detail in Chapter 2. Specifically related to the geriatric patient, agitation can point towards potential life-threatening medical illnesses, with not surprisingly higher mortality rates in delirious and demented patients.[48] These patients may not be able to communicate what they are experiencing to the clinician. Unmanaged agitation can compromise the patient's safety and medical care, as well as the safety of others. Initial focus should be on finding a safe way to evaluate the patient. Actions include: establishing firm behavioral limits, verbal redirection, ensuring provider safety (sufficient space between provider and patient, easy and rapid egress, use of security personnel), placing the patient in a quiet setting to calm down first, and ensuring ability to provide chemical or physical restraints for the severely psychotic or threatening patient.

After ensuring a safe clinical environment for both the clinician and the patient, more detailed history, physical exam, and laboratory tests can be conducted. For the geriatric, agitated patient, small doses of haloperidol 0.5–2 mg PO or IM administered with benztropine 1 mg (if anticholinergic treatment is required) may be well tolerated, as long as total dose does not exceed more than 5 mg of haloperidol in a two-hour period.[41] Higher doses of neuroleptics are associated with dystonias. Low doses of atypical antipsychotics are also helpful at reducing agitation in the geriatric patient. Lorazepam is available IM and is used in combination with haloperidol in the general population. However, geriatric patients with agitation related to delirium or dementia can become disinhibited with administration of lorazepam or other benzodiazepines, and thus, worsen their agitation. Finally, a withdrawal syndrome from benzodiazepines may be a source of acute confusion and agitation, particularly for older patients taking short-acting benzodiazepines such as alprazolam. Access to and reconciliation with home medication lists is critical and may guide treatment.

The depressed elderly patient

Treatment of MDD at times involves acute management in the ED setting combined with arrangements for long-term medication treatment, psychotherapy, and somatic and psychosocial interventions. The first intervention is identifying MDD and suicide risk factors in the elderly, which are sometimes missed in this population.[20] Factors that point to poor prognosis in the geriatric patient with depression include: history of multiple episodes and psychiatric admissions, death of a partner or relative, an ill or disabled spouse, multiple or significant medical illnesses, and psychotic or catatonic symptoms.[20] The ED physician should try to ensure a protective and supportive environment for the patient including either an observer (sitter) in the ED, or continuous close supervision by a caregiver or family member (if appropriate) of the non-suicidal patient in the home and appropriate psychiatric follow-up, and/or inpatient admission.

The mnemonic SIGECAPS is a quick screening tool for symptoms of depression. These symptoms include Sleep (disordered), Interest (lack of), Guilty feelings, Energy (low), Concentration (poor), Appetite (disordered), Passive death wish, and Suicidal thoughts, ideation, or plan.

Antidepressants are the standard of care for moderate to severe MDD. Choice of antidepressant, given the different classes, is often based upon side effect profile and the specific features that accompany the illness. A large-scale clinical trial conducted by the NIMH showed that nortriptyline, a tricyclic antidepressant, is one of the most effective maintenance treatments for recurrent depression in adults older than 60.[49] Fluoxetine, an SSRI has also been specifically approved by the FDA for the treatment of geriatric depression.[50] A series of meta-analyses and comparisons of side effect profiles tend to support fluoxetine and other SSRI classes of antidepressants over nortriptyline.[22,35] The majority of these studies looked at long-term use as an outpatient. Antidepressant medication should not be started in the ED, unless follow-up with a treating physician or other provider has been established and a treatment plan agreed upon by the patient, any relevant caregivers, and all providers involved.

In the emergency setting, depression in the elderly can be heterogeneous, and associated with dementia, delusions, and/or anxiety in over 45% of cases.[51] Randomized clinical trials show that a combination of SSRIs with a low dose effect profile and an atypical neuroleptic medication was effective in treated delusional depression in the elderly.[52]

Medical vs. psychiatric hospital admission

Determining the appropriate inpatient care setting for a geriatric patient with both psychiatric and medical issues can be a challenge. A patient's initial presentation can change over time and sometimes the accurate diagnosis is not revealed until the patient has been observed for an extended period of time. In the case of delirium, older patients admitted to psychiatric units are less likely to undergo complete medical diagnostic assessments than delirious elderly patients admitted to medical units.[30,39] Thus, it is recommended that delirious patients be admitted to a medical service with psychiatric consultation, unless the available psychiatric service or hospital has sufficient medical management resources. In a series of studies, 2.3% of the elderly, delirious patients referred to psychiatric units required medical intervention within the first 12 hours of hospitalization.[30] Symptoms of delirium appear more likely to be incorrectly attributed to psychiatric illness in patients with a history of mental illness (over 66.7% of these patients) than in patients without such a history (26.7%).

Outpatient follow-up with clearly communicated instructions

Follow-up after an emergency visit is important for the geriatric patient and the patient with a psychiatric history. Whenever possible, the clinician should contact the primary care provider and treating psychiatrist or arrange for them to receive copies of any discharging documents. Involvement of the patient's caregiver is also important to facilitate proper understanding of the patient's diagnosis and treatment rationale, in addition to solidifying the outpatient follow-up visit with their primary physician.[53] Despite being connected to multiple services across a variety of institutions and agencies, geriatric patients tend to return to the ED more frequently with the same chief complaint than the general population.[54] Clear communication with a central caregiver or central health care professional should help to decrease repeat emergency visits by establishing more aggressive and closely monitored outpatient care.

Conclusions: evaluation and management of Mr. J.

The assessment of geriatric patients with psychiatric concerns in the ED requires a multi-disciplinary approach and very close scrutiny of all the available data to make the correct diagnosis and treatment decisions. In the geriatric patient, signs of dementia and delirium can be subtle, as can the signs and symptoms of depression or anxiety. On the other hand, symptoms in the elderly may not be characteristic or classic in the textbook sense, and can mislead the treating team toward an incorrect diagnosis. Because these patients are medically fragile and psychiatrically vulnerable, an accurate diagnosis is critical and often requires serial observations, collateral information, and time-intensive ED evaluations.

Mr. J's symptoms in the clinical scenario represent typical symptoms of a geriatric patient who warrants a psychiatric evaluation. His gender, age, and marital status place him at a statistically high suicide risk. His underlying cardiovascular condition may be contributing to his current symptoms of agitation and aggression. He should have an ECG to rule out a new myocardial infarction or other cardiac etiology, as well as other workup to rule out a pulmonary process or a new stroke. His cardiac status makes him more prone to clinical depression. He has a brain that is vulnerable to delirium because of his past stroke and he is more susceptible to mood and behavioral changes related to a urinary tract infection, pneumonia, and polypharmacy. His chronic pain may be treated with an opiate, so he may be experiencing withdrawal or even overdose. His headache could be an indication of a subdural hematoma, as he has been engaging in more physical activity and may be subject to falls because of his motor dysfunction. His social withdrawal may be related to a major depressive episode, with characteristic changes in sleep, interests, low energy, appetite, and mood. His aggression may be related to an underlying delirium, his inability to accurately interpret stimuli, his frustration with his current physical rehabilitation, and/or miscommunication with the staff member. The emergency setting is the most appropriate place for a detailed assessment and to provide the patient with the necessary mental support and medical evaluation and treatment.

References

1. Centers for Disease Control and Prevention, Mental health and aging. Available at: http://www.cdc.gov/aging/pdf/mental_health.pdf. Accessed August 28, 2011.

2. Thienhaus OJ, Piasecki MP. Assessment of geriatric patients in the psychiatric emergency service. *Psychiatr Serv.* 2004; 55(6):639–642.

3. Hybels CF, Blazer DG. Epidemiology of late-life mental disorders. *Clin Geriatr Med.* 2003;19(4):663–696.

4. Newman SC, Bland RC, Orn HT. The prevalence of mental disorders in the elderly in Edmonton: a community survey using GMS-AGECAT. Geriatric Mental State-Automated Geriatric Examination for Computer Assisted Taxonomy. *Can J Psychiatry.* 1998;43(9):910–914.

5. He W, Sengupta M, Velkoff VA, DeBarros KA. *U.S. Census Bureau, Current Population Reports, P23–209, 65+ in the United States: 2005.* Washington, DC: US Government Printing Office, 2005.

6. Lebowitz BD, Pearson JL, Schneider LS, et al. Diagnosis and treatment of depression in late life. Consensus statement update. *JAMA* 1997;**278**(14):1186–1190.

7. Butters MA, Bhalla RK, Mulsant BH, et al. Executive functioning, illness course, and relapse/recurrence in continuation and maintenance treatment of late-life depression: is there a relationship? *Am J Geriatr Psychiatry.* 2004;**12**(4): 387–394.

8. Ferrando S, ed. Geriatric Psychiatry, *Psychiatry in Review*, ETAS, 2008.

9. Colenda CC, Greenwald BS, Crossett JH, Husain MM, Kennedy GJ. Barriers to effective psychiatric emergency services for elderly persons. *Psychiatr Serv.* 1997; **48**(3):321–325.

10. Folstein MF, Maiberger R, McHugh PR. Mood disorder as a specific complication of stroke. *J Neurol Neurosurg Psychiatry.* 1977;**40**(10):1018–1020.

11. Robinson RG, Price TR. Post-stroke depressive disorders: a follow-up study of 103 patients. *Stroke.* 1982;**13**(5): 635–641.

12. Robinson RG, Starr LB, Kubos KL, Price TR. A two-year longitudinal study of post-stroke mood disorders: findings during the initial evaluation. *Stroke.* 1983;**14**(5): 736–741.

13. Robinson RG, Szetela B. Mood change following left hemispheric brain injury. *Ann Neurol.* 1981;**9**(5):447–453.

14. Frasure-Smith N, Lesperance F, Talajic M. Depression and 18-month prognosis after myocardial infarction. *Circulation.* 1995; **91**(4):999–1005.

15. Parakh K, Thombs BD, Fauerbach JA, Bush DE, Ziegelstein RC. Effect of depression on late (8 years) mortality after myocardial infarction. *Am J Cardiol.* 2008;**101**(5): 602–606.

16. Thombs BD, Bass EB, Ford DE, et al. Prevalence of depression in survivors of acute myocardial infarction. *J Gen Intern Med.* 2006;**21**(1):30–38.

17. Ziegelstein RC. Depression after myocardial infarction. *Cardiol Rev.* 2001;**9**(1):45–51.

18. Clerici M, Arosio B, Mundo E, et al. Cytokine polymorphisms in the pathophysiology of mood disorders. *CNS Spectr.* 2009;**14**(8): 419–425.

19. Godbout JP, Johnson RW. Age and neuroinflammation: a lifetime of psychoneuroimmune consequences. *Immunol Allergy Clin North Am.* 2009;**29**(2):321–337.

20. Fiske A, Wetherell JL, Gatz M. Depression in older adults. *Annu Rev Clin Psychol.* 2009;**5**:363–389.

21. Families USA. http://www.familiesusa.org/. Accessed August 28, 2011.

22. Bruce, ML, Ten Have TR, Reynolds CF 3rd, Katz, II, Schulberg HC, Mulsant BH, et al. Reducing suicidal ideation and depressive symptoms in depressed older primary care patients: a randomized controlled trial. *JAMA* 2004;**291**(9):1081–1091.

23. Conwell Y. Suicide in later life: a review and recommendations for prevention. *Suicide and Life Threatening Behavior.* 2001;**31**(Suppl):32–47.

24. Wiktorsson S, Runeson B, Skoog I, Ostling S, Waern M. Attempted suicide in the elderly: characteristics of suicide attempters 70 years and older and a general population comparison group. *Am J Geriatr Psychiatry.* 2010;**18**(1):57–67.

25. Centers for Disease Control and Prevention, National Center for Injury Prevention and Control. Web-based Injury Statistics Query and Reporting System (WISQARS): www.cdc.gov/ncipc/wisqars. Accessed August 28, 2011.

26. Puryear DA, Lovitt R, Miller DA. Characteristics of elderly persons seen in an urban psychiatric emergency room. *Hosp Community Psychiatry.* 1991;**42**(8): 802–807.

27. Shulman RW, Marton P, Fisher A, Cohen C. Characteristics of psychogeriatric

patient visits to a general hospital emergency room. *Can J Psychiatry.* 1996; **41**(3):175–180.

28. Kefer A. *Elderly Living With Family.* http://www.livestrong.com/article/95828-elderly-family/#ixzz1TGypamt0. Accessed February 9, 2013.

29. Alexopoulos GS, Jeste DV, Chung H, Carpenter D, Ross R, Docherty JP. The expert consensus guideline series. Treatment of dementia and its behavioral disturbances. Introduction: methods, commentary, and summary. *Postgrad Med.* 2005;*Spec No:*6–22.

30. Han, JH, Shintani A, Eden S, Morandi A, Solberg LM, Schnelle J, et al. Delirium in the emergency department: an independent predictor of death within 6 months. *Ann Emerg Med.* 2010;**56**(3):244–252.e1.

31. Folstein MF, Folstein SE, McHugh PR.. "Mini-mental state". A practical method for grading the cognitive state of patients for the clinician. *J Psychiatr Res.* 1975; **12**(3):189–198.

32. Nasreddine ZS, Phillips NA, Bedirian V, et al. The Montreal Cognitive Assessment, MoCA: a brief screening tool for mild cognitive impairment. *J Am Geriatr Soc.* 2005;**53**(4):695–699.

33. Abernethy V. Compassion, control, and decisions about competency. *Am J Psychiatry.* 1984;**141**(1):53–58.

34. Preskorn SH, Flockhart D. 2010 guide to psychiatric drug interactions. *Primary Psychiatry.* 2009;**16**(12):45–74.

35. Olfson M, Marcus SC. National patterns in antidepressant medication treatment. *Arch Gen Psychiatry.* 2009;**66**(8): 848–856.

36. Linde K, Berner M, Egger M, Mulrow C. St John's wort for depression: meta-analysis of randomised controlled trials. *Br J Psychiatry.* 2005;**186**:99–107.

37. Woo BK, Chen W. Substance misuse among older patients in psychiatric emergency service. *Gen Hosp Psychiatry.* 2010;**32**(1):99–101.

38. Rabins PV, Fitting MD, Eastham J, Fetting J. The emotional impact of caring for the chronically ill. *Psychosomatics.* 1990;**31**(3):331–336.

39. Fong TG, Tulebaev SR, Inouye SK. Delirium in elderly adults: diagnosis, prevention and treatment. *Nat Rev Neurol.* 2009;**5**(4):210–220.

40. Cohen-Mansfield J. Nonpharmacologic interventions for psychotic symptoms in dementia. *J Geriatr Psychiatry Neurol.* 2003;**16**(4):219–224.

41. Bernstein CA, Ishak WW, Weiner ED, Ladds BJ. *On Call Psychiatry.* 2nd ed. Philadelphia, PA: W.B. Saunders, 2001.

42. Breitbart WR, Marotta R, Platt MM, Weisman H, Derevenco M., Grau C, et al. A double-blind trial of haloperidol, chlorpromazine, and lorazepam in the treatment of delirium in hospitalized AIDS patients. *Am J Psychiatry.* 1996; **153**(2):231–237.

43. Jeste DV, Blazer D, Casey D, Meeks T, Salzman C, Schneider L, et al. ACNP White Paper: update on use of antipsychotic drugs in elderly persons with dementia. *Neuropsychopharmacology.* 2008;**33**(5): 957–970.

44. Ballard C, Waite J. The effectiveness of atypical antipsychotics for the treatment of aggression and psychosis in alzheimer's disease. *Cochrane Database Syst Rev.* 2006;(**1**):CD003476.

45. FDA Public Health Advisory. *Deaths with Antipsychotics in Elderly Patients With Behavioral Disturbances.* April 11, 2005. http://www.fda.gov/Drugs/DrugSafety/PostmarketDrugSafetyInformationfor PatientsandProviders/DrugSafety InformationforHeathcareProfessionals/PublicHealthAdvisories/UCM053171. Accessed August 28, 2011.

46. Salzman C, Jeste DV, Meyer RE, et al. Elderly patients with dementia-related symptoms of severe agitation and aggression: consensus statement on treatment options, clinical trials methodology, and policy. *J Clin Psychiatry.* 2008;**69**(6):889–898.

47. Cheong JA. An evidence-based approach to the management of agitation in the geriatric patient. *Focus.* 2004;**2**:197–205.

48. Zal MH. Agitation in the elderly. *Psychiatric Times*. 2006. http://www.psychiatrictimes.com/dementia/content/article/10168/51791. Accessed August 29, 2011.

49. Reynolds, CF 3rd, Frank E, Perel JM, et al. Nortriptyline and interpersonal psychotherapy as maintenance therapies for recurrent major depression: a randomized controlled trial in patients older than 59 years. *JAMA* 1999;**281**(1):39–45.

50. Tollefson GD, Bosomworth JC, Heiligenstein JH, Potcin JH, Holman S. A double-blind, placebo-controlled clinical trial of fluoxetine in geriatric patients with major depression. The Fluoxetine Collaborative Study Group. *Int Psychogeriatr*. 1995;7(1):89–104.

51. Meyers BS, Klimstra SA, Gabriele M, et al. Continuation treatment of delusional depression in older adults. *Am J Geriatr Psychiatry*. 2001;**9**(4):415–422.

52. Meyers BS, Flint AJ, Rothschild AJ, et al. A double-blind randomized controlled trial of olanzapine plus sertraline vs olanzapine plus placebo for psychotic depression: the study of pharmacotherapy of psychotic depression (STOP-PD). *Arch Gen Psychiatry*. 2009;**66**(8): 838–847.

53. Mace NL, Rabins PV. *The 36-Hour Day: A Family Guide to Caring for Persons With Alzheimer Disease, Related Dementing Illnesses, and Memory Loss in Later Life*. Baltimore, MD: Johns Hopkins Press, 2011.

54. Bassuk EL, Minden S, Apsler R. Geriatric emergencies: psychiatric or medical? *Am J Psychiatry*. 1983;**140**(5): 539–542.

Appendix

Geriatric Depression Scale

1. Are you basically satisfied with your life?

2. Have you dropped many of your activities and interests?

3. Do you feel that your life is empty?

4. Do you often get bored?

5. Are you hopeful about the future?

6. Are you bothered by thoughts you can't get out of your head?

7. Are you in good spirits most of the time?

8. Are you afraid that something bad is going to happen to you?

9. Do you feel happy most of the time?

10. Do you often feel helpless?

11. Do you often get restless and fidgety?

12. Do you prefer to stay at home, rather than going out and doing new things?

13. Do you frequently worry about the future?

14. Do you feel you have more problems with memory than most?

15. Do you think it is wonderful to be alive now?

16. Do you often feel downhearted and blue?

17. Do you feel pretty worthless the way you are now?

18. Do you worry a lot about the past?

19. Do you find life very exciting?

20. Is it hard for you to get started on new projects?

21. Do you feel full of energy?

22. Do you feel that your situation is hopeless?

23. Do you think that most people are better off than you are?

24. Do you frequently get upset over little things?

25. Do you frequently feel like crying?

26. Do you have trouble concentrating?

27. Do you enjoy getting up in the morning?

28. Do you prefer to avoid social gatherings?

29. Is it easy for you to make decisions?

30. Is your mind as clear as it used to be?

This is the original scoring for the scale: One point for each of these answers. Cutoff: normal 0–9; mild depressives 10–19; severe depressives 20–30.

1. no 6. yes 11. yes 16. yes 21. no 26. yes

2. yes 7. no 12. yes 17. yes 22. yes 27. no

3. yes 8. yes 13. yes 18. yes 23. yes 28. yes

4. yes 9. no 14. yes 19. no 24. yes 29. no

5. no 10. yes 15. no 20. yes 25. yes 30. no

http://www.stanford.edu/~yesavage/GDS.english.long.html

Issues in pediatric psychiatric emergency care

Emily Frosch and Patrick Kelly

Introduction

Approximately 10% of the population under age 18 have a psychiatric illness that warrants treatment, yet only half of those with an identified serious mental disorder actually obtain an appointment with a child mental health specialist, and even fewer receive specialty treatment.[1] By comparison, the marked growth nationally in the number of emergency department (ED) visits for psychiatric problems in those under 18 years of age suggests that this has become an alternate source of mental health care for youths.[2-6] Given the persistent increase in these volumes, it is imperative that ED care settings develop strategies to address the concerns of these youths and families in an efficient and effective manner. This chapter describes strategies for evaluating youths with emotional and behavioral conditions seeking acute care in EDs.

Assessing a child with mental health issues requires several steps. In the discussion that follows, each of the steps are explored in greater detail. These steps can be completed sequentially or concurrently, depending on the situation, but whichever method is used, a careful consideration of each step is warranted.

Understanding the guardian's motivation for seeking care

It has long been recognized that adults bring youths to the ED not only for severe psychiatric illness but also for poor social adjustment, psychosocial problems, and disconnects in the systems of care that surround the youth and family.[3,7-9] It is rare that a youngster decides to seek emergency mental health services on his/her own. More typically, an adult in his/her life – a parent, teacher, or relative – makes the decision to seek acute care. The reasons adults make that decision can be sorted into three primary domains: *Anxiety*, *Anger*, and *Adequacy*. These can be present independently, or in any combination.

Adults may become *anxious* about how a youngster is acting or feeling. Perhaps the child seems different from other youths or from his/her "regular self" or perhaps he/she has said something about their distress or done something that causes the adult to take notice, such as writing sad or upsetting stories, or refusing to leave their room or go to school; perhaps others have alerted the adult about concerning behavior. An example might be teachers noting increasing isolation at school. Something raises the adult's level of worry across a threshold that leads them to believe that an urgent assessment is needed, and so

Emergency Psychiatry, ed. Arjun Chanmugam, Patrick Triplett, and Gabor Kelen. Published by Cambridge University Press. © Cambridge University Press 2013.

care is sought in an ED setting. One of the initial steps is to assess if the adult's level of worry is appropriate and warranted.

An adult may become *angry* – either directly at the child or at his/her actions. Perhaps the child is destructive of property, disobedient of rules, or directly sassy and back-talking in a way that infuriates adults. Coming to an ED setting may represent the hope that others will intervene as the adult feels too angry to deal with the situation aptly. In some cases, the ED visit may be part of the consequence or punishment for the action or attitude. In this situation, one of the first steps is to determine who needs the intervention, (the adult(s), the child, or both) and what approaches may be available to manage the situation.

At other times, there can be a mismatch between the ability of the parent to *adequately* supervise and provide for a youngster's needs. Perhaps the child is extremely challenging to manage, e.g., constantly running into the street, wandering off with strangers, etc., and "industrial-strength" parenting skills are needed but not yet developed. Or, perhaps the caretaker has his or her own limitations and challenges – psychiatric, medical, cognitive, substance-related, financial, overwhelming family caregiver responsibilities, etc. – and simply cannot attend to what may be reasonably normal developmental needs of the youngster. In this case, providers must determine on which side of the equation this problem lies and identify appropriate resources and interventions.

Optimizing the evaluation in an ED setting

Providing care to children, adolescents, and families experiencing acute disturbances in their emotions and behaviors is a challenge for a care setting typically designed for acute medical concerns. Safety of the patient must be a primary concern. The rooms in many ED settings are not designed for mental health visits, and thus some thought as to the details of the rooms and other resources is helpful in being optimally prepared to care for these patients.

Physical setting

Patient rooms for psychiatric crisis are ideally as free of medical equipment as possible. Young children may be very active in the room, opening drawers, emptying contents of cupboards, and tossing things around that could cause harm to themselves or to others. Sharps, liquids, and other materials should be removed from the room. Security is an important consideration for multiple reasons – to ensure that patients do not elope from the ED setting, to observe and intervene regarding any conflict within the family in the room, and even to ensure that the youngster does not do anything to harm his/herself or staff. Generally, it is best to have two portals of entry to areas where psychiatric patients are evaluated so that staff have an escape egress and cannot be trapped by a suddenly violent patient. Security should have additional training if their primary role will be working with youths and families. Working with these youths and families requires some different tactics and approaches including training in behavioral de-escalation. In addition, there should be adequate space for families to be seen – enough chairs and space in the room so that everyone can sit with staff to discuss the problems and the plans.

Consultation resources

Social work support for ED providers in such cases is vital and having an identified subgroup of staff who develop skills and feel comfortable working with this population is optimal. Once a subgroup of staff is identified to take the lead in working with this population, it is important to create a resource book of some sort that all of the ED staff can access. Lists of frequently used outpatient care programs and providers, inpatient hospitals, crisis response teams, and other such services in the local and regional community with important contact numbers, program leaders, and requirements/limits for enrollment can be a valuable resource.

Contextualizing the situation

Each of the above mentioned reasons for using an ED setting, whether alone or in combination, emerges from the concept that children come attached to adults and are thus embedded within systems. A child cannot be fully assessed alone, especially when in psychiatric crisis. The primary goal of an ED evaluation is to determine the optimal route to ensure safety. When working with youngsters, that process must include not only an assessment of an individual child's safety, but also an assessment of their safety in the **context** of their world with adults – their family, their school, and their community.

While most crises in youngsters' lives are handled by their caretakers, their school, and their community, an ED-level assessment may lead to interventions that allow other external providers to help find new ways to identify, contain, or resolve a problem. Parents may be more open to suggestions and resources during an acute crisis. They may be more willing to communicate, listen, and resolve conflicts with professional support and guidance. With this opportunity comes the responsibility to share knowledge of child development and childhood psychopathology as part of the evaluation. The goal is to utilize skills in interviewing and managing strong emotions while at the same time monitoring one's own attitudes towards the young patient and the concerned adult(s) seeking help, all the while sustaining a sense of hopefulness in order to create the optimal environment for a positive outcome.

Schools and communities

In addition to assessing the family functioning, it is critical to assess the other key components of a youngster's daily living: school and community. Where and with whom the family/patient is living, the characteristics of their neighborhood, and their involvement with city agencies (department of social services, child protective services, etc.) can all point to antecedents to the current crisis, and also identify potential assets or problems that will affect their disposition.

Similarly, school is a large part of most children's lives, so a detailed educational history can help explain a given presentation. Information on (1) current grade, (2) academic performance, (3) attendance, (4) relationship with teachers/administrators, (5) disciplinary problems, (6) relationship with peers (taking note of bullying and other social relationships), (7) honors/awards, and (8) testing or special services should all be reviewed systematically. At times, such information can explain a number of problems such as school refusal, aggression, or academic failure.

Connection to mental health care

Youths presenting to an ED are likely to already be known to the mental health care system – either through outpatient treatment connections or prior hospitalizations.[10]

Youths presenting with behavior problems (aggression, runaway, threatening, disruptive, etc.) are more likely than those presenting with suicide-related events (ideation or attempts) to report existing connections to community mental health services,[11] and those who repeatedly use the ED are also more likely to be connected with a community mental health provider at the time of the ED visit.[12] Psychiatric ED assessment of youngsters and their caregivers needs to consider not only the specific clinical issues in a developmental and social context, but also the larger backdrop of known patterns of care and resource use. Contacting the identified provider, to both understand the events leading to the ED visit but also to plan for post-ED care, can be very helpful.

Age-specific presentations and considerations

Any assessment should include a review of developmental and medical issues, school and social functioning, the presenting concern and past interventions; the ED assessment, by necessity, must have a focused and targeted approach due to time constraints. This section focuses on age-specific presentations and clinical care considerations, to offer ED providers guidance as they consider age-specific concerns that might present for care.

Preschoolers

The use of the ED for emotional and behavioral concerns in preschoolers is fairly rare – they represent only 10% of all youths seen in emergency care settings for emotional/behavioral problems.[6] The types of problems this age group can have fall into four main categories: (1) developmental disabilities, (2) attentional/activity level concerns, (3) anxiety/trauma related issues, and (4) parental challenges. When such youngsters do present, the evaluation of the familial interaction is critical. Connecting families to developmentally appropriate resources that address not only the youngster but also the parents and the family relationships will likely be the focus of these assessments.

Although autism spectrum disorders (ASDs) are estimated to be increasingly more common (as many as 1 in 150 children are currently thought to meet criteria), an ASD by itself does not usually cause the type of disturbance that would lead a parent to seek an emergency evaluation in this age group. Parents can, however, grow frustrated with the challenges of parenting these children. Assessing the youngster's developmental capacity and the parents' understanding of that capacity can be helpful in determining the type of intervention that might best benefit the family.

Attention deficit hyperactivity disorder (ADHD) is being identified earlier in children, in part because of the increasing enrollment of preschoolers in a variety of structured care settings. Some of these youngsters can be extremely difficult to parent and supervise. Their activity level and impulsive behaviors (darting into the street, running away from the parent in public places, hitting parents or other children, etc.) can lead to parents seeking an evaluation. In this situation, again, the alignment of parental capacity, inclination, and attitude towards the child and towards the behaviors need to be included in the assessment.

Anxiety and other responses to traumatic events can bring young children to an ED for evaluation – sometimes without any pathological symptoms on the part of the child. A three year old witnessing the death of a parent, who then goes on to develop nightmares, could easily prompt an "emergency" evaluation. Some children experience single traumatic events, such as a car wreck. For others, it is part of their daily lives as in the case of domestic violence. In addition, parental trauma can directly impact the child, particularly younger children, as mediated through their availability and ability to parent.[13]

Children experience the same symptom clusters after traumatic events as adults: reexperiencing, avoidance/numbing, and arousal.[14] Youngsters may not have the cognitive maturity to express their concerns in words, so play may become the mode of communication. Aggressive play or play that reenacts an event can be seen in some children, while others may become more distant and disconnected to their surroundings. Longer-term consequences of trauma may include difficulties with cognitive functioning, self-esteem, and impulse control.[15] In turn, these can lead to impulsive or disruptive behaviors which may put the child at direct risk for harm. It is important to assess the overall context not only of the child's immediate presenting behaviors and emotions but also of his/her larger world and how the adults might be managing the crisis. It is equally important to consider the emotional safety of the youngster in such situations. In general, proper treatment of trauma in an emergency care setting should focus on keeping the child safe and calm while developing a disposition that includes connecting the family with appropriate mental health services.

Elementary school age

School age children are more likely than preschoolers to present for an emergency evaluation. In these instances, other adults (teachers, coaches, etc.) may recommend emergency assessments to assist with a difficult or concerning child. The types of problems that this age group can have are similar to those seen in preschoolers but additional considerations include the onset of mood disorders as well as increased disruptive behavior.

The prevalence of ADHD in 5–11 year olds is 5%.[16] These youths can be referred for evaluation as they are often off-task, underachieving, and disruptive in a classroom setting, but typically ADHD, in and of itself, does not lead an adult to seek emergency care for a child. Learning disorders, also present in about 5% of children, can begin to be seen at this time, as school becomes more demanding. This setting can then lead to increased frustration and ultimately disruptive behavior as the child tries to conceal their insecurities, lack of understanding, or mistakes. For many children, it can seem better to be viewed as "naughty" than as "dumb," though of course neither is accurate. This could lead a youngster to be brought for an emergency evaluation as the disruptive classroom behavior may be unmanageable for teachers.

Anxiety becomes more prevalent in this age group – the median age of onset of separation anxiety (leading to problems such as school refusal, avoidance, tantrums, etc.) is seven years old, with a prevalence of about 4%.[17] This can seem like a "new" problem in a previously well-adjusted toddler/preschooler at home and could cause concern for parents if going to, and staying in, school is not easy.

Although only about 1% of children in this young age group have depression, it should not be discounted as a possibility. A young child who is constantly tearful and says that he/she wants to die can certainly lead a caregiver to bring him/her to the emergency department.

Perhaps the biggest challenge in an ED care setting is the school age youngster who is brought in for "aggression" or "disruptive behavior." The youth may not have any clear problem with worries, attention, or mood but is openly defiant, disruptive, and difficult to manage. For many of these children brought to the ED, they have calmed down and seem adequately behaved by the time the evaluation occurs, making the diagnostic assessment more challenging. Parent-child interactions driven by power struggles, modeling of aggressive behavior in the home, and reinforcement of maladaptive behavior by inconsistent limits, can all lead to significant defiance and disruption. Evaluation must include an assessment of the interaction, the parental view of the behavior, and the parental interventions that have been attempted to interrupt it. Also, a careful review of mood, anxiety, attentional, and learning issues that might be causing undue frustration in a youngster with limited coping is essential. Further discussion of acute management of aggression is in the special topics section later in this chapter.

Evaluation of school age children should include time with the family and also with the youngster alone. It is important to observe how the family negotiates the situation together as the best indicator for how they are likely to handle it at home. It is, however, equally important to allow the youngster some time and space to discuss his/her feelings and actions without the parent in the room. Concerns about worries, safety, or consequences of behavior may all emerge when talking alone, and that information will directly impact decision-making about disposition. Bringing the adults back into the discussion as one develops the aftercare plan is then a critical step and must be done in a way that ensures the youngster's safety.

Adolescence

During adolescence, the risk increases for substance use, mood disorders including depression and bipolar disorder, and in very rare cases, psychotic illnesses. Although problems such as ADHD and learning disorders would have been present in this population since earlier in their lives, the added academic and social stress of middle and high school can lead them to develop maladaptive behaviors.

The diagnosis of bipolar affective disorder in youth is still controversial; accordingly, estimates of prevalence are at best fairly rough. About 20% of adults with bipolar disorder had their first manic or mixed episode in adolescence, and about 10–15% of children diagnosed with "depression" went on to develop bipolar disorder as adults.[18] This puts the estimate of prevalence at about 0.4% or lower, but the intensity of the psychopathology associated with bipolar affective disorder likely makes this a highly overrepresented population in most EDs. Assessment must include a review not only of the youngster's phenomenology but also of the parental capacity for supervision.

Substance use is more prevalent in adolescents than in younger children – although the average age of drug use in the US continues to lower. The issues that adolescents face with substance use, intoxication, dependence, and withdrawal are similar to adults and will not be covered here specifically. However, it is important to consider the vulnerability of those substance-using youths who are developmentally immature or cognitively limited as they are at greater risk for being exploited. Questions in the assessment should consider such risks for any young person using substances.

Aggression as the primary problem, either leading to the use of the ED setting or in the ED itself, is a serious concern. Aggression may be the result of another illness that requires direct intervention aimed at the underlying disorder, including potential medication use and hospitalization. At other times, however, the aggression has less obvious causes and needs to be handled directly and quickly. Aggressive behaviors can exist in the context of a disorder of thinking, anxiety, or mood; however, they can also exist independently. Careful review of the symptoms should include assessing the degree of aggression, prior outbursts and their consequences, current mental state and intentions, and options for resolution and redirection both alone and in conjunction with the family. Inpatient hospitalization may be required for some aggression, even if it is not clearly in the context of other psychiatric dysfunction if the acute behavior and conflict cannot be safely resolved in the ED setting. Specific approaches to aggression are addressed in the special topics section.

Family assessment

Since youngsters do not typically present alone to the ED, assessment of the family and family interactions is a critical component of the evaluation. There are several domains of questioning that are important, including (1) family psychiatric history to understand the risks and biological vulnerabilities that the youngster might have, (2) family interactional style to understand the modes of communication and problem solving, and (3) family attitudes and beliefs regarding the nature of the problem and potential solutions.

Family psychiatric history

Reviewing the family psychiatric history, with particular attention to the parents and siblings, can lend clues not only to biological vulnerabilities for certain psychiatric disorders, but also to the stability and predictability of the home environment. Active mental illness in a caregiver can precipitate any number of crises and can sabotage the most carefully planned disposition. The same can be said of other parental issues such as substance abuse, domestic violence, or agitation/aggression. Any condition which may impair a caregiver's emotional stability or judgment (mental illness, intellectual dysfunction, substance abuse, medical conditions, etc.) can impair parental functioning.

Family interactional style

It is also important to evaluate the internal relationships in a family. The connection between the child and parents/caregivers, and the relationships between the caregivers themselves, the child to his or her siblings, and the siblings to the parents, can all be potential sources of strength, or problems, in determining a safe discharge. Strength in verbal communication and problem solving abilities can also be good prognostic factors for a safe discharge from the emergency setting. External support for the family members, such as friends, religious communities, social agency involvement, or non-nuclear family members, can be important in managing a crisis. Prior successful engagement with resources or adherence to treatment can suggest an increased likelihood of re-engaging with outpatient resources.

Family attitudes and beliefs

The family's belief as to the nature of the problem and the appropriate solution is critical to understand. Do they see it as: a focal, time-limited concern; a longstanding problem that will require broad-based interventions; a medical problem that has a medication-only fix; a problem not within the child but related to external forces such as the school, the neighbors, childhood friends, etc? The assumptions and beliefs of the parents/caregivers are the main determining factors as to whether they are likely to adhere to the ED aftercare plan.[19] The family of an actively suicidal teenager who thinks the child is "showing off" to get attention may not fully appreciate the risk and thus may not be able to provide the needed supervision for a safe discharge home. Paying careful attention to the strengths and weaknesses of a family, and using this information to develop a well thought out plan, will increase the chance for a successful outcome.

Specific situations

This section focuses on those domains that require specific and/or additional considerations in children and adolescents, including aggression, suicide, psychosis, and trauma.

Aggression

School aged youths and adolescents can present to an ED after aggressive or disruptive events. They may arrive with family or with police. They may be in handcuffs or with security guards. While many of these quickly calm down on arrival in the ED, some do not and may require acute management. Apart from specifically addressing treatable underlying conditions, measures to ensure the physical safety of not only the patient but also the staff include setting limits, de-escalation techniques, and physical and/or chemical restraints. Where appropriate, medication to treat an underlying problem (e.g., psychosis or mania) or to augment an existing medication regimen (e.g., an antipsychotic regimen with recent missed doses) will often prove useful and may obviate or shorten the need for other measures.

For those situations where the disruptive behavior is less severe, de-escalation techniques should be considered. These include speaking to the patient directly using clear, simple language in a soft voice, reducing the stimulation by lowering the lights, having fewer people in the room, allowing space for the patient if he/she needs to pace, removing anything that could be thrown, maintaining a safe distance in a non-threatening body stance, and ensuring that adjunct support staff are aware of the situation and available.

The use of emergency medications for acute management of aggression or otherwise disruptive behaviors is considered chemical restraint. The American Academy of Child and Adolescent Psychiatry Practice Parameter defines chemical restraint as "involuntary [by the patient] use of psychoactive medication in a crisis situation to help a patient contain out of control aggressive behavior."[20] Use of physical and chemical restraints require documentation of the order and the reason for its use, and requirement of monitoring protocols depending on the means used.

Limited data are available regarding how often medication interventions are used, either in addition to or in place of behavioral strategies. One study reported that nearly 7% of all ED child psychiatric evaluations required use of restraint – however, it included both physical and chemical restraints.[21] A review of pediatric ED training programs revealed that for agitated youths, benzodiazepines (71%), haloperidol (46%), and antihistamines (25%), were the mostly commonly used agents.[22] Unfortunately there was a lack of clarity regarding indications, responses, and longer-term outcomes.

There are currently no research studies comparing acute medication use in youngsters in ED settings. Limited empirical data in the adult literature and anecdotal reporting in the pediatric literature suggests that the following concepts may be helpful:[23]

1. Medication familiar to the patient/already prescribed should be used whenever possible.
2. Knowledge of previous effects of medications should be used as a guide.
3. Anticipate and prepare for any potential adverse effects of medication.

In particular, benzodiazepines have been reported to disinhibit young children, making them more agitated rather than less agitated.

4. Oral medication is preferable whenever safe and possible.
5. The following can be considered:
   a. PO or IM diphenhydramine: 1mg/kg/dose
   b. PO risperidone: 0.25mg–2mg
   c. PO or IM lorazepam: 0.05mg/kg/dose *(with caveat as noted above)*
   d. PO or IM haloperidol: 0.025–0.075mg/kg/dose.

Unfortunately, there is no clear algorithm for such emergency medication use in youths in crisis. It is best for each care setting to obtain expert consultation and develop guidelines or protocols for a standardized approach to such situations.

Suicide-related

Suicide remains the third leading cause of death for children aged 10–19 in the United States.[24] While negligible in the very young, completed suicide accounts for 7% of deaths in children aged 10–14 and 12% of deaths in children aged 15–19, with one completed suicide per 13,000 teenagers. For every completed suicide, however, there are many more attempts. Three percent of the adolescent population will make a suicide attempt requiring medical attention every year. An additional 30% of the adolescent population will have suicidal ideation at some point in any given year. Thus, although completion is a rare event, the precursors to suicide are much less rare and ED care settings need to be prepared to provide immediate and effective assessment and intervention to these youths and their families.[25]

While adolescent girls are more likely than boys to attempt suicide (21–31% versus 13–20%),[26] adolescent boys are more likely to succeed.[27] Most studies relate the differences in completion rates to the method chosen – girls tend to choose less lethal means, such as overdose or cutting, whereas boys tend to choose firearms and hanging.[28]

There are certain risk factors which may make a child more likely to attempt or complete suicide. Most youths who complete suicide have an underlying mental disorder and half have had recent contact with a mental health clinician.[28] Suicidal ideation can occur in the context of major mental illness, and therefore any assessment needs to thoroughly and thoughtfully consider signs and symptoms suggestive of an underlying disease state that requires specific treatment. While serious affective illnesses are addressed elsewhere in this text, it is also important in younger patients to consider the role of anxiety and humiliation, including the effects of bullying. A number of other factors should also be considered in the child with suicide attempt or ideation. Substance abuse and alcohol use, particularly preteen alcohol initiation, are important risk factors for both suicide ideation and suicide attempt.[29] Substance abuse can negatively affect mood and also disinhibit the youngster so that he or she is more likely to act on suicidal thoughts. In one study examining health risk behaviors of 12 to 13 year olds (n=2090), the authors concluded that all health risk behaviors were associated with suicidal ideation and attempts. In this study, health risk behaviors included disruptive (shoplifting, physical fighting, damaging property, fighting with a weapon, carrying a knife, and gambling), sexual (petting below the waist and sexual intercourse), and substance use behaviors (smoking cigarettes, consuming alcohol, marijuana or hash, and glue or solvents).[30]

Suicidal ideation, and even suicide attempts, can also occur in the context of maladaptive behavior patterns particularly in significant relationships in the youngster's life. Careful review of these issues is critical to assessing the child's intent, plan, and access to means. All of these issues are relevant in considering successful discharge planning and aftercare options.

Of those youths presenting to ED care settings with emotional or behavioral concerns, approximately 10% present after a suicide attempt. These, however, represent a high risk group as they are not only more likely to have made a prior suicide attempt, but also are less likely to be connected to outpatient treatment.[11] Aftercare planning with this high risk group is thus a critical component of an ED assessment.

Being aware of the developmental stage of the child is particularly important in the assessment of suicide-related concerns. Until they are about seven or eight years old, children do not fully appreciate the concept that death is permanent. Therefore, a six year old who states that he/she is going to kill him/herself is more likely expressing strong affect of sadness or frustration or perhaps imitating others than actually seeking a permanent escape via death. However, this lack of understanding is two-sided – young children can also be more prone to impulsivity, taking suicidal actions and not appreciating that they will not be able to "take it back" later.

These concepts also apply to older children with developmental disabilities or mental retardation. Questions such as, "What do you think will happen to you after you die?" can be very revealing in this population, and answers like, "My mommy will forgive me then we'll be alright" can tell one a lot about a child's conception of death and the impact of their actions. Even though some children are developmentally incapable of understanding the irreversibility of death, it is important to review the seriousness of any actions to end their life, e.g., never seeing parents or friends again, and making their family very sad. Trying to understand why they want to die, what they actually desire to achieve by this action, and discussing alternate means of reaching this goal, can sometimes prevent future ED visits.

Homicidal ideation

The evaluation of suicidal ideation is somewhat analogous to the evaluation of "homicidal ideation" in young people. In order to fully evaluate the seriousness of any threat, it is important to review (1) intent, (2) plan, (3) access to means, (4) expectation of outcome, (5) prior aggression, and (6) quality of adult supervision. Although a seven year old may be brought to an ED for "homicidal ideation" it is more likely that he/she is expressing frustration and anger rather than that he/she has a plan to actually kill anyone. Trying to understand the motivation behind the threat, and emphasizing the seriousness and consequences of making such a threat, can minimize future threats.

Typically, if a youngster in the ED expresses homicidal ideation towards a specific target, that target is already aware as it is frequently his/her parents/guardian, teacher, and may well be the reason for the ED visit. Such patients should be considered for inpatient hospitalization, which (along with informing the receiving team of the intent) executes the duty to protect. In other circumstances, it would be helpful to consult with the hospital's legal department or an experienced provider to ensure that the duty to warn is executed in the proper manner before the patient is discharged. The details of the Tarasoff Act are covered elsewhere in this text as it is much more common in the evaluation and aftercare planning for adult patients.

Psychosis or psychotic-like presentations

True psychosis in pre-pubertal children is extremely rare, about 1 in 10,000.[31] It is far more common for such youngsters to be suffering from another process such as intoxication, delirium, extreme anxiety, or mood disorders than to have a primary psychotic illness.

Children with mental retardation or other developmental disabilities can at times create rich imaginary worlds which, if not carefully investigated, can seem to be permanent delusions rather than imagination. The "story telling" behaviors or "imaginary friends" which would be seen as normal developmental stages in younger children can persist to much older ages in disabled children or adolescents. These children may experience increased attention when reporting such stories and thus they are unintentionally reinforced for telling them.

Anxiety in young children can present with seemingly psychotic, and at times aggressive, behaviors that might lead to an ED visit. Heightened threat awareness and hyper-arousal may lead a youngster to believe that there are dangers where none exist or feel so scared that they will fight to get away from the perceived threat. Many anxiety-ridden children will complain of seeing things in their room at night, or hearing voices calling them in the house when they are alone and frightened, or even seeing a person looking in their window. These are typically illusions (misperceptions of an actual sensory stimulus, such as seeing a figure in the shape of a coat on a coat rack), the result of an overactive imagination combined with fright.

In adolescents, the risk of true psychotic symptoms becomes more pronounced. However, even in this population, mood disorders are far more common than schizophrenia. True psychotic symptoms are more likely due to an underlying psychotic depression, bipolar disorder, or substance use than schizophrenia. Schizophrenia is more likely to present in adolescent boys than girls, as men typically have earlier onset of symptoms than women. Of the three core symptom clusters in schizophrenia (cognitive, positive, and negative)*, the positive symptoms (hallucinations and delusions) are the most likely to lead to a presentation in the ED.[32] In adolescence, other prodromal symptoms of schizophrenia may emerge such as a decline in attention or school performance, a decreased ability to perform activities of daily living, decreased organizational skills, social isolation or withdrawal, or low mood;[33] however, these findings are less likely to present to an ED setting for acute care.

Another possible cause of a psychotic-like presentation is delirium. Delirium is always caused by (an) underlying medical condition(s) but often presents as an acute change in mental status. Fundamentally a waxing and waning pattern of arousal and attention, delirium tends to present acutely or subacutely and can include changes in behavior, mood, and thinking. Clinically, patients may present with the hyperactive form of delirium (agitation, mood lability, and abnormal perceptual phenomena) or with the hypoactive form (excessive sleepiness, difficulty staying awake, and poor attention). The hyperactive youngsters can appear to be psychotic, severely anxious, or aggressive and

---

* Cognitive symptoms include an impaired ability to absorb and interpret information and make decisions based on that information. Negative symptoms include inexpressive faces, blank looks, monotone and monosyllabic speech, few gestures, seeming lack of interest in the world and other people, and inability to feel pleasure or act spontaneously.

require much staff support and management while the hypoactive youngsters tend to be the quietly confused children who may seem disinterested, cognitively limited, or depressed. Some portion of youth will exhibit both types of presentations and are considered "mixed."

The most common etiologies in children and adolescents include infection, illicit drug intoxication or withdrawal, medications (e.g., pain medications or certain antibiotics), hypoxia (such as from a severe asthma attack), and trauma or other CNS pathology (such as a tumor). Other, rarer causes include nutritional deficit (vitamin deficiencies, starvation, or severe dehydration), acute metabolic changes, endocrine abnormalities, heavy metal exposure, or stroke.

When a patient comes in to the ED with an acute onset of severely disturbed behavior, the ED staff must consider delirium before assuming it is a primary psychiatric illness, particularly if it is a first time or new behavior presentation. The medical history should focus on possible predisposing factors or obvious etiologic agents. Asking other informants about recent hospitalizations or injuries, more longstanding medical concerns, and substance or medication use (with an eye toward sources of intoxication or potential withdrawal) can quickly suggest a cause for the current presentation. Repeat examinations of the patient to try to capture the waxing and waning quality of the presentation is important. Although there are some scales for assessing delirium in the literature, none have been evaluated for a one-time diagnostic assessment in the ED. Other biological assessments for delirium (such as EEG) are so non-specific as to be limited in usefulness, and usually not readily available in most acute care settings.

Management of delirium hinges upon identifying and treating the underlying cause. A patient with hyperactive delirium, however, may be so behaviorally disruptive that further evaluation for the etiology is impossible. In this case, acute behavioral management can generally follow the incremental interventions used for other aggressive patients, beginning with behavioral interventions to minimize noxious stimuli. Should additional interventions be required, benzodiazepines should be avoided (unless alcohol withdrawal is suspected), as should diphenhydramine, as both of these agents can worsen non-alcohol-withdrawal related delirium. Haloperidol is generally a safe choice, and is included in the Society of Critical Care Medicine's guidelines for sedatives and anesthesia for treatment of delirium.[34]

Legal considerations

Nowhere in the emergency psychiatric provider's experience is the law more relevant, or more complicated, than in its relationship to children. Fundamentally, it revolves around: (1) under what circumstances do children have the right to make medical decisions for themselves, and (2) if the child does not have such authority, who does? Cases will appear in which many parties are fighting for the right to make child care decisions, and also in which parties are trying to hand off that responsibility to one another with no clear responsible party. The purview of these laws includes: consent for treatment or medications, confidentiality, hospitalization in a psychiatric facility, and finally, mandated reporting laws for providers. Laws vary from state to state so the reader is encouraged to consult with a knowledgeable professional or peer in his/her own care setting or region. There are, however, some general guidelines to the approach that can be helpful to consider.

Consent for care

Typically, ED professionals have the right to treat children if they are suffering from life-threatening medical conditions and no guardian is available. However, when an emergency exists but immediate medical attention is not required, the provider must make "all reasonable efforts" to obtain official consent before proceeding. Most psychiatric emergencies may be initiated/evaluated without consent of the guardian; however, obtaining informed consent for treatment (as compared to evaluation) is usually necessary. Most children are brought to the ED by their legal guardian specifically for the mental health assessment. Challenges may arise when:

(1) The child is unaccompanied by their guardian (brought in by police, school, etc.).
(2) Legal guardianship is unclear.
(3) Legal guardians disagree with the proposed treatment.
(4) The legal guardian is the State.

In these cases, scrupulous documentation regarding the attempts to clarify guardianship and consent must be followed, and consultation with an ED/hospital/institution setting's legal staff can be of great help in determining who can do what in each circumstance.

In some states, minors may consent to their own treatment. These laws typically fall under three categories: (1) emancipated minor laws, (2) mature minor laws, (3) age of consent laws (to medical treatment, commitment to a hospital, outpatient treatment). Emancipated minors are considered to have a level of responsibility above that of the typical minor, usually because they live independently, are married, or have children. "Mature minor" laws cover those adolescents who have demonstrated a level of maturity that they should be allowed to consent to treatment, without the involvement of the court system. Most states also have certain types of treatment that do not require parental involvement, including substance use treatment and reproductive health care. Mental health treatment may also be included under these laws.

Admissions

In many states, "voluntary" admission to a psychiatric hospital is based entirely on the guardian's decision. A few states (e.g. Iowa, Texas, etc.) prevent the voluntary admission of a minor without the minor's express consent (depending on age). Other states have made exceptions in which a minor can sign him or herself in for treatment, without parent/guardian consent, at varying ages.

An involuntary admission to a hospital for a minor is similar to the process used with adults. In general, the child must meet certain minimum "substantive requirements for admission." The American Academy of Child and Adolescent Psychiatry issued a policy statement in 1989 regarding the use of involuntary hospitalization in the continuum of child psychiatric care:

(1) The psychiatric disorder must be of such severity as to cause significant impairment of daily functioning in at least two important areas of the adolescent's life.
(2) The treatment proposed must be relevant to the problems diagnosed and adjudged likely to benefit the patient.
(3) A less restrictive alternative must have been considered and found to be not available, inappropriate, or not successful in the past.[35]

Summary

Despite the fact that most ED care settings do not have access to sub-specialty child psychiatry consultation, there are skills and strategies that ED providers can develop that will facilitate caring for youth and families in crisis. Understanding the developmental differences and the importance of contextual factors such as family and school, knowing the prevalence of different disorders and options for acute interventions, and recognizing the provider's role and responsibility in advocating for and protecting youths can increase comfort with and confidence in caring for these youths.

References

1. Merikangas KR, He JP, Brody D, et al. Prevalence and treatment of mental disorders among US children in the 2001–2004 NHANES. *Pediatrics*. 2009; **125**(1):75–81.

2. Breslow RE, Erickson BJ, Cavanaugh KC. The psychiatric emergency service: where we've been and where we're going. *Psychiatr Q*. 2000;**71**(2):101–121.

3. Edelsohn GA, Braitman LE, Rabinovich H, Sheves P, Melendez A. Predictors of urgency in a pediatric psychiatric emergency service. *J Am Acad Child Adolesc Psychiatry*. 2003;**42**(10): 1197–1202.

4. Haugh R. A crisis in adolescent psych. *Hosp Health Netw*. 2003;**77**(1):38–41.

5. Page D. Pediatric psychiatry. More blues in ED? *Hosp Health Netw*. 2000;**74**(8):24.

6. Sills MR, Bland SD. Summary statistics for pediatric psychiatric visits to US emergency departments, 1993–1999. *Pediatrics*. 2002;**110**(4):e40.

7. Burks HL, Hoekstra M. Psychiatric emergencies in children. *Am J Orthopsychiatry*. 1964;**34**:134–137.

8. Mattson A, Hawkins J, Sees L. Child psychiatric emergencies: clinical characteristics and follow-up results. *Arch Gen Psychiatry*. 1967;**17**:584–592.

9. Morrison G. Therapeutic intervention in a child psychiatry emergency service. *J Am Acad Child Adolesc Psychiatry*. 1969;**8**: 542–558.

10. Healy E, Saha S, Subotsky F, Fombonne E. Emergency presentations to an inner-city adolescent psychiatric service. *J Adolesc*. 2002;**25**(4):397–404.

11. Frosch E, McCulloch J, Yoon Y, Dosreis S. Pediatric emergency consultations: prior mental health service use in suicide attempters. *J Behav Health Serv Res*. 2011;**38**(1):68–79.

12. Goldstein AB, Frosch E, Davarya S, Leaf PJ. Factors associated with a six-month return to emergency services among child and adolescent psychiatric patients. *Psychiatr Serv*. 2007;**58**(11): 1489–1492.

13. Scheeringa MS, Zeanah CH, Drell MJ, Larrieu JA. Two approaches to the diagnosis of posttraumatic stress disorder in infancy and early childhood. *J Am Acad Child Adolesc Psychiatry*. 1995;**34**(2):191–200.

14. Coates S, Gaensbauer TJ. Event trauma in early childhood: symptoms, assessment, intervention. *Child Adolesc Psychiatr Clin N Am*. 2009;**18**(3):611–626.

15. Nader K, Stuber M, Pynoos R. Posttraumatic stress reactions in preschool children with catastrophic illness: assessment needs. *Comprehensive Mental Health Care*. 1991;**1**(3):223–229.

16. Polancyzk G, de Lima MS, Horta BL, Biederman J, Rohde LA. The worldwide prevalence of ADHD: a systematic review and metaregression analysis. *Am J Psychiatry*. 2007;**164**(6):942–948.

17. Shear K, Jin R, Ruscio AM, Walters EE, Kessler RC. Prevalence and correlates of estimated DSM-IV child and adult separation anxiety disorder in the National Comorbidity Survey Replication. *Am J Psychiatry*. 2006;**163**(6):1074–1083.

18. McClellan J, Werry J. Practice parameters for the assessment and treatment of children and adolescents with bipolar

disorder. American Academy of Child and Adolescent Psychiatry. *J Am Acad Child Adolesc Psychiatry*. 1997;**36**(10 Suppl): 157S–176S.

19. Olaniyan O, dosReis S, Garriett V, et al. Community perspectives of childhood behavioral problems and ADHD among African American parents. *Ambul Pediatr*. 2007;**7**(3):226–231.

20. American Academy of Child and Adolescent Psychiatry. Practice parameter for the prevention and management of aggressive behavior in child and adolescent psychiatric institutions with special reference to seclusion and restraint. *J Am Acad Child Adolesc Psychiatry*. 2002; **41**(Suppl):4s–25s.

21. Dorfman DH, Mehta SD. Restraint use for psychiatric patients in the pediatric emergency department. *Pediatr Emerg Care*. 2006;**22**(1):7–12.

22. Dorfman DH, Kastner B. The use of restraint for pediatric psychiatric patients in emergency departments. *Pediatr Emerg Care*. 2004;**20**(3):151–156.

23. Hilt RJ, Woodward TA. Agitation treatment for pediatric emergency patients. *J Am Acad Child Adolesc Psychiatry*. 2008;**47**(2):132–138.

24. National Institute of Mental Health. *Suicide in the U.S.: Statistics and Prevention. A fact sheet of statistics on suicide with information on treatments and suicide prevention*. 2009. http://www.nimh.nih. gov/health/publications/suicide-in-the-us-statistics-and-prevention/index.shtml.

25. Grunbaum JA, Kann L, Kinchen S, et al. Youth risk behavior surveillance – United States, 2003. *MMWR Surveill Summ*. 2004;**53**(2):1–96.

26. Centers for Disease Control and Prevention. Fatal and nonfatal suicide attempts among adolescents – Oregon,

1988–1993. *MMWR Morb Mortal Wkly Rep*. 1995;**44**(16):312–315,321–313.

27. Brent DA, Baugher M, Bridge J, Chen T, Chiappetta L. Age- and sex-related risk factors for adolescent suicide. *J Am Acad Child Adolesc Psychiatry*. 1999; **38**(12):1497–1505.

28. Shaffer D, Craft L. Methods of adolescent suicide prevention. *J Clin Psychiatry*. 1999;**60**(Suppl 2):70–74; discussion 75–76, 113–116.

29. Swahn MH, Bossarte RM. Gender, early alcohol use, and suicide ideation and attempts: findings from the 2005 youth risk behavior survey. *J Adolesc Health*. 2007; **41**(2):175–181.

30. Afifi TO, Cox BJ, Katz LY. The associations between health risk behaviours and suicidal ideation and attempts in a nationally representative sample of young adolescents. *Can J Psychiatry*. 2007;**52**(10):666–74.

31. Remschmidt H. Early-onset schizophrenia as a progressive-deteriorating developmental disorder: evidence from child psychiatry. *J Neural Transm*. 2002;**109**(1):101–117.

32. Remschmidt H. Psychosocial milestones in normal puberty and adolescence. *Horm Res*. 1994;**41**(Suppl 2):19–29.

33. Asarnow JR, Tompson MC, Goldstein MJ. Childhood-onset schizophrenia: a follow up study. *Schizophr Bull*. 1994;**20**(4):599–617.

34. Jacobi J, Fraser GL, Coursin DB, et al. Clinical practice guidelines for the sustained use of sedatives and analgesics in the critically ill adult. *Crit Care Med*. 2002;**30**(1):119–141.

35. American Academy of Child and Adolescent Psychiatry. *Policy statement on inpatient hospital treatment of children and adolescents*. Washington, DC: American Academy of Child and Adolescent Psychiatry, 1989.

Chapter 13

The evaluation of intellectual and developmental disabilities

Lisa S. Hovermale, Theodosia Paclawskyj, Dyanne Simpson, and Eric Samstad

Introduction

Emergency departments (EDs) must anticipate and prepare for the presentation of people with intellectual and developmental disabilities (PWIDD) to their facilities. Following the June 22, 1999 *Olmstead* Supreme Court decision,[1] the national expectation is that PWIDD will live in the least restrictive and most integrated setting that can meet their needs. As more states move toward closing institutions where many people from this population formerly lived, it is the common expectation that medical and psychiatric care will be delivered though mainstream (including outpatient) services.[2] The literature has clearly established that the prevalence of somatic illness and psychiatric illness is unequivocally greater in PWIDD, as compared to the general population.[3,4] Unfortunately, the extent of specialized knowledge in community settings remains uneven and sometimes only marginally capable of meeting the needs of PWIDD, particularly in the realm of psychiatric services.[2,5] Medical professionals often readily admit their lack of training, experience, and compromised comfort level in working with this group of people.[6-9] Given this set of circumstances, in combination with the role of the ED as the safety net for gaps in the medical care delivery system, proactive planning that anticipates the needs of PWIDD will improve efficiency in the acute care environment and avoid long stays in the ED.

The purpose of this chapter is to provide guidance to ED personnel and other acute care providers as they cope with the many challenges that accompany the care of PWIDD. A series of topics are addressed: proactive acquisition of system knowledge, impact of the clinical environments including EDs, consent issues, communication and information collection strategies, and a strategy for clinical assessment.

People-first language

The acceptance of persons with disabilities in society has improved significantly in recent times. However, stigma still persists. Advocates, professionals, and family members have all promoted use of "people-first" language in recent years.[10] This is intended to focus on the person first and the disability second. In addition, people-first language helps counter the notion that the disability defines PWIDD's potential. Therefore, appropriate phrasing consists of stating "a person with (disability)" rather than the use of vocabulary such as "an autistic," "a paraplegic," "the handicapped," or "deaf and dumb." Instead, the following phrases can be substituted for those terms: "a person with autism," "a person with

Emergency Psychiatry, ed. Arjun Chanmugam, Patrick Triplett, and Gabor Kelen. Published by Cambridge University Press. © Cambridge University Press 2013.

paraplegia," "people with disabilities," and "a person who is deaf/hearing impaired," respectively. The goal here is not one of political correctness, rather recognition that use of language helps shape our attitudes, beliefs, and behaviors. Although it is impossible to avoid all bias in the care of patients, the use of appropriate language can improve awareness and help minimize the potential bias associated with stigmatizing labels. Furthermore, the term "intellectual disability" will be used in lieu of "mental retardation" throughout this chapter except when using exact quotes from earlier literature. The authors acknowledge "intellectual disability" as the more appropriate term.

Proactive understanding of the local developmental disabilities system

One of the first steps in improving the emergency assessment and care of PWIDD is to have a working knowledge of the Developmental Disabilities system of supports and local services, which varies by state, region, and municipality. It is equally important to provide durable links to this knowledge and resources in a way that is independent of staff changes. It is most effective to do this in anticipation of crisis situations and should be part of any surge or disaster planning. Advance understanding of the available systems can greatly enhance efficiency and decrease the emotional toll of learning complicated systems of care in the midst of delivering emergency services. Some EDs commit the knowledge obtained to a specific stepwise policy containing names and contact information that results in a procedural algorithm for the use of the staff of the ED. Meeting with personnel providing the local oversight of the system can clarify expectations, uncover gaps in the system of care, create opportunities to advocate for addressing those system gaps, and may lead to the creation of memos of understanding. These actions not only foster a collaborative spirit, but can improve the efficiency of transfer of care issues. One of the more common assumptions, that there are government agencies or resources that are readily available for the PWIDD who may have an urgent need, is just not valid in most circumstances. It cannot be assumed that because a patient appears to have a developmental disability based on the clinical assessment of the clinician, a government agency will be available to assume responsibility for meeting the needs of that person. Access to services and degree of available wrap-around supports (e.g., 24/7 live-in assistance) varies widely across localities. Some places have developed specialized teams and respite services that can be used to facilitate evaluation and disposition while other places have very limited options at best.[11] Knowing the availability of these resources will allow the episodic care provider to efficiently craft the most appropriate treatment plan.

Consent issues

Although consent issues are less of a concern in emergency treatment situations, in treating adults whose competency to consent may be in question, clinicians require a working knowledge of the community standard. Although not easily accomplished, guardianship or the status of surrogate decision-makers should be established as quickly as possible, preferably at triage or the intake stage. A key point is that PWIDD should be considered to be their own legal guardian, even when they may present as people who require much support and have great difficulty communicating, unless legal documentation of guardianship or surrogacy is provided.[12] In some localities, consent to psychiatric treatment including admission to a psychiatric facility cannot be given by a guardian and requires involuntary admission even if PWIDD appear to agree with the admission. Families whose adult PWIDD live with them may assume that they are the person's guardian when in fact they are not legally designated to act in that capacity.

Guardianship is a complicated, time-consuming, and expensive endeavor. Having the legal paperwork establishing guardianship or surrogate decision-maker status located on the medical chart makes conversations about the authority and limitations of these roles more effective. Establishing a surrogate decision-maker is a very important step but has its limitations. In some states, surrogate decision-makers cannot give consent for psychotropic medications, reproductive health decisions, or anything that PWIDD do not agree to accept. Proactively understanding the many legal nuances of guardianship in the state involved, as well as the provider's policies and procedures impacted by these nuances, will provide a return in efficiency and reduce the complications that are often associated with competency discussions.

Evaluation and assessment

Physicians providing episodic care as may occur in the acute setting have to provide a significant degree of leadership when assessing PWIDD, because of the complexity surrounding their social and medical condition and the resulting emotional impact they may have on the staff. PWIDD are a highly heterogeneous population. Impairments may range from severe physical and communication deficits to much milder impairments in adaptive functioning. Practitioners may feel overwhelmed by the degree of disability when managing those at the severe limitation end of the spectrum, while other PWIDD need little or no accommodation of practice. High-intensity behaviors such as aggression and self-abusive behaviors, or any behavior that threatens the safety of PWIDD or their caregivers, are common reasons for presentation to the ED,[12,13] and typically represent the primary concern for the ED. For these reasons, acute care providers must actively use their leadership capabilities to foster partnerships with PWIDD, their caregivers, and the system of care; all while conducting the necessary diagnostic and treatment interventions.

ED setting concerns

PWIDD will frequently view the ED setting as frightening and unfamiliar. Associated with past negative experiences such as injections, blood draws, temporary isolation, or other painful or uncomfortable procedures, the ED may be a difficult if not potentially threatening environment. The lack of comprehension among PWIDD for the majority of the procedures in the ED naturally results in increased fear and anxiety, which often manifests by some form of agitation. For all these reasons, the typical appearance and behavior of health care professionals may need to be modified to provide a sense of comfort and reassurance to the person.

Episodic care providers should consider the following strategies to optimize the setting for PWIDD who present with an urgency or emergency. First, it is best to avoid wearing a lab coat if possible. This will minimize the likelihood of PWIDD becoming agitated in the presence of the staff they associate with previously painful experiences. Second, PWIDD may have significant discrepancies in their expressive language as compared to their receptive language; they may comprehend more than they can communicate. Therefore, conversations about PWIDD in their presence should be carefully considered unless the discussion is neutral or on preferred topics. Third, despite communication difficulties, most PWIDD readily recognize facial expressions and emotions in others. To maintain a reassuring presence, it may be helpful to make eye contact and smile both during and outside of direct interaction with the person, regardless of the context or ongoing procedure.[12]

Numerous simple interventions can be considered with the goal of decreasing the stimulation of the environment and, consequently, reducing the likelihood of agitated behavior. Generally, the patient should be put in a relatively quiet area. The room should be empty of portable equipment, especially if the patient is having difficulty sitting still. For some PWIDD, bright room lights should be dimmed or turned off entirely. For others, a well lit area is preferred but fluorescent lights may be agitating. Many EDs have standard protocols for psychiatric patients that often include having the patient change into hospital attire, frequently paper scrubs. Many PWIDD are hypersensitive to the texture of paper scrubs and the discomfort can lead to increased agitation. It is often helpful to offer these patients cloth hospital gowns, cloth scrubs, or even allow them to remain in their own clothes.

Communication and interaction strategies

In addition to environmental modifications, there are multiple communication and inter-action strategies that can make the ED experience more manageable and comfortable for the patient and staff. Being mindful of language is a critical component of successful interaction that engenders compliance in the patient. To enhance the opportunity for better understanding, staff should communicate clearly and with simple one to two step requests when speaking to the patient. Even ordinary terms used with patients, such as, "Are you comfortable?" may be too abstract and not clearly understood by PWIDD. Instructions should be phrased as polite one-step requests such as, "Please sit up," or "Open your mouth please." Instructions as questions should be avoided, as the person could justifiably refuse (e.g., say "Show me your finger" instead of "Could you show me your arm?"). "First-then" instructions can be helpful in communicating that requests and examinations will soon be completed (e.g., "first needle, then rest"). Finally, modeling often can improve both comprehension and compliance. With modeling, gestures or simulation are used to demonstrate the procedure that is about to be performed. If available, the procedure can be simulated on a doll; alternatively, the procedure can be simulated on another adult in the room. This can significantly reduce anxiety over unfamiliar procedures.

It is preferable to avoid "yes/no" questions until a caregiver confirms that the person can reliably answer such questions. Many PWIDD have a history of being eager to please. The PWIDD may say "yes" without understanding the meaning of the situation; alternatively, for some PWIDD who find themselves in a fearful situation, the default answer to every question may be "no." If it is not clear that PWIDD are responding consistently, the examiner can assess their understanding by asking two questions: one in which the answer is affirmative (e.g., "Are you (person's name)?"), and one in which the answer is negative (e.g., "Are you (state incorrect age)?"). The key point is that the provider must assess the PWIDD's ability to appropriately answer questions, especially yes/no questions, before beginning the search for information regarding the presenting complaint.

In general, the caregiver is the best source of information regarding PWIDD's modality of communication. Although many PWIDD communicate verbally, others may use one of three forms of augmentative communication: sign language, picture cards, or assistive technology devices. Picture cards are typically index card-sized drawings of an item or activity paired with the written word. Over the past decade, many individuals with autism in particular have been taught communication strategies in school that involve exchanging picture cards with another person in order to request an item, make a comment, or in general, hold a conversation. Assistive technology devices utilize the same concept in the form of computerized voice-output devices. Such devices may be as simple as a button that when pressed, says the word "help," or can be as complex as a voice-output typewriter. If a caregiver is present, they may be able to do the following: provide an understanding of the person's basic communicative abilities, assist the method of augmentative communication, interpret idiosyncratic signs or gestures, clarify the speech of a person with oral motor impairment, and help to confirm that communication to the person has been understood. Overall, clinicians must be sensitive to PWIDD's capability and be prepared to employ a variety of communication techniques.

Information collection strategies

Paid direct service professionals (DSPs) or family caregivers should be contacted early in the information gathering process if they are not present in the ED or the acute care setting. DSPs can of course provide useful information if they have known the person longitudinally. Turnover rates among professional caregivers can be quite high,[14] thus, it is important to know the duration of contact between the DSP and the PWIDD. In addition, DSPs may have a distinct agenda, one that may differ from that of PWIDD or the acute care team. The physician and other caregivers would do well to assess the DSP's agenda to avoid potentially confounding biases.

When PWIDD are in community placements, voluminous records may be available, but no succinct summary may exist. Working up the chain of supervision to house managers or agency nurses can be useful in understanding the timeline of events. Some community agencies employ or have close relationships with medical and psychiatric clinicians who serve PWIDD. Contact with these clinicians often proves invaluable. Accessing information from previous ED visits allows the opportunity to build on information previously acquired.

Reverse application of the multiaxial system in emergency evaluation of PWIDD

Although it is not possible to eliminate bias, an understanding of the biases that may exist in a clinical setting is important. One bias, "diagnostic overshadowing," typically refers to the clinical tendency to allow the presence of significant cognitive deficits to negate productive assessment of emotional disturbances.[15,16] It can be extended to the tendency to attribute atypical expression of symptoms of somatic illness to the behavioral manifestations of severe disability.[17] In order to avoid the common pitfall of diagnostic overshadowing, the clinician should try to keep a specific diagnostic strategy in mind. This can be accomplished by utilizing the diagnostic structure that many psychiatric clinicians employ, i.e., the multiaxial assessment system.[18]

The multiaxial assessment system provides a structure with which to evaluate PWIDD holistically. In this system, there are five domains that are used to assess a patient. Axis I (psychiatric illness), Axis II (well established behavioral coping strategies/temperamental characteristics – perhaps manifesting a baseline exaggeration), Axis III (somatic illness), Axis IV (psychosocial stressors), and Axis V which represents how well a person functions overall by employing a rating scale called the Global Assessment of Functioning (GAF). The GAF scale ranges from 0 to 100 and provides a way to summarize in a single number just how well the person is functioning overall at a particular point in time.

Developmental disabilities do not typically wax and wane as other disease processes do. Intellectual and developmental disabilities are generally considered long-term static conditions requiring accommodation and habilitation rather than treatment. If PWIDD experience a deterioration of adaptive skills, then a superimposed process, or combination of superimposed processes, must be sought to account for the change. These superimposed processes typically fall into one or more of the categories represented by Axis I, II, III, and IV. The strategy here, however, is to begin with Axis V as the initial assessment rather than with Axis I. In fact, in this strategy, it is optimal to proceed from Axis V to Axis I in reverse sequence (V, IV, III, II, I).

The *Diagnostic Manual – Intellectual Disability: A Textbook of Diagnosis of Mental Disorders in Persons with Intellectual Disability,* published by the National Association for the Dually Diagnosed (2007)[19] (DM-ID) may provide additional insights into how typical DSM criteria may be adapted for PWIDD as well as additional tips on strategy for arriving at a diagnosis. For instance, Hurley have emphasized the need to avoid a rush to definitive diagnosis by maintaining skepticism and openness to constantly reassess the diagnostic formulation as more information is acquired.[20]

Axis V: Establishing optimal baseline. In psychiatric diagnostic systems, global assessment of function (GAF) resides in Axis V. This provides the clinician's assessment of the person's current level of psychological, social, and occupational functioning as expressed by GAF scores. Axis V can also include a GAF score for the highest level of functioning within the past year. Although clinicians may question the day-to-day usefulness of GAF due to its subjective nature, the emphasis here is in understanding how the current presentation of PWIDD compares with their best presentation within recent history. Considering the optimal baseline of PWIDD is critical to avoiding the pitfall of diagnostic overshadowing. Knowing that the person before you was successfully living, and working in his/her community at some point in the past, provides an entirely different perspective on the person who may now present as aggressive and affectively dysregulated. Alternatively, knowing that PWIDD have a long history of challenging trademark behaviors helps to frame the fundamental key question of "What is different now?" Informants may need reassurance that discussing PWIDD's past optimal presentation does not lessen the emphasis on the current emergency, but rather puts it in context.

A GAF scoring system has been developed specifically for PWIDD. GAF assessment instructions specifically state that consideration of impairments in physical functioning should not be included. Hurley has created equivalents for GAF scores specific to the PWIDD population,[20] which have been recreated in Table 13.1. The DM-ID can provide greater detail for the adaption of the GAF to PWIDD.

Axis IV: Psychosocial stressors. This axis is reserved for estimation of the effect that environmental stressors or psychosocial difficulties can have in the presentation of the case. It has been suggested that one explanation for the increased prevalence of mental illness in this group of people is lowered coping skills resulting from limited cognition and adaptive functioning deficits that establish the designation of developmental disability.[21] Acknowledging this particular vulnerability to stress clarifies the importance of knowing if there are psychosocial or environmental setting events. The greater impact of ordinary psychosocial events like job/day placement changes, staff changes, residential moves, and roommate changes tend to be undervalued in this group. Hurley has summarized these stressors in Table 13.2.

NOTE: Although modern values in the field hold that the person should have as much control as possible over these facets of their life, currently this remains more of a goal than a reality in the culture of the care system. The very definition of developmental disability[22]

Table 13.1. Axis V Global Assessment of Functioning combined Social and Occupational Functioning Assessment Scale (GAF combined SOFAS) with suggested general modifications for individuals with mental retardation developmental delay

Rating	Description	Natural supports effective	Behavior supports needed	Psychiatric supports
100	**Superior functioning**, many positive qualities, adapts to life's problems easily; special behavioral or psychiatric supports are never necessary.	×		
90	**Absent or minimal** symptoms, situation specific, independent or cooperates with ADLs; minor problems at school/work or in social realms occasionally; all problem areas are easily addressed by natural supports, special behavioral or psychiatric supports are never necessary.	×		
80	**Transient** symptoms normal for social stressors, satisfied with life, ordinary problems; infrequent interpersonal conflicts, work/school problems in achievement; problems can be addressed through natural supports and occasional informal meetings of supporters; behavioral or psychiatric supports are never necessary.	×		
70	**Mild** symptoms, slightly affecting functioning at work/home, social relationships, or ADLs; behavioral or psychiatric supports are considered; interventions are positive based on reinforcement; psychotherapy is considered; antipsychotic medication is not considered.	×	×	×
60	**Moderate** symptoms, difficulty in adapting to life, minor conflicts with others, few friends, or minor effect on ADLs; positive behavioral support plans are needed; psychiatric interventions are considered; psychotherapy is considered; antipsychotic medication is not considered.	×	×	×
50	**Serious** impairment in ADLs, social, work or school functioning; unable to function well with supports in at least one environment; positive and decelerating behavioral plans are considered; supporters beyond those naturally available are necessary; consultants or formal team meeting are necessary; all psychiatric interventions		×	×

Table 13.1. (cont.)

Rating	Description	Natural supports effective	Behavior supports needed	Psychiatric supports
	considered, including antipsychotic medication.			
40	**Major** impairment in **several areas**: work/school, relationships, or ADLs; in more than one area, positive and decelerating behavioral plans are considered; supports beyond those naturally available are necessary; consultants or formal team meeting are necessary; psychiatric interventions considered, including antipsychotic medication.	×		×
30	**Serious** impairment, psychotic symptoms unable to function in all areas, independently or with supports consistent with developmental level: psychotic symptoms, inability to function and needs major increase in support level; positive and decelerating behavioral plans are considered; formal team support meetings necessary for all areas; all psychiatric interventions considered, including antipsychotic medication and inpatient hospitalization.	×		×
20	**Some danger** of hurting self or others, serious thought disorder; occasionally cannot maintain or cooperate with ADLs and seriously jeopardizes health or safety; specialized new levels of support are needed for all areas; behavioral plans are considered to not be adequate, all psychiatric interventions considered including inpatient hospitalization.	×		×
10	**Persistent danger** of severely hurting self or others, cannot maintain/cooperate with basic care at all; behavioral plans are considered to be inadequate in themselves; specialized 24-hour supports are needed, to be provided in specialized unit or inpatient psychiatric hospital; all levels of psychiatric interventions considered.			×

From Hurley AD. Axis IV and Axis V: Assessment of persons with mental retardation and developmental disabilities. *Mental Health Aspects of Developmental Disabilities*. 2001;**4**(1):21.

Table 13.2. Axis IV: Psychosocial and environmental problems with suggested general considerations for individuals with mental retardation developmental delay

Dsm category and examples	Suggested general considerations for mental retardation and development disabilities
Primary support group: meant for family and partners, death, divorce, abuse, discord with other family members	Long-term relationships with peers, staff/supports, and house mates should considered to apply to this category.
Social environment: loss of friends, living alone. Discrimination, life-cycle stresses such as retirement	Living independently may be a particular stressor, discrimination is a severe and persistent condition for people with disabilities; stresses in change in service and lack of state available service should apply to this category.
Education/occupation. Performance issues in school, work, difficult classroom or work conditions, discord with peers at school/work	School environments are often extremely stressful for special needs students; peers in school and at work sites may either have disrupting behavior due to disabilities, or severe social rejection from intellectually normal peers; dissatisfaction with actual job tasks available to adult MR/DD workers should be considered a major stressor.
Housing: homelessness, unsafe neighborhood, discord with neighbors	For those living independently, especially in cities, there is an increased level of unsafe conditions.
Access to health care, health insurance, transportation	For those with HMO regulated plans, access to needed mental health and evaluation services may be considerable; ability to access available health care providers may be lessened due to dependence on caregivers, or lack of specialists in the area familiar with MR/DD.
Legal system/crime: arrest, victimization	Those with MR/DD have major barriers in the criminal justice system; victimization is more prevalent, especially for those living independently in cities; sexual victimization of adults is more prevalent for MR/DD.
Other: local disasters, discord with non-family caregivers such as social worker, physician, social service agencies	Access to agency support and relationship with agency personnel is frequently less than needed; discord with agency staff, including supervising staff of residential of day service should be considered to be a major stressor for those with MR/DD due to dependence for basic functioning and advocacy.

From Hurley AD. Axis IV and Axis V: Assessment of persons with mental retardation and developmental disabilities. *Mental Health Aspects of Developmental Disabilities*. 2001;**4**(1):21.

implies that there will be a degree of dependence on others and consequently a vulnerability to perturbations in those support systems. Changes in the primary support system, social environment, education or occupation, housing, benefits such as health care, legal involvement, or other relevant changes should be investigated. An ED clinician inquiring into this domain may learn that it is really the system of care that is in crisis rather than the PWIDD.[2] This is important in framing the pertinent issues and crafting the appropriate intervention in such a way that does not inappropriately further ascribe pathology to PWIDD.

An area of special concern for the episodic care clinician should be the increasing awareness of the high risk of physical and sexual abuse in children and adults with intellectual and developmental disability.[23,24] This line of inquiry may reveal a psycho-social stressor as the basis for a diagnosis of PTSD[23] and may dictate a clinical pathway involving child or adult protective services. Having an already established algorithm for this eventuality involving appropriate social service agencies and government entities would be helpful.

Axis III: Medical concerns. Medical comorbidities are common among PWIDD[25] and symptoms can appear to be psychiatric rather than somatic in origin. The underlying cause of intellectual and developmental disabilities is known in as little as 25% of the affected population, but when known, can point to pertinent associated medical conditions.[5] For instance, the association between Down's syndrome and multiple medical comorbidities such as cardiac disease, thyroid dysfunction, and Alzheimer's disease is well known. These should be part of the differential diagnosis in the presentation of behavioral difficulties in someone with this syndrome.[26,27]

The background information obtained from PWIDD and caregivers will permit a more focused and meaningful approach. The following structured approach may be helpful:

(1) An accurate list of PWIDD's previously recognized medical problems and medications should be obtained.

(2) Any new or emergent medical issues or exacerbations of chronic conditions, recent medication changes, or seizure activity should be sought.

(3) Informants should be questioned regarding any changes in PWIDD's day-to-day functioning: overall energy level, bowel and bladder habits, level of orientation ("confusion"), refusal or avoidance of usual activities, and complaints of pain or discomfort.

(4) Potential for trauma, including the possibility of head trauma (falls, head-banging), should be ascertained.

It should be appreciated that presenting behaviors may be suggestive of localized pain. Focus of the physical exam, as with other medical conditions, is directed by history of the caregiver and PWIDD interviews. Physical contact should initially involve non-threatening areas, moving slowly and calmly, asking permission ("Can I press on your belly?"), and allowing the PWIDD to "help" where possible. If an agitated patient will not cooperate for a physical exam, mild sedation is generally less traumatic and a better option in most situations than physical restraints.

Certain basic laboratory studies are indicated for all patients, particularly if a transfer to a psychiatric inpatient facility is likely. This would include a complete blood count with differential, comprehensive metabolic panel, and urinalysis. Obtaining blood serum values of level-based antiepileptics (e.g., valproate, carbamazepine), and other medications (e.g., lithium, digoxin) should also obtained if the patient is on these medications. An ECG will generally be required in cases of suspected toxicity. The decision to draw serum ethanol and urine toxicology will be based upon the history, but these are requirements for some psychiatric facilities. There should be a high index of suspicion for ingestions, either intentionally (suicide attempt or impulsive act), or unintentionally (e.g., curiosity, error). The history and basic labs may suggest the need for acetaminophen and salicylate levels or other toxicological studies and interventions. These are usually indicated in cases of suspected deliberate poisonings. A history of acute change in mental status, unusual symptoms (such as visual hallucinations, new-onset seizures), or reports of head-banging or other trauma, indicate the need for head CT. EEG, although rarely indicated in the emergency setting, may be helpful in assessing suspected non-convulsive status epilepticus. Studies of B12, folate, or RPR are generally not necessary unless indicated by the history or required by the receiving psychiatric facility.

It is not unusual for PWIDD to have comorbid seizure disorders[5,28] that are treated with valproate or other agents that also effectively function as mood stabilizers. In the context of an emergency psychiatric visit, family and care providers may not recognize the psychiatric and neurologic utility of such medications (anticonvulsants) and may neglect to mention any changes made by other physicians or a lack of compliance. Emergency physicians should ask targeted questions to ascertain whether there are any neurological issues or medications that may be confounding the acute presentation. If, for example, a neurologist recently decreased the patient's valproate dose, the lower dose could potentially destabilize the patient's mood.

The emergent evaluation of PWIDD should always include a thorough evaluation of the patient's current medications. Evaluating practitioners should pay particular attention to the patient's compliance with medications, any recent medication changes, current drug levels, underlying medical problems, and possible drug-drug interactions. Despite the fact that most PWIDD have some degree of support from DSPs, medications may or may not be handled by the person. Thus, informants should be asked about any possibility of missed or erroneous dosages. Illegal substance abuse is possible in this population. Thus, it is important to determine whether caregivers have any related concerns. Finally, as in the general population, many PWIDD are addicted to either caffeine or nicotine, and changes in the availability of such substances (e.g., as advised in the interest of health by the primary care doctor) may contribute to a presentation of agitation.

Medication issues:

Polypharmacy is commonly seen in PWIDD.[25,28] While this may be necessary due to the complexities of their underlying conditions, it may also lead to interactions that present as target behavioral concerns. Much like a geriatric population, PWIDD can be particularly sensitive to psychotropic medications and, consequently, often quite sensitive to medication changes that might otherwise seem like minor adjustments. Increased agitation, irritability, or aggressive behaviors are common presenting problems that can be related to medications and medication interactions. SSRIs can be activating and small increases may lead to increased agitation or aggressive behavior.[29] Antipsychotics can be sedating and may lead to increased fatigue, decreased focus, and irritability.[30] Benzodiazepines can be overly sedating or paradoxically lead to increased agitated behavior.[31]

If the patient is taking a medication that requires therapeutic drug level monitoring, then a level should be obtained to check for toxicity or sub-therapeutic levels. When obtaining a drug level, it is critically important to question the patient or care provider about the timing of the patient's last dose of that particular medication. To monitor medications like valproic acid and lithium, a trough level needs to be obtained. Generally, to obtain a trough level, the blood must be drawn and tested approximately 12 hours after the last dose of that particular medication. (The 12-hour rule does not necessarily hold true to accurately measure the trough level of some extended release formulations of medications.) This is of particular importance in an ED where patients may present within minutes or just a few hours of their last dose of medications. As a rule, when documenting a therapeutic, sub-therapeutic, or supratherapeutic drug level in a chart, it is always helpful to write both the level and the time of the last dose. By noting both, it helps keep the laboratory data in context for anyone who may be reviewing the chart in the future. It can be especially helpful if the patient needs to be admitted to the hospital for that episode.

Along with a thorough review of the patient's psychiatric and neurologic medications, the emergency physician should be attentive to recent changes in the patient's somatic medication regimen. There are well-known drug-drug interactions between many antibiotics and psychiatric medications. The recent addition of an antibiotic should alert the physician not only to possible underlying medical conditions, but also to drug interactions that could potentially affect therapeutic drug levels of psychotropic medicines. A history of asthma should prompt more questions about the use of inhalers or prednisone, both of which can lead to increased agitation, irritability, and anxiety.[32] The physician should be attentive to medications that might indicate specific medical problems that might contribute to psychiatric decompensation. For example, if the patient reports that he takes levothyroxine, the evaluator might consider the need to determine TSH level.

The use of "PRN" medications should be avoided if possible. Because PWIDD can be sensitive to medications, they may experience greater side effects (e.g., increased sedation) or paradoxical reactions (e.g., increased agitation with benzodiazepines).[31] The use of an IM injection may be overstimulating to patients with tactile sensitivity and can add to agitation. If PRN medication is necessary and indicated, oral-disintegrating tablets can be useful alternatives to IM medicines. The use of IM PRNs often requires physical restraint to administer, which typically worsens the agitation. If the patient will accept an oral-disintegrating medication, there is more opportunity to build rapport with the patient, which helps with the overall process of de-escalation. If the patient is unwilling or unable to take oral medications, the parenteral option should be exercised.

Table 13.3 provides a check-list of questions to ask caregivers.

Axis II: What is behavioral communication versus disease entity? In considering this facet of presentation, it is important to have an agreed-upon understanding of what the word "behavioral" means. Applied Behavioral Analysis (ABA) is a method employed by trained professionals in working with PWIDD with communication deficits. In this context, an action is behavioral if it serves as communication to achieve a goal. While there may be many potential goals, they can be conceptualized into four major categories: seeking attention, task or situation avoidance, obtaining a tangible item, and self-stimulation/self-soothing (stereotypy). If a behavior achieves any one of these goals in a maladaptive fashion, a behavioral plan can be developed to teach an alternative non-maladaptive behavior that allows PWIDD to achieve the same goal and appropriately control their interface with the environment. This use of the term behavioral is in contrast to the typical use of the term in psychiatry where affective dysregulation, the inability to express emotions adaptively, and poor impulse control, are batched into the "behavioral" category with implied volitional and secondary gain components. Distinguishing between the two concepts is critically important. Using the available history to construe if the behavior is communicating a goal or if it is a manifestation of illness is often the crux of the evaluation. When considered in the context of the ABA concept of four major categories of behavioral communication goals, the usefulness of biologic markers of psychiatric illness, such as weight loss and sleep disruption, becomes more apparent. Loss of sleep and weight is most often causally ineffective in achieving the potential goals considered by ABA. Of course, there are the potential exceptions such as PWIDD sleeping during the day in order to have the exclusive attention of the night staff. Knowing the usual pattern of sleep in a 24-hour period helps to

Table 13.3. Checklist of items to ask caregivers

Vegetative changes (sleep, appetite, energy)

Recent seizure activity

Recent changes in health

Recent medication changes

Verify lists of medications and medical problems

Bowel/bladder habit changes

Interest in usual activities

Degree of communication/social interaction/best ways to communicate

Avoidance of certain people or situations

Where/when problem behaviors occur

Any possibility of injury (especially head trauma)

Medication compliance

Suspicion of toxin ingestion

Changes in staff/residence/work/peers, or losses in patient's life

Changes in orientation or other "confusion"

Changes in caffeine/nicotine

Substance abuse

Pain symptoms or behaviors

Suicidal statements or threats

Agitation or other new problem behaviors (note antecedents and consequences)

clarify whether this is a sleep phase shift suggesting a behavioral origin versus true sleep loss representing a change from baseline therefore suggesting a psychiatric illness. If the target behavior is self-stimulation/self-soothing (stereotypy) in nature or a trademark maladaptive behavior frequently employed by the individual, the history should reveal it to be long-standing. The question then becomes whether there has been a change in intensity. A change in intensity of a well-established behavior (he used to tap his face with his fingers, now he uses his fist and leaves a bruise) should also prompt a search for a superimposed process in Axis IV through Axis I.

Although personality disorders are not frequently diagnosed,[33] people meeting the criteria for any of the personality disorders certainly exist in the intellectual and developmental disability population.[34] It is possible for visits to the ED (and psychiatric admission) to become unintentionally reinforcing. PWIDD may learn to express suicidality or "homicidality" when they are angry or frustrated in order to avoid a difficult situation. This lack of mature coping skills should be seen as a behavioral communication perhaps requiring a non-pharmacologic intervention such as a behavioral intervention with a plan for behavioral follow-up. With calm and caring discussion, verbal patients will often own up to the source of their "suicidal" ideation (e.g., "They wouldn't let me go outside"); brief mediation between the staff and the patient can often help build the person's sense of control over their environment and avoid an unnecessary (and potentially detrimental) admission. A period of "cooling off" in the ED, to the extent allowable, can also be helpful in distinguishing a patient in genuine need of psychiatric admission from a person who would best return home with supports and outpatient follow-up. Whenever safety allows, behavioral problems due to life situations or personality vulnerabilities are best handled within the person's home environment coupled with behavioral intervention, outpatient, and/or day-hospital treatment.

Axis I: Psychiatric Illness. Determining an accurate psychiatric diagnosis becomes increasingly difficult as the degree of intellectual disability increases.[35] Making an accurate diagnosis of a new-onset or exacerbated Axis I condition in the ED may well exceed the resources available and in the acute setting may not be as important as recognizing that an Axis I disorder is contributing to the patient's presentation. If so, it should be acknowledged and the appropriate setting sought, based on the available information and consultation. Regardless, making a psychiatric diagnosis in PWIDD should only occur after careful consideration of the other four DSM axes. The importance of this cannot be overemphasized. Most psychiatric facilities are primarily focused on the treatment of acute danger stemming from Axis I problems. Apart from a few, rare specialized units, most facilities have sparse experience with handling PWIDD and their specialized behavioral challenges and treatments. Admission of PWIDD to a general psychiatric facility may be the "path of least resistance" in the ED setting, but often leads to overuse of medication management and development of maladaptive coping mechanisms on the part of the patient. Making a careful diagnosis and disposition in the ED is a tremendous service in the care of PWIDD and can be instrumental in the appropriate allocation of scarce resources.

PWIDD will often arrive with previous Axis I diagnoses that are misleading or inaccurate. The presentations of PWIDD often do not conform well with the criteria of DSM-IV (which was developed for a population without intellectual and developmental disabilities). Thus, patients may receive a "closest fit" diagnosis (e.g., Mood NOS) or a non-traditional diagnosis (e.g., Intermittant Explosive Disorder). For example, if PWIDD with a history of, say, bipolar disorder present to the ED, do not assume that someone has established that the patient has a clear history of classic depressive and manic cycles and that the agitation observed in the ED must therefore be "mania."

In evaluating Axis I, the key is determining if there has been a change from baseline. Many patients at their baseline may appear to "respond to internal stimuli," are "socially withdrawn," have "disrupted sleep," or have other symptoms suggestive of an Axis I disorder. Chronic issues are best evaluated and handled in an outpatient setting. Caregivers should be queried regarding *changes* in the patient's baseline functioning, particularly with regard to vegetative symptoms, interest in usual activities, interactions with others, avoidance of familiar people or situations, irritability, agitation (and associated antecedents and consequences), communication changes, and expressions of mood. The interview with the patient or caregiver will be guided by the history and the differential diagnosis. Sleep and weight logs, if available, are extremely helpful. Significant changes in these markers are valuable indicators of biologic process suggesting an Axis I diagnosis and are useful in differentiating behavior as a communication from psychiatric illness requiring treatment. PWIDD may look markedly different in the ED than they do in their home environment, either for the better or worse. A trip to the ED can be overwhelming for some, or a calming "vacation" from home stresses for others. Thus, while the mental status exam is important, it must be tempered with reports from caregivers.

It bears repeating that the presentations of the major mental illnesses can differ in PWIDD versus the general adult population. Assessing symptoms must be done through the lens of the disability. For instance, new onset stripping behavior may suggest hyper-sexuality for PWIDD who are limited in their ability to express sexuality. New-onset leaving-without-staff-knowledge "behaviors" may suggest the restless wanderlust of mania in PWIDD unable to access any other form of transportation. The DM-ID is a useful reference in thinking through how symptoms may translate.[19] Some comments regarding common symptoms are included in the sections that follow.

Depression. In assessing depression, neurovegetative signs and loss of participation in the activities that normally engage the patient's interest are perhaps the most reliable indicators (no longer enjoying their favorite food, only coloring with somber colors). Some patients may express sadness, but a fair number of patients lack the ability to verbalize their internal emotional state (due to alexithymia or simply poor verbal or introspective skills). Attention and concentration problems are often chronic and therefore have limited diagnostic usefulness.

Suicidality/violent ideation. Though many PWIDD lack the capacity to plan out a completed suicide, the risk of impulsive injury (e.g., drinking bleach or cutting) is still present and, if manifested, may be an indication of suicidal ideation.

Mania. In assessing the manic state, neurovegetative changes, particularly a decreased need for sleep, are most helpful. An increase in goal-directed activity, psychomotor agita-tion, or irritability are suggestive if they span more than a day or so in duration and are not clearly precipitated by situational factors. Irritability precipitated by situational factors should be assessed in comparison to a baseline (e.g., in the past, waiting was not a problem but now it is). Mood lability is common in many patients and may reflect an extended manic or mixed state (appropriate for inpatient management if severe) or personality vulnerabilities (best managed behaviorally at home with outpatient follow-up, or in day hospital). A careful history, along with neurovegetative assessment, can usually distinguish between the two.

Catatonia. While relatively rare in the general population, catatonia (in conjunction with a mood or psychotic disorder) may be more common in PWIDD, particularly in patients with autistic spectrum disorders.[36] Catatonia may present in a variety of ways, from a deficit in activity and speech, so-called "waxy-flexibility" and odd posturing, to purpose-less movements and repetitive utterances. A 1–2 mg IM or IV test dose of lorazepam can help distinguish catatonia (i.e., symptoms should improve, though seizure activity will remain in the differential). Patients with catatonic symptoms should generally be admitted to a psychiatric facility unless the symptoms are non-life-threatening (e.g., the patient is accepting normal meals), are chronic, and are already being managed on an outpatient basis. Use of antipsychotics should generally be avoided in catatonic patients as this can worsen symptoms.[37]

Psychosis. It can be a difficult to assess psychosis in PWIDD. Some PWIDD may have learned to report "voices" in the absence of true psychosis as a maladaptive strategy. In other cases, "voices" or "seeing things" can be recollections of bad memories or past abuse rather than true hallucinations; these are often chronic, situational-exacerbated, and don't necessarily benefit from acute admission. People with very significant intellectual disabilities may simply not be able to understand what you are asking in regard to paranoia and hallucinations. A question such as, "Do you ever hear people talk to you when no one is there" may elicit a positive response simply because of a patient's active internal life (e.g., imaginary friends). Follow-up questions such as, "Do they say nice things or mean things?" and obtaining further characterization may help in the differentiation. Appropriately phrased questions should be used to assess the person's fears and sense of safety. Asking caregivers about any behaviors that would suggest recent fearfulness, self-talk, or self-absorption can be suggestive. A change in the symptomatology, lasting more than a day or so, without a clear secondary-gain or evidence of a behavioral communication should raise suspicion of psychosis.

Anxiety. Many PWIDD will not understand the meaning of words like "anxious," "nervous," and "worried." Be sure to inquire about the patient's understanding when asking such questions. Inquiring "What are you thinking about?" may elicit some worries. Showing the patient drawings of faces in various emotional states may help elicit mood and anxiety symptoms ("Which picture is like you?").

PTSD: There is a growing body of research that demonstrates that people with developmental disabilities are at greater risk for sexual and physical abuse.[24,38] Staff should be thoughtful about potential triggers in the ED environment causing a reexperiencing of past trauma. Finding skilled professionals to address this diagnosis in PWIDD remains challenging but good review articles offering strategies that can be used outside the urgent or emergent setting can be found in the literature.[39,40] Depending on the locality, there is some awareness of the need to develop this expertise in the clinical workforce. This diagnosis is often missed in the acute care setting because PWIDD can be so limited in describing their life stories and their emotional responses to their life experience. Caretakers may not know the details of PWIDD's past life or may not see those past experiences as relevant to present events. The work that is done outside the acute care setting will often determine the impact that can be made in the midst of an emergency.

Attention-related problems. Attention problems are common, and span the range from "too much" (OCD) to "too little" (ADD/ADHD). Behavioral problems associated with attention are common and the ED clinician or ED psychiatrist should be aware of this in assessing the events leading to an ED visit. Internally focused or obsessive patients can become frustrated and agitated when external events force their attention to shift. Overstimulation can similarly lead to agitation. Many "disputes" between patients and caregivers occur because of the inability of patients to maintain focus on necessary tasks or because of their difficulty with reluctance to transition between activities.

Autism. Autistic traits are best considered along a continuum, from small degrees in the "typical" population, to Asperger's disorder, to more "classic" autism. Autism is not to be confused with intellectual disability – patients may have a much higher IQ or even superior IQ than suggested by their presentation – though the two disorders of autism and intellectual disability often coexist. Patients with autism will typically have deficits in verbal expression, but may have good understanding. Some patients with limited spoken communication understand some sign language, an important factor to ascertain in this population. Engaging the patient during the interview may be difficult; redirect the patient's attention to the clinician when needed, but yield if the patient starts to show agitation. People with autistic spectrum disorders can be particularly sensitive to overstimulation; a quiet environment should be provided and inquiries regarding hearing deficits or sound-sensitivity should be sought to help guide the clinician's and staff's volume and type of speech. Providing a video game or other diversion may calm some patients. A heavy blanket will calm some patients (improves proprioception). A certain amount of "rocking," light self-tapping, verbal utterances, or other self-stimulatory behaviors may be normal for the patient and should not necessarily cause concern. Hospital staff should be adequately trained to understand that many people with autistic spectrum disorders will display repetitive actions or motions that function as self-soothing behaviors. Typically, this is seen as hand wringing, hand flapping, or rocking back and forth. Unless these behaviors have reached a level where significant injury to self or others is a concern, staff should not attempt to restrain patients from these behaviors. Physical attempts to prevent patients from engaging in their typical self-soothing actions will almost always lead to increased agitation. However, increases in these behaviors likely indicate increased anxiety or discomfort and efforts should be made to address the underlying cause of the patient's anxiety. Care providers and family members can usually provide hospital staff with very useful information about the patient's typical self-soothing behaviors.

Summary points for the clinician

- Proactively learn the system that serves PWIDD in the catchment area of the ED.
- Proactively understand the legal considerations of guardianship and surrogate decision-makers that are relevant to PWIDD with compromised ability to consent to treatment.
- Pay careful attention to the ED environment and the emotional tone of interactions with PWIDD. Use "people-first" language.
- Collect collateral information, with careful attention to potential bias, and be sure to place emphasis on understanding the evolution of the current target problem.
- Using the multiaxial system as a guide, begin with Axis V establishing optimal baseline functioning and when it last occurred. Use this as the baseline point from which to track the trajectory of the current target behavior.
- Work through Axis V through I seeking superimposed processes that may account for deterioration necessitating an ED visit.
- Be tolerant of some behaviors as they may be adaptive mechanisms, but ensure safety and provide as calm an environment as possible for PWIDD.

References

1. Cottrell RP. The Olmstead decision: landmark opportunity or platform for rhetoric? Our collective responsibility for full community participation. *Am J Occup Ther.* 2005;**59**(5):561–568.

2. Lunsky Y, Gracey C, Gelfand S. Emergency psychiatric services for individuals with intellectual disabilities: perspectives of hospital staff. *Intellect Dev Disabil.* 2008; **46**(6):446–455.

3. Borthwick-Duffy SA. Epidemiology and prevalence of psychopathology in people with mental retardation. *J Consult Clin Psychol.* 1994;**62**(1):17–27.

4. Borthwick-Duffy SA, Eyman RK. Who are the dually diagnosed? *Am J Ment Retard.* 1990;**94**(6):586–595.

5. Grossman SA, Richards CF, Anglin D, Hutson HR. Caring for the patient with mental retardation in the emergency department. *Ann Emerg Med.* 2000;**35**(1): 69–76.

6. Gill F, Stenfert Kroese B, Rose J. General practitioners' attitudes to patients who have learning disabilities. *Psychol Med.* 2002; **32**(8):1445–1455.

7. Lian WB, Ho SK, Yeo CL, Ho LY. General practitioners' knowledge on childhood developmental and behavioural disorders. *Singapore Med J.* 2003;**44**(8):397–403.

8. Friedlander R. Mental health for persons with intellectual disability in the post-deinstitutionalization era: experiences from British Columbia. *Isr J Psychiatry Relat Sci.* 2006;**43**(4):275–280.

9. Lennox N, Chaplin R. The psychiatric care of people with intellectual disabilities: the perceptions of trainee psychiatrists and psychiatric medical officers. *Aust N Z J Psychiatry.* 1995;**29**(4):632–637.

10. La Forge J. Preferred language practice in professional rehabilitation journals. *Journal of Rehabilitation.* 1991;**57**(1):49–51.

11. VanderSchie-Bezyak JL. Service problems and solutions for individuals with mental retardation and mental illness. *Journal of Rehabilitation.* 2003;**69**(1):53.

12. Bradley E, Lofchy J. Learning disablity in the Accident and Emergency Department. *Adv Psychiatric Treatment.* 2005;**11**:45–57.

13. Weiss J, Lunsky Y, Gracey C, Canrinus MMS. Emergency psychiatric services for individuals with intellectual disabilities: caregivers' perspectives. *JARID.* 2009;**22**:354–362.

14. Hewitt A, Larson S. The direct support workforce in community supports to individuals with developmental disabilities: issues, implications, and promising practices. *Ment Retard Dev Disabil Res Rev.* 2007;**13**(2):178–187.

15. Reiss S, Levitan GW, Szyszko J. Emotional disturbance and mental retardation: diagnostic overshadowing. *Am J Ment Defic.* 1982;**86**(6):567–574.

16. Jopp DA, Keys CB. Diagnostic overshadowing reviewed and reconsidered. *Am J Ment Retard.* 2001;**106**(5):416–433.

17. Hovermale L. When people with developmental disabilities present to community practitioners. *Md Med J.* 1997;**46**(7):363–366.

18. American Psychiatric Association. *Diagnostic and Statistical Manual of Mental Disorders, Fourth Edition, Text Revision.* Washington, DC: American Psychiatric Association, 2000.

19. Fletcher R, Loschen E, Stavrakaki C, First M (Eds.), *Diagnostic Manual – Intellectual Disability.* Kingston, NY: NADD Press/ National Association for the Dually Diagnosed, 2007.

20. Hurley AD. Axis IV and Axis V: Assessment of persons with mental retardation and developmental disabilities. *Mental Health Aspects of Developmental Disabilities.* 2001;**4**(1):21.

21. Rush KS, Bowman LG, Eidman SL, Toole LM, Mortenson BP. Assessing psychopathology in individuals with developmental disabilities. *Behav Modif.* 2004;**28**(5):621–637.

22. The Developmental Disabilities Assistance and Bill of Rights Act of 2000. 2000;**42** USC:**102**(8).

23. Ryan R. Posttraumatic stress disorder in persons with developmental disabilities. *Community Ment Health J.* 1994;**30**(1): 45–54.

24. Sobsey D. *Violence and Abuse in the Lives of People with Disabilities: The End of Silent Acceptance.* Baltimore, MD: Paul H. Brookes Publishing Co., 1994.

25. Beange H, McElduff A, Baker W. Medical disorders of adults with mental retardation: a population study. *Am J Ment Retard.* 1995;**99**(6):595–604.

26. Zigman WB, Devenny DA, Krinsky-McHale SJ, et al. Alzheimer's disease in adults with Down syndrome. *Int Rev Res Ment Retard.* 2008;**36**:103–145.

27. Smith DS. Health care management of adults with Down syndrome. *Am Fam Physician.* 2001;**64**(6):1031–1038.

28. Wilson DN, Haire A. Health care screening for people with mental handicap living in the community. *BMJ* 1990;**301**(6765): 1379–1381.

29. King BH, Hollander E, Sikich L, et al. Lack of efficacy of citalopram in children with autism spectrum disorders and high levels of repetitive behavior: citalopram ineffective in children with autism. *Arch Gen Psychiatry.* 2009;**66**(6):583–590.

30. Matson JL, Bamburg JW, Mayville EA, et al. Psychopharmacology and mental retardation: a 10 year review (1990-1999). *Res Dev Disabil.* 2000;**21**(4):263–296.

31. Kalachnik JE, Hanzel TE, Sevenich R, Harder SR. Benzodiazepine behavioral side effects: review and implications for individuals with mental retardation. *Am J Ment Retard.* 2002;**107**(5):376–410.

32. Beshay H, Pumariega AJ. Sertraline treatment of mood disorder associated with prednisone: a case report. *J Child Adolesc Psychopharmacol.* 1998;8(3):187–193.

33. Holden P, Neff JA. Intensive outpatient treatment of persons with mental retardation and psychiatric disorder: a preliminary study. *Mental Retardation* 2000;38(1):27–32.

34. Hurley AD, Sovner R. Six cases of patients with mental retardation who have antisocial personality disorder. *Psychiatr Serv.* 1995;46(8):828–831.

35. Rush AM, Frances AM. Expert Consensus Guideline Series: Treatment of psychiatric and behavioral problems in mental retardation. *Am J Ment Retard.* 2000; 105(3):159–226.

36. Dhossche DM, Reti IM, Wachtel LE. Catatonia and autism: a historical review, with implications for electroconvulsive therapy. *JECT* 2009;25(1):19–22.

37. Fink M, Taylor MA. The catatonia syndrome: forgotten but not gone. *Arch Gen Psychiatry.* 2009;66(11):1173–1177.

38. Sullivan PM, Knutson JF. Maltreatment and disabilities: a population-based epidemiological study. *Child Abuse Negl.* 2000;24(10):1257–1273.

39. Focht-New G, Barol B, Clements PT, Milliken TF. Persons with developmental disability exposed to interpersonal violence and crime: approaches for intervention. *Perspect Psychiatr Care.* 2008;44(2):89–98.

40. Focht-New G, Clements PT, Barol B, Faulkner MJ, Service KP. Persons with developmental disabilities exposed to interpersonal violence and crime: strategies and guidance for assessment. *Perspect Psychiatr Care.* 2008;44(1):3–13.

Emergency management of eating disorders

Graham W. Redgrave, James Harrison, and Angela S. Guarda

Introduction

Eating disorders are common, complicated, and highly morbid illnesses. These are disorders characterized by extreme disturbances in eating behaviors that result in either a reduction in caloric intake, extreme over-eating, or extreme distress about body weight or shape. Eating disorders have become one of the most medically consequential psychiatric conditions, because individuals engaged in eating disorder behaviors are, by definition, altering normal physiology in the pursuit of various goals. These goals usually include weight loss or prevention of weight gain – but could also include regulation of mood and anxiety. The manipulation of normal physiological functions that occurs in eating disorders can have lethal effects on multiple organ systems, including the cardiac, neurologic, metabolic, and gastrointestinal systems. The alteration in normal caloric intake can also adversely impact pre-existing or more chronic, but nevertheless problematic, impairments of the musculoskeletal and endocrine systems. In addition, eating disorders commonly co-occur with, and can complicate, the management of more easily recognized psychiatric conditions such as mood and anxiety, personality, and substance use disorders and suicide. Early diagnosis and proper management will help to limit the impact of these disorders; acute care providers can improve their role in decreasing morbidity and mortality of eating disorders with a greater understanding of the diagnostic criteria and management of these conditions.

Patients with eating disorders will often not be forthcoming about the nature or extent of their behaviors for several reasons. First, these behaviors are rewarding to patients, which mitigates their desire to seek behavioral change. Second, many patients will have poor insight regarding their condition and their behaviors. Third, even when patients are aware of their condition, eating disorders are so stigmatized by society that there is a reluctance by patients to be forthcoming. Though it is tempting to think it easy to recognize someone with an eating disorder because of presumed extreme emaciation, the majority of patients with eating disorders are normal weight or overweight. Thus, about half of those with eating disorders in the general population go unrecognized.[1] Accordingly, there is reliance on acute care clinicians and other providers to make the appropriate diagnosis, manage complications, and make timely referrals. Failure to do so often leads to repeat visits to the emergency department, increased morbidity and mortality, and the loss of an opportunity to make a definitive intervention.

Emergency Psychiatry, ed. Arjun Chanmugam, Patrick Triplett, and Gabor Kelen. Published by Cambridge University Press. © Cambridge University Press 2013.

Most patients do not present to the emergency department for treatment of their eating disorders, but rather because of associated complications. Certain presentations should suggest further evaluation for an eating disorder especially in young women with either hypokalemia, brittle diabetes with recurrent diabetic ketoacidosis, seizures, syncope, or abdominal pain, to name a few of the many possible presentations. To help improve early recognition and appropriate management, this chapter is presented in four main parts: (1) brief overview of the conceptual model, diagnosis, and management of eating disorders; (2) acute and life-threatening presentations; (3) chronic problems presenting in emergency settings; (4) special issues, such as working with minors and families, coercion and involuntary hospitalization, and locating appropriate eating disorder resources.

Conceptual model, diagnosis, and workup

Conceptual model: eating disorders are motivated behavioral disorders

Understanding the nature of eating disorders is vital to avoiding the two most common mistakes in management: (1) overemphasis on symptomatic management without addressing the underlying disorder, and (2) blaming patients and/or families. Treating symptoms alone colludes with patients' denial of the nature and severity of the problem and the desire to avoid behavior change. Although symptom treatment may initially and temporarily stabilize the patient, ignoring the underlying disorder will likely result in the continuation of the behaviors that caused the initial symptom complex. Blaming patients who often feel intensely ashamed and guilty often produces hostility or hopelessness and does not effect change; blaming families alienates potential allies in the treatment of the eating disorder. By regarding eating disorders as **disorders of motivated behavior**, clinicians can take a clear, supportive, but effective approach that addresses the underlying cause of the immediate presentation.

The motivated behaviors are those that are governed by *drives*, and include sleep, sexual, and eating drives. These behaviors are central to the survival of individuals and species. All animals must seek adequate amounts of sleep, food satiation, and sex in order to maintain an evolutionary advantage.

Motivated behaviors take place in cycles. Over time, we become hungry, seek out food, eat until we are satiated, and, after some time, we become hungry and repeat these behaviors (Figure 14.1).[2] In time we learn by conditioning from the consequences of our behavior what and when to eat. Similar cycles exist for sleep and sexual behaviors. Because these behaviors are so vital for our survival, complex neurohormonal mechanisms have evolved that drive us to eat, sleep, and engage in sexual activity (procreate). In the case of eating, there are at least 25 different hormones that participate in the drive mechanism.[3]

The phenomenon for humans is further complicated by the fact that we are deeply social creatures, and our behavior is strongly influenced by the cultures and social environment within which we live. The societal value of thinness, the availability of leisure time to exercise and eat, and the contemporary overabundance of cheap, calorie-dense food in many Western societies all combine to increase the risk for vulnerable individuals to develop eating disorders.

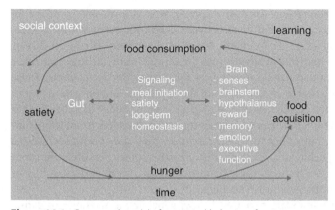

Figure 14.1. Conceptual model of motivated behavior of eating.
The cycle begins with hunger, followed by the acquisition and consumption of food, and finally satiation. Learning's arc goes in the opposite direction of time's arrow because we learn from the consequences of our behavior. Multiple neural and hormonal mechanisms facilitate communication between gut and brain to ensure that we eat as much energy as we burn (homeostasis). Eating disorder patients, through a combination of aberrant biology, social influences, and maladaptive learning, engage in repeated bouts of excessive eating or dieting, purgation, overexercise, and other behaviors. Seeing eating disorders as disorders of motivated behaviors allows clinicians to be sympathetic (because of how difficult eating disordered urges are to resist, as they are based on the same biological reward mechanisms as normal eating), but clear that as long as the behaviors persist, the eating disorder and all of its complications cannot be effectively treated. (Figure adapted with permission from McHugh and Slavney, 1998.[2])

Seen from this perspective, those with eating disorders are at war with their physiology, a conflict that produces multiple physical and psychological symptoms. Consider the extreme discomfort of breath holding until stars appear, or avoidance of urinating with a full bladder. In this light it is much easier to understand the distress of those engaged in complex behaviors that are appreciated as harmful, but which at another level are as rewarding as an illicit drug.

Viewing eating disorders as motivated behavior disorders allows the emergency clinician to avoid the pitfalls of excessive focus on symptoms or blaming the patient. Treating symptoms alone relieves short-term suffering but does nothing to interrupt the behaviors and therefore nothing to treat the illness. Blaming the patient ignores the large body of evidence showing that once an eating disorder is established, biological mechanisms as strong as instinctual drives make it difficult to resist urges to engage in eating disorder behaviors. Instead, the clinician should emphasize the fact that, though the patient did not choose the illness, they must resist the urges and initially make difficult choices to eat healthily because the medical (and in some cases social) consequences of the eating disorder will not go away without behavioral change.

Diagnosis

There are three main eating disorders: anorexia nervosa (AN), bulimia nervosa (BN), and binge eating disorder (BED). There is also a large, catchall diagnostic category called eating disorder not otherwise specified (EDNOS). For the emergency clinician it is more important to make the diagnosis of "eating disorder" and to ascertain what behaviors the patient is doing, rather than worrying too much about in which diagnostic category the patient is best placed. This approach is advantageous for two reasons. First, the nosology of eating disorders is flawed (patients move back and forth between diagnostic categories over time, and many clinically significant eating disorders do not meet diagnostic criteria for AN or BN). Second, it is the cycle of abnormal behaviors and the thoughts and feelings that cause and are caused by the behaviors that have consequences for eating disorder patients. These complications are related to the degree of restriction of dietary intake and purgation and to other behaviors such as excessive exercise or failure to dose insulin, rather than to whether the patient has AN, BN, or EDNOS. The key to diagnosing eating disorders is not ruling out all conceivable medical causes, but rather to take a careful history and specifically ask the patient about his or her eating behaviors. A careful history may require persistent inquiries to both the patient and other sources until the diagnostician has a clear understanding of the type of behaviors in which the patient is engaging.

While two screening instruments are reviewed below, generally, a diagnosis of eating disorder can be made if the presentation is attributable to repetitive engagement in abnormal eating or eating-related behaviors paired with strong fears or desires related to food, weight, or shape. Those fears or desires have been called "morbid fear of fatness" or a "drive for thinness"[4,5] and manifest themselves in a variety of ways. These manifestations include worrying about what the number reads on the scale, how clothes fit, how lean they are, the shape of particular parts of their bodies (especially stomach, hips, thighs, and upper arms), wanting to look a certain way in comparison to others, wanting to eat excessively healthily, and so forth.

The abnormal behaviors in which patients engage include dietary restriction (which might include skipping meals, only eating a certain number of calories, eliminating as much dietary fat as possible, eating only "safe" foods, and others), binge eating (eating an excessive amount of food, usually greater than 1000 kcal, in a discrete period of time while simultaneously feeling out of control), purging (vomiting, laxative abuse), diuretic, diet pill, or ipecac abuse, excessive exercising, chewing and spitting food, regurgitation and rumination of food, and others.

For completeness sake, we will briefly review the diagnostic criteria for eating disorders as delineated by the American Psychiatric Association.[6] The diagnosis of AN requires that the patient be at or below a weight 85% of that expected, roughly a body mass index (BMI) of <18 kg/m^2 in adults; intense fear of gaining weight or becoming fat, even though underweight; disturbance in the way in which one's body weight or shape is experienced, undue influence of body weight or shape on self-evaluation, or denial of the seriousness of the current low body weight; and, in postmenarcheal females, amenorrhea, i.e., the absence of at least three consecutive menstrual cycles. Patients with AN may or may not engage in binge eating or purging. (AN is sometimes further classified as one of two types – restricting AN and bingeing or purging AN. Restricting AN refers to those patients who restrict their caloric intake, and do not engage in bingeing and purging. Purging or bingeing AN refers to those patients who induce vomiting or misuse laxatives, emetics, enemas, or diuretics.)

The diagnosis of BN requires twice-weekly binge eating for at least three months; recurrent inappropriate compensatory behavior in order to prevent weight gain (e.g., self-induced vomiting; misuse of laxatives, diuretics, enemas, or other medications; fasting; or excessive exercise), again, at least twice-weekly for three months; self-evaluation unduly influenced by body shape and weight; and the disturbance does not occur exclusively during episodes of AN. The diagnosis of BED is made when binge eating occurs without inappropriate compensatory mechanisms being employed.

There are some patients who become significantly underweight or engage in self-induced vomiting or other behaviors for reasons other than fear of fatness. These patients, with so-called "atypical" eating disorders, are still at risk for complications as much as those with more classic eating disorder symptoms, and are probably more likely to go undiagnosed in the general population. Again, counseling about the consequences of behavior, irrespective of underlying mindset, is crucial.

Screening

Two screening instruments in general use are the SCOFF[7] and ESP[8] (see Table 14.1). Both have comparable sensitivity and specificity and are easy to administer. A positive screen (two or more positive responses on either instrument) warrants some brief follow-up questions, such as, "What would you like to weigh?", "What did you eat yesterday for breakfast, lunch and dinner?", as well as asking about time spent exercising, frequency of bingeing, vomiting, laxative diuretic and diet pill abuse in the past month, etc. The patient's actual height and weight should be measured and the BMI calculated from these data (or see the online BMI calculator at http://www.nhlbisupport.com/bmi/). There should not be a reliance on the patient's self-reported weight or height. Most women with AN or BN will have desired weights that are below the normal weight for their height. BED is associated with obesity (BMI >30), but not everyone with BED is obese. Other behaviors suggestive of an eating disorder include recent change to vegetarianism, refusal to eat meals with others, social isolation, and dressing to conceal the body.[9] Two questions which have been shown to be very sensitive when posed by primary care physicians are "Do you ever eat in secret?" and "How satisfied are you with your eating habits?"[10] Additional signs and symptoms of eating disorders are presented in Table 14.2.

Table 14.1. Two screening instruments for eating disorders

SCOFF[7]	ESP (Eating Disorder Screen for Primary Care)[8]
Do you make yourself **Sick** because you feel uncomfortably full?	Are you satisfied with your eating patterns?
Do you worry you have lost **Control** over how much you eat?	Do you ever eat in secret?
Have you lost more than **One** stone* over the last three months?	Does your weight affect how you feel about yourself? Has anyone in your family ever suffered with an eating disorder?
Do you believe yourself to be **Fat** when others say you are thin?	Do you currently suffer with or in the past have you suffered with an eating disorder?
Would you say that **Food** dominates your life?	
*One stone is 14 lbs., or 6.4 kg.	
*One stone is 14 lbs., or 6.4 kg. Cut off: two or more abnormal responses has sensitivity of 100%, specificity of 87.5% for an eating disorder	Cut off: two or more abnormal responses has sensitivity of 100%, specificity of 71% for an eating disorder

Table 14.2. Signs and symptoms of eating disorders related to starvation or purgation

Starvation-related signs and symptoms	Purging-related signs and symptoms
Dry skin, lanugo hair, scalp hair loss	Perioral acne
Cold intolerance, hypothermia	Parotid gland enlargement
Acrocyanosis	Dental caries and erosion (lingual surface of teeth)
Weakness, fatigue, or low energy (despite high physical activity)	Orthostatic hypotension and dehydration
Sinus bradycardia, orthostatic hypotension	Presyncope and syncope
Presyncope and syncope	Heartburn, gastroesophageal reflux
Early satiety	Muscle cramps and paresthesias (from electrolyte abnormalities)
Bloating	Diarrhea and constipation (laxative abusers)
Constipation	Cardiac arrhythmias
Primary or secondary amenorrhea	Oligomenorrhea or amenorrhea
Peripheral neuropathy	
Decreased bone density, fractures	
Muscle wasting and cachexia	
Nose bleeds, bruising (thrombocytopenia)	

Acute or life-threatening presentations of eating disorders

The mortality of AN has been consistently shown to be very high, with a recent study showing a standardized mortality ratio of 6.2, meaning that AN patients are more than six times more likely to die than age-matched peers.[11] In BN, the evidence is more mixed, but a recent study found increased all-cause mortality in a large sample.[12] Morbidity in eating disorders is related directly to weight status (underweight, obesity, or rapid weight loss into a normal weight range) or purging behaviors.

Patients who die with AN do so from cardiac and endocrine mechanisms, renal and pulmonary infections (mostly pyelonephritis and pneumonia), or from suicide or complications of substance abuse. One reason infectious causes may play a large role in the mortality of AN is that patients with AN may not be able to mount an adequate fever response, so diagnosis may be delayed.[13] AN patients may also be more susceptible to sepsis and opportunistic infections because of immunosuppression from malnutrition.

Unless otherwise noted, the medical management of these conditions does not differ for eating disorder patients and the general population.

Severely underweight patients

Patients who present with a BMI ≤ 14 kg/m^2 are emergently ill and should be hospitalized for treatment when possible both because of the medical morbidities associated with this state and also because patients this underweight are more likely to suffer from serious complications of refeeding syndrome including hypophosphatemia and pulmonary edema among others. Patients may require involuntary treatment (see section below on coercion and involuntary treatment).

Cardiovascular

Dysrhythmias

The three most significant cardiovascular concerns in patients with eating disorders are dysrhythmias, cardiomyopathy, and heart failure.[14] Dysrhythmias are seen in patients who are underweight and/or engaged in significant purgation (vomiting, or laxative or diuretic abuse). Patients with restricting AN are often found to have significant bradycardia, often in the severe range of 30–40 beats per minute. This may be due to increased vagal tone and usually corrects with refeeding.[15] AN and BN have both been associated with prolonged QT interval, which increases risk for ventricular arrhythmias, including ventricular tachycardia and sudden cardiac death.[14] There is also evidence that heart rate variability may play a role in cardiac morbidity in AN.[16] Dysrhythmias do not appear to be associated with any specific prodromal symptoms, and care is warranted in the management of the severely underweight patient who also purges, since this group is at highest risk as a consequence of electrolyte abnormalities.[17] Correction of electrolyte imbalances and repletion of magnesium are required to minimize the likelihood of dysrhythmias in the short term, while refeeding is vital in the middle and long term. In the patient who is significantly underweight, care should be taken not to rapidly or injudiciously hydrate lest the volume repletion cause fluid overload conditions such as congestive heart failure or pulmonary edema. Asymptomatic hypotension is best managed conservatively with very careful and judicious use of IV hydration or oral repletion alone.

Cardiomyopathy

The two main causes of structural cardiac changes in eating disorders are starvation and ipecac abuse. Starvation alters cardiac structure, reducing left ventricular size, septal thickness, the cardiac index, and cardiac output.[14,18] Syrup of ipecac was once a widely used cough syrup and emetic. Its active ingredient, emetine, is toxic to cardiac myocytes. Accordingly, since 2003, the American Academy of Pediatrics has recommended that it not be kept in the house and that supplies be destroyed. It has subsequently become difficult to obtain in the US.[19] Nevertheless, ipecac is still used by some to induce emesis as part of purging type AN or BN, and emergency clinicians should be mindful of this method of purgation when assessing patients with eating disorders, particularly since it has been associated with cardiac morbidity and sudden cardiac death.[14] Management of cardiomyopathy includes avoidance of fluid overload (either from refeeding or aggressive hydration) in the short term, and weight restoration and cessation of ipecac use in the long term. Both of these measures will increase the likelihood that the heart will return to normal size and function.

Heart failure

Heart failure in eating disorders is more common in patients during refeeding than in the acutely starved or purged state, so it is less likely that it will present de novo in the emergency setting. However, occasionally very compliant patients will develop refeeding syndrome with heart failure during outpatient treatment. (See below for a discussion of refeeding syndrome.)

Metabolic: acid-base imbalances and the refeeding syndrome

Metabolic disturbances in eating disorders generally present as a direct response to purgation but are exacerbated by being extremely underweight. Patients who vomit or abuse laxatives are at risk for developing a hypokalemic, hypochloremic metabolic alkalosis.[20] It is possible for these patients to have chronically low serum potassium levels of well below 3, or even 2 mEq/L. Furthermore, there is some evidence that repleting potassium in patients with eating disorders may be more difficult because patients are often in a state of excess cortisol.[21] These patients usually require intensive potassium repletion, but the usual rule of thumb of repleting 10 mg of KCl per mEq/L of deficiency may not be sufficient. Repeat measurement of electrolytes should guide to repletion. It should be kept in mind that undernourished patients with hypokalemia will often have total body potassium depletion as well and will likely require days of potassium replacement in a hospitalized setting. Patients with resistant hypokalemia may be hypomagnesemic and will require magnesium repletion before their serum potassium repletion is effective.

Refeeding syndrome is a potentially life-threatening complication of the treatment of anorexia nervosa and consists of hypomagnesemia, hypophosphatemia, and hypoglycemia. It may be accompanied by elevated liver transaminases. Though it is more usually seen in inpatients undergoing refeeding, it may be seen in patients in outpatient treatment as well, and it is therefore important for emergency clinicians to be aware of this condition. Treatment includes supportive management and reduction in the rate of caloric intake to more modest levels (e.g., for patients whose BMI is <16, initial caloric intake of no more than 17–20 kcal/lb).[22] Several risk factors are thought to raise the risk of refeeding syndrome, including BMI <16 kg/m^2, weight loss of >15% in the previous 3–6 months, little or no nutritional intake for >10 days, low levels of potassium, phosphorus, or magnesium before refeeding, or history of alcohol or drug misuse, including insulin, chemotherapy, antacids, or diuretics.[22]

Neurologic

Central pontine myelinolysis

Central pontine myelinolysis (CPM) is a potentially fatal syndrome, occurring in patients with severe or prolonged hyponatremia and particularly associated with overly rapid correction of hyponatremia that results in the demyelination of the pons.[23] Risk factors include malnutrition, alcoholism, liver disease (particularly post-operative patients with liver transplant), and severe hypoglycemia. Patients are unlikely to present to the emergency department with a CPM presentation. Rather, the emergency presentation is likely to be depressed level of consciousness or delirium associated with a low serum sodium level. If sodium repletion occurs at a rapid rate the patient may improve in the short run, but within two to three days there is neurologic deterioration as a result of CPM. CPM should be considered in such patients. Presentation includes depressed level of awareness (confusion) and pseudobulbar palsy (head and neck weakness, dysarthria, and dysphagia). Symptoms may progress over one to two weeks to include impaired thinking, weakness, spastic quadriplegia, and balance problems. Coma and even death may ensue.[24] One key finding pointing to this diagnosis is horizontal gaze paralysis. Magnetic resonance imaging (MRI) will show significant demylelination of the pons.

Clinicians must recognize the potential for CPM in all patients with severe or prolonged hyponatremia and avoid it by correcting hyponatremia in a slow, carefully monitored fashion. The initial goal is to raise serum sodium to 125 mmol/L at a rate of only 1–2 mmol/h.

Hypoglycemia

In severely underweight patients, intravenous administration of 5% dextrose (D5W) continuously and slowly (roughly 75cc per hour) should proceed until blood sugars normalize. (A suggested protocol involves fingerstick blood glucose (FSBG) measurements at 10am, 3pm, 10pm, and 3am, while administering D5W until 48 hours of FSBG >70 has been achieved. Once that has been reached, IV fluids may be discontinued, but FSBG are monitored for a further 8 hours.)

Wernicke-Korsakoff syndrome

Wernicke encephalopathy is caused by low thiamine levels and has been characterized classically as a triad of ophthalmoplegia, ataxia, and confusion that may progress to a chronic encephalopathy called Korsakoff syndrome. The condition is difficult to identify because only 16% of cases present with the classic triad. MRI (specifically T2 and fluid-attenuated inversion recovery (FLAIR) sequences) may be the best diagnostic test.[25] It is vital that severely underweight patients, with a body mass index under 15 kg/m^2, be administered thiamine 100 mg intramuscularly or intravenously immediately – but especially before ingestion or administration of IV glucose – if they present with findings consistent with Wernicke-Korsakoff syndrome. Thiamine should then be continued orally on a daily basis during refeeding.

Seizures

Patients who drink excessive amounts of water to transiently increase their weight (and thereby avoid consequences imposed by family or physicians) are at risk of developing seizures, secondary to dilutional hyponatremia. Also at risk for seizures are patients in states of starvation with resulting severely low dips in blood sugar. Seizures may develop in undernourished patients who develop hypophosphatemia during refeeding as well.[26,27]

In general, acute management of seizures in patients with eating disorders does not differ from the general medical patient with seizures. Ensuring the physical safety of the patient is the first step. Most seizures are likely to be self-limited. However, multiple seizures and status epilepticus will of course require pharmacologic control. A systematic and careful search for the immediate cause with close monitoring should be undertaken. As with other sequelae conditions in this chapter, recognition of the role of the eating disorder in the pathogenesis of the seizures is vital because treatment of the eating disorder will be the best way to prevent recurrence of the condition.

Gastrointestinal

Superior mesenteric artery syndrome

The superior mesenteric artery (SMA) syndrome occurs when the SMA and the aorta intermittently compress the third part of the duodenum because of loss of normal mesenteric fat.[28] Patients with SMA syndrome present with intermittent pain after eating, nausea, vomiting, and weight loss. Symptoms may go undiagnosed for years until they escalate but may also develop acutely or subacutely, particularly after rapid weight loss. Historically, barium swallow was the diagnostic method of choice, though more contemporary techniques like computed tomography (CT) with oral contrast are also used. The difficulty in making the diagnosis of SMA syndrome in patients with eating disorders is that all of the symptoms of SMA syndrome are also seen in eating disorders.[29] Clinicians must therefore think carefully about this diagnosis, especially in patients with very rapid weight loss. Treatment is either conservative or surgical, usually involving division of the ligament of Treitz.

Acute gastric dilatation

Acute gastric distention or dilatation is a rare side effect of binge-eating and may be more common in early rapid refeeding or binge eating in very underweight patients. It can result in gastric necrosis, perforation, shock, and death.[30] Diagnosis is usually made by abdominal radiography and/or CT. Treatment should include emergent nasogastric decompression but may require gastrostomy of necrotic tissue.

Mallory Weiss tear

Recurrent, forceful vomiting can cause longitudinal dissections of the distal esophagus and proximal stomach, otherwise known as a Mallory Weiss tear. While the amount of blood lost by this mechanism is usually small and self-limited, it can be large and life-threatening. Treatment is endoscopic repair by any of a variety of means and supportive treatment: about half of cases will require blood transfusion. Predictors of a complicated course are active bleeding and hematemesis.[31,32] Eating disorders are one of five identified risk factors for gastroesophageal intussusception, a frequent precursor of Mallory Weiss tears.[33]

Psychiatric

Suicide

The main acute, life-threatening psychiatric complication of eating disorders is suicide, the most significant non-natural cause of death in patients with eating disorders. The standardized mortality ratio is estimated to be 13–28.[11,34,35] In a recent study, suicide accounted for 20–30% of all deaths in AN.[11] Careful assessment of suicide risk and direct questioning regarding suicidal ideation is important. A sympathetic stance is crucial as patients notoriously underreport or deny suicidal thinking if they feel they are not going to be taken seriously. Of note, patients with eating disorders may be otherwise functional at work or school, so family and friends may not know the extent of suicidal thinking. All complaints of suicidal ideation in eating disorders should be taken very seriously.

Chronic eating disorder problems presenting in the emergency setting

Eating disorders cause chronic medical and psychiatric morbidity in addition to the acute and life-threatening conditions noted above. As stated above, in helping manage these conditions, emergency clinicians should emphasize to the patient that symptomatic relief provides a short-term solution but will not treat the underlying problem. Successful management will require interruption of abnormal eating and related behaviors (such as over-exercise or under-dosing insulin in a type I diabetic) and weight restoration if underweight. Repeated presentations with multiple eating disorder-related complaints suggest that patients will need a higher level of care for their condition, such as intensive outpatient treatment, partial hospitalization, or inpatient treatment (see below for finding referral sources).

Cardiovascular

The most frequent cardiovascular complaint associated with eating disorders is syncope. Syncope may occur because of hypovolemia (caused by severe fluid restriction or purgation), autonomic instability, or arrhythmia (as may occur with hypokalemia). Fluid resuscitation may be warranted but should be carefully considered in the context of possible cardiac dysfunction noted above. In the case of autonomic instability, fluid resuscitation may not correct vital sign abnormalities. Again, the mainstay of treatment is treatment of the underlying eating disorder. Following emergency department management, patients who continue to exhibit autonomic instability despite adequate fluid repletion, hypokalemia and other electrolyte disturbances, arrhythmias, and ECG changes (particularly left bundle branch block, fascicular blocks, or prolonged QT) should be admitted for monitoring and further management.

Gastrointestinal

As should be expected, there are a number of chronic gastrointestinal complaints associated with eating disorders, including gastroesophageal reflux, constipation, bloating, diarrhea, pain, gastroparesis, and rectal prolapse. Eating disorders, whether AN or BN, cause delayed gastric emptying, decreased small bowel follow through, and delayed colonic transit time, resulting in early satiety, constipation, bloating, and abdominal pain.[36–38] In discussing these conditions with the patient in the emergency department, it should be emphasized that treatment of the eating disorder, while often physically uncomfortable at first (constipation transiently worsens, for example), is the best way to improve a whole host of gastrointestinal symptoms.[39]

Standard therapy for reflux is appropriate. In treating constipation, stimulant laxatives should be avoided whenever possible. Hydration and osmotic agents like polyethylene glycol, given every two hours, or soap suds/mineral oil/glycerin enemas are appropriate first line therapies. Diarrhea is managed by discontinuation of laxatives and gentle hydration. Gastroparesis, which in these patients is almost always secondary to dietary restriction or purgation (except in the case of longstanding type I diabetes), should preferentially be addressed by normalization of eating patterns rather than through the use of pro-motility agents.

Musculoskeletal

Female patients with AN who have been amenorrheic for as little as six months are at risk for developing osteopenia, and such patients remain at elevated risk of significant fractures for decades after the diagnosis of AN.[21,40] There is evidence that treatment with estrogen does not improve bone mineral density. Bisphosphonates should be avoided in women of child-bearing age because they are stored in bone, are teratogenic in animals, and are apparently ineffective in AN. Finally, weight restoration appears to be the only consistent mechanism for improvement of bone mineral density.[41]

Psychiatric

There are a variety of effects of eating disorder behaviors on mood and anxiety. Starvation causes many symptoms of depression, including apathy, diminished energy, poor sleep, and worsening obsessiveness, among others.[42] Patients with BN frequently report a short-term euphoria or numbness before or during binge eating and purging, but further questioning usually reveals poor mood as a consequence of the behaviors in the long term.

Patients with eating disorders are more likely to have other psychiatric disorders as well, although this phenomenon is non-specific. Persons with one psychiatric diagnosis are more likely to have a second or third diagnosis.[43,44] Patients with eating disorders are generally at elevated risk for alcohol and drug abuse and dependence (particularly those engaged in purging behaviors, either binge/purge AN or BN), mood and anxiety disorders, personality disorders, and self-injury[45–51] In our experience, patients with multiple diagnoses require concurrent treatment for all clinically significant conditions. Mood and anxiety tends to worsen early in treatment for eating disorders. Patients with other problem behaviors such as self-injury or substance abuse tend to increase these behaviors when attempting to stop eating disorder behaviors. Without adequate support for, and treatment of, these other conditions, simply focusing on arresting eating disordered behavior will likely be ineffective in the long term.

Special issues in the emergency management of eating disorders

There are several issues in the treatment of eating disorders that require special mention. This section will address: working with children and families in the emergency setting, using coercion and involuntary hospitalization, and locating inpatient and outpatient referrals for appropriate patients.

Working with children and families

Children and adolescents with eating disorders present an opportunity and a challenge for the emergency clinician. On the one hand, patients are likely to have been ill for a shorter time; this is a good prognostic indicator. On the other hand, children and adolescents frequently use differences of parental opinion to "divide and conquer" their parents' efforts to obtain treatment. Often one parent is more cautious about the diagnosis and requires more convincing that there is, in fact, an eating disorder present. Alternatively a parent may believe that the patient should simply be able to stop on his/her own. This is truer in broken and otherwise dysfunctional families, where step-parents and animosities may exacerbate otherwise relatively minor disagreements about treatment planning. Whatever the family situation, it is crucial to explain to parents, grandparents – and anyone involved in the care of the patient – that they must parent the child with one voice, because the patient will be ambivalent about recovery and will therefore require firm limit-setting and clear consequences for failing to behave within those limits. Minors who have been ill less than three years may be well-suited to family-based treatment, known as the "Maudsley method," in which parents are coached to set firm limits and guide their children to eat in a healthy manner.[52]

Coercion and involuntary hospitalization

Ambivalence towards treatment is a core feature of eating disorders. Eating disorders are by definition rewarding, and the more patients engage in associated behaviors, the more narrow their behavioral repertoire becomes and the more limited their view of their world. Because eating disorders are so morbid, and because mortality is so high, patients must sometimes be pressured into treatment. This can range from having parents refuse to pay for college unless their child completes treatment all the way to involuntary hospitalization in a psychiatric facility. Such steps are justified because patients tend to feel better about accepting treatment once they have had some treatment, even if initially coerced. For example, in one study, 40% of the group of patients who felt most coerced into treatment ultimately recognized their need for treatment and agreed they needed to stay in the hospital after completing two weeks of inpatient treatment on a specialty unit for eating disorders.[53] Weight gain in involuntarily hospitalized treatment has been shown to be equivalent to voluntary patients, suggesting that once hospitalized, involuntary patients are willing and able to comply with treatment when provided within an expert eating disorders behavioral program.[54,55] Eating disorder behaviors affect cognitive function and worldview, and therefore patients tend to have a much different outlook once they have been weight restored and are "clean and sober" from behaviors such as excessive exercise and purgation. Furthermore, group therapy in a behavioral eating disorder program is especially effective in helping patients recognize the impact of their eating disorder and in motivating them to change their behavior.

Finding inpatient and outpatient referrals for eating disorders

If the resources are available, probably the most common outpatient treatment model is the team approach. This approach, as the name suggests, will involve a number of providers, ideally including: a psychiatrist responsible for managing medications, a primary care physician for medical complications, a nutritionist managing the meal plan, and a therapist (master's or doctoral level psychologist or social worker) managing the behaviors, thoughts, and feelings, and possibly a family therapist, particularly when adolescents are involved. This is a comprehensive model but one that puts a high demand on practitioners in terms of clear and frequent communication. In many cases, assessment and treatment planning with patients and families requires multiple visits per week. In another model, the psychiatrist/ therapist team manages most of the nutrition and family interactions.

There is no one right model. Whichever model is used, the evidence supports a limited number of approaches to eating disorder treatment, namely cognitive-behavioral therapy for AN and BN in adults, and family-based therapy (sometimes known as the Maudsley method, after the Maudsley Hospital in London, UK, where the treatment was developed). Appropriate treatment referrals for patients can be found by searching the websites of two organizations, the Academy of Eating Disorders (www.aedweb.org) and the National Eating Disorders Association (www.nationaleatingdisorders.org). We recommend geographically convenient therapists who take a behavioral approach to therapy for patients with eating disorders. We also believe it is extremely helpful for such therapists to weigh the patient, although some therapists are uncomfortable doing so. In the case of adolescents and families, experts in family-based treatment are highly desirable. If there are no appropriate practitioners available, referral to an out-of-region, academic, behaviorally based facility with an eating disorders program for a comprehensive consultation is recommended. A good resource for parents that provides support and guidelines for refeeding a child with AN is www.maudsleyparents.org.

Acknowledgements

The authors would like to acknowledge the help of our patients and colleagues in learning how to care for women and men, adolescents and adults, with eating disorders. We would like to thank Ms. Linda Ryan for providing critical organizational support in running the Eating Disorders Program at Johns Hopkins.

References

1. Becker AE, Grinspoon SK, Klibanski A, Herzog DB. Eating disorders. *N Engl J Med.* 1999;**340**(14):1092–1098.

2. McHugh PR, Slavney PR. *The Perspectives of Psychiatry*. 2nd ed. Baltimore, MD: The Johns Hopkins University Press; 1998.

3. Shin AC, Zheng H, Berthoud HR. An expanded view of energy homeostasis: neural integration of metabolic, cognitive, and emotional drives to eat. *Physiol Behav.* 2009;**97**(5):572–580.

4. Russell G. Bulimia nervosa: an ominous variant of anorexia nervosa. *Psychol Med.* 1979;**9**(3):429–448.

5. Bruch H. Perceptual and conceptual disturbances in anorexia nervosa. *Psychosom Med.* 1962;**24**:187–194.

6. American Psychiatric Association. *Diagnostic and Statistical Manual of Mental Disorders.* 4th ed. Washington, DC: American Psychiatric Press, 1994.

7. Morgan JF, Reid F, Lacey JH. The SCOFF questionnaire: assessment of a new screening tool for eating disorders. *BMJ.* 1999;**319**(7223):1467–1468.

8. Cotton MA, Ball C, Robinson P. Four simple questions can help screen for eating disorders. *J Gen Intern Med.* 2003;**18**(1): 53–56.

9. Rome ES. Eating disorders. *Obstet Gynecol Clin North Am.* 2003;**30**(2):353–377.

10. Freund KM, Graham SM, Lesky LG, Moskowitz MA. Detection of bulimia in a primary care setting. *J Gen Intern Med.* 1993;**8**(5):236–242.

11. Papadopoulos FC, Ekbom A, Brandt L, Ekselius L. Excess mortality, causes of death and prognostic factors in anorexia nervosa. *Br J Psychiatry.* 2009;**194**(1):10–17.

12. Crow SJ, Peterson CB, Swanson SA, et al. Increased mortality in bulimia nervosa and other eating disorders. *Am J Psychiatry.* 2009;**166**(12):1342–1346.

13. Brown RF, Bartrop R, Beumont P, Birmingham CL. Bacterial infections in anorexia nervosa: delayed recognition increases complications. *Int J Eat Disord.* 2005;**37**(3):261–265.

14. Casiero D, Frishman WH. Cardiovascular complications of eating disorders. *Cardiol Rev.* 2006;**14**(5):227–231.

15. Swenne I. Heart risk associated with weight loss in anorexia nervosa and eating disorders: electrocardiographic changes during the early phase of refeeding. *Acta Paediatr.* 2000;**89**(4):447–452.

16. Koschke M, Boettger MK, Macholdt C, et al. Increased QT variability in patients with anorexia nervosa – an indicator for increased cardiac mortality? *Int J Eat Disord.* 2010;**43**(8):743–750.

17. Garner DM, Garner MV, Rosen LW. Anorexia nervosa "restricters" who purge: implications for subtyping anorexia nervosa. *Int J Eat Disord.* 1993;**13**(2): 171–185.

18. Vazquez M, Olivares JL, Fleta J, Lacambra I, Gonzalez M. [Cardiac disorders in young women with anorexia nervosa]. *Rev Esp Cardiol.* 2003;**56**(7):669–673.

19. American Academy of Pediatrics Committee on Injury Violence and Poison Prevention. Poison treatment in the home. *Pediatrics.* 2003;**112**(5):1182–1185.

20. Whittier WL, Rutecki GW. Primer on clinical acid-base problem solving. *Dis Mon.* 2004;**50**(3):122–162.

21. Mehler PS, Andersen AE. *Eating Disorders: A Guide to Medical Care and Complications.* Baltimore, MD: The Johns Hopkins University Press, 1999.

22. Mehler PS, Winkelman AB, Andersen DM, Gaudiani JL. Nutritional rehabilitation: practical guidelines for refeeding the anorectic patient. *J Nutr Metab.* 2010 Epub 2010 Feb 7.

23. Bando N, Watanabe K, Tomotake M, Taniguchi T, Ohmori T. Central pontine myelinolysis associated with a hypoglycemic coma in anorexia nervosa. *Gen Hosp Psychiatry.* 2005;**27**(5):372–374.

24. Patel AS, Matthews L, Bruce-Jones W. Central pontine myelinolysis as a complication of refeeding syndrome in a patient with anorexia nervosa.

J Neuropsychiatry Clin Neurosci. 2008; **20**(3):371–373.

25. Saad L, Silva LF, Banzato CE, Dantas CR, Garcia C Jr. Anorexia nervosa and Wernicke-Korsakoff syndrome: a case report. *J Med Case Reports.* 2010;**4**:217.

26. Birmingham CL, Puddicombe D, Hlynsky J. Hypomagnesemia during refeeding in anorexia nervosa. *Eat Weight Disord.* 2004;**9**(3):236–237.

27. Santonastaso P, Sala A, Favaro A. Water intoxication in anorexia nervosa: a case report. *Int J Eat Disord.* 1998;**24**(4): 439–442.

28. Merrett ND, Wilson RB, Cosman P, Biankin AV. Superior mesenteric artery syndrome: diagnosis and treatment strategies. *J Gastrointest Surg.* 2009;**13**(2): 287–292.

29. Adson DE, Mitchell JE, Trenkner SW. The superior mesenteric artery syndrome and acute gastric dilatation in eating disorders: a report of two cases and a review of the literature. *Int J Eat Disord.* 1997;**21**(2): 103–114.

30. Tweed-Kent AM, Fagenholz PJ, Alam HB. Acute gastric dilatation in a patient with anorexia nervosa binge/purge subtype. *J Emerg Trauma Shock.* 2010;**3**(4):403–405.

31. Knauer CM. Mallory-Weiss syndrome. Characterization of 75 Mallory-weiss lacerations in 528 patients with upper gastrointestinal hemorrhage. *Gastroenterology.* 1976;**71**(1):5–8.

32. Kortas DY, Haas LS, Simpson WG, Nickl NJ 3rd, Gates LK Jr. Mallory-Weiss tear: predisposing factors and predictors of a complicated course. *Am J Gastroenterol.* 2001;**96**(10):2863–2865.

33. Gowen GF, Stoldt HS, Rosato FE. Five risk factors identify patients with gastroesophageal intussusception. *Arch Surg.* 1999;**134**(12):1394–1397.

34. Keel PK, Dorer DJ, Eddy KT, et al. Predictors of mortality in eating disorders. *Arch Gen Psychiatry.* 2003;**60**(2):179–183.

35. Harris EC, Barraclough B. Excess mortality of mental disorder. *Br J Psychiatry.* 1998;**173**:11–53.

36. De Caprio C, Pasanisi F, Contaldo F. Gastrointestinal complications in a patient with eating disorders. *Eat Weight Disord.* 2000;**5**(4):228–230.

37. Hadley SJ, Walsh BT. Gastrointestinal disturbances in anorexia nervosa and bulimia nervosa. *Curr Drug Target CNS Neurol Disord.* 2003;**2**(1):1–9.

38. Zipfel S, Sammet I, Rapps N, et al. Gastrointestinal disturbances in eating disorders: clinical and neurobiological aspects. *Auton Neurosci.* 2006;**129**(1–2): 99–106.

39. Waldholtz BD, Andersen AE. Gastrointestinal symptoms in anorexia nervosa. A prospective study. *Gastroenterology.* 1990;**98**(6):1415–1419.

40. Lucas AR, Melton LJ 3rd, Crowson CS, O'Fallon WM. Long-term fracture risk among women with anorexia nervosa: a population-based cohort study. *Mayo Clin Proc.* 1999;**74**(10):972–977.

41. Vescovi JD, Jamal SA, De Souza MJ. Strategies to reverse bone loss in women with functional hypothalamic amenorrhea: a systematic review of the literature. *Osteoporos Int.* 2008;**19**(4):465–478.

42. Keys AB. *The Biology of Human Starvation.* Minneapolis, MN: University of Minnesota Press, 1950.

43. Kessler RC, Crum RM, Warner LA, et al. Lifetime co-occurrence of DSM-III-R alcohol abuse and dependence with other psychiatric disorders in the National Comorbidity Survey. *Arch Gen Psychiatry.* 1997;**54**(4):313–321.

44. Regier DA, Farmer ME, Rae DS, et al. Comorbidity of mental disorders with alcohol and other drug abuse. Results from the Epidemiologic Catchment Area (ECA) Study. *JAMA.* 1990;**264**(19):2511–2518.

45. Wonderlich SA, Mitchell JE. Eating disorders and comorbidity: empirical, conceptual, and clinical implications. *Psychopharmacol Bull.* 1997;**33**(3):381–390.

46. Bulik CM, Sullivan PF, Fear JL, Joyce PR. Eating disorders and antecedent anxiety disorders: a controlled study. *Acta Psychiatr Scand.* 1997;**96**(2):101–107.

47. Lilenfeld LR, Kaye WH, Greeno CG, et al. A controlled family study of anorexia nervosa and bulimia nervosa: psychiatric disorders in first-degree relatives and effects of proband comorbidity. *Arch Gen Psychiatry*. 1998;**55**(7):603–610.

48. Sinha R, O'Malley SS. Alcohol and eating disorders: implications for alcohol treatment and health services research. *Alcohol, Clinical and Experimental Research*. 2000;**24**(8):1312–1319.

49. Bulik CM, Klump KL, Thornton L, et al. Alcohol use disorder comorbidity in eating disorders: a multicenter study. *J Clin Psychiatry*. 2004;**65**(7):1000–1006.

50. Svirko E, Hawton K. Self-injurious behavior and eating disorders: the extent and nature of the association. *Suicide Life Threat Behav*. 2007;**37**(4):409–421.

51. Strober M, Freeman R, Lampert C, Diamond J. The association of anxiety disorders and obsessive compulsive personality disorder with anorexia nervosa: evidence from a family study with discussion of nosological and neurodevelopmental implications. *Int J Eat Disord*. 2007;**40**(Suppl):S46–S51.

52. Eisler I, Dare C, Hodes M, et al. Family therapy for adolescent anorexia nervosa: the results of a controlled comparison of two family interventions. *J Child Psychol Psychiatry*. 2000;**41**(6): 727–736.

53. Guarda AS, Pinto AM, Coughlin JW, et al. Perceived coercion and change in perceived need for admission in patients hospitalized for eating disorders. *Am J Psychiatry*. 2007;**164**(1):108–114.

54. Ramsay R, Ward A, Treasure J, Russell GF. Compulsory treatment in anorexia nervosa. Short-term benefits and long-term mortality. *Br J Psychiatry*. 1999;**175**: 147–153.

55. Russell GF. Involuntary treatment in anorexia nervosa. *Psychiatr Clin North Am*. 2001;**24**(2):337–349.

Chapter 5

The acute management of patients with psychiatric complications of chronic illness or chronic pain

Michael Clark and Glenn Treisman

Introduction

Patients with chronic medical problems often present to emergency departments (EDs) for acute management of psychiatric or psychological complications of their medical conditions. HIV, which can be considered a prototypical chronic illness, provides an example of the complexity of the acute evaluation and treatment of patients with chronic illness. In this chapter, HIV will serve as the chronic illness model, and the principles used to evaluate the psychiatric manifestations of HIV should serve as a reasonable illustration for the management of other chronic conditions.

The psychiatric manifestations of a chronic illness such as HIV can be due to the virus itself, related to secondary opportunistic disorders in the face of immunosupression, or expressions of other problems that tend to be comorbid with HIV infection. Patients with chronic pain present with similar challenges in that their complaints can be the result of progression of underlying disease(s) that is/are the root of the pain, behavioral complications due to chronic pain itself, or comorbid disorders associated with chronic pain.

Patients with chronic illness often present with psychiatric complaints that are often labeled as acute mental status changes, cognitive decline, mood problems and suicidal ideation, insomnia, pain, and sensory abnormalities. These terms and other labels can be misleading as they denote different states when used by different people. Because the terms lack specificity, terms like acute mental status change should be considered as umbrella terms that encompass conditions such as confusion, cognitive impairment, agitation, hallucinations, delusions, delirium, catatonia, irritability, and problematic management. The first step in evaluation of these patients is to seek clarification and have a better understanding of the baseline condition of the patient. A description of **what has changed in terms of subjective and objective findings as well as the duration of time** in which these changes have occurred can help to better define the patient's condition rather than using terms with multiple connotations.

The psychiatric problems that present in these patients can be thought of as falling into four categories: diseases of the brain (such as dementia, depression, and mania), problems of personality (such as borderline and antisocial personality disorders), problems of addiction (both illicit use and prescribed medications), and psychosocial problems (such as

---

Emergency Psychiatry, ed. Arjun Chanmugam, Patrick Triplett, and Gabor Kelen. Published by Cambridge University Press. © Cambridge University Press 2013.

homelessness, family upheaval and crisis needing intervention, or psychological maladaptation to the current medical problem).

Disease states associated with HIV and chronic pain

Several psychiatric conditions have been shown to be provoked by HIV infection, including AIDS dementia and AIDS mania. Major depression is particularly prevalent in HIV patients. Depression increases the risk of HIV infection, and HIV infection increases the vulnerability of the brain to the development of depression. Other psychiatric conditions also increase the risk for becoming infected with HIV, including schizophrenia, bipolar disorder, brain injury, and dementia.

We begin our discussion with delirium, because it mimics other disorders, is difficult to diagnose, and because of the frequent friction between providers over the most appropriate disposition of the patients (also see Chapter 6).

Delirium

The hallmarks of delirium are a change in the level of consciousness, a waxing and waning course, and confusion. Delirium is the result of global brain dysfunction, usually related to the combination of a vulnerable brain and metabolic factors, intoxication, or poisoning. Elderly patients, and those with increased medical burdens, previous brain injuries, or those requiring multiple medications, are particularly vulnerable. In terms of medications, opiates, benzodiazepines, and anticholinergic drugs have the greatest association with delirium. Patients with delirium represent a very diverse group; those with chronic conditions are particularly vulnerable and can present with manifestations that can range from mild to profound dysfunction.

A common finding in patients with delirium is altered mood; their mood is often labile with episodes of either elevated or depressed feelings which can be misdiagnosed as depresssion or bipolar disorder. Hallucinations and delusions may be present. One important distinction is that visual hallucinations are more likely to occur with delirium than with schizophrenia or affective psychosis.

As stated above, there may be many factors associated with delirium, and this is particularly true in patients with HIV. Precipitating factors in these patients include hypoxia (often with *Pneumocystis* pneumonia), malnutrition, CNS infections and neoplasms, systemic infections (e.g., mycobacteria, CMV, bacterial sepsis), acute renal failure (associated with HIV nephropathy, heroin nephropathy, or certain HIV medications), substance intoxication and withdrawal, medication toxicity, and polypharmacy. Variations in hydration or electrolyte status also may profoundly affect patients with HIV who already have cerebral compromise. HIV infection itself is associated with a high prevalence of neuropsychiatric disorders.[1]

Patients with chronic pain are also at increased risk for delirium. This is particularly true for the patient who presents to the ED with an exacerbation of their chronic pain or states that they are no longer able to tolerate their chronic pain. Patients who have chronic pain may present with a decreased ability to manage their pain or a complaint of new pain as a subtle manifestation of delirium. Such complaints are often indications that the patient's coping skills have been compromised by a subtle yet dangerous global brain dysfunction. As opposed to a classic waxing and waning level of consciousness, these patients will present with an overt inability to cope with pain. Acute care providers should be aware that a chronic pain patient who reports an exacerbation of their pain or a new pain may in fact be suffering from a mild delirium. Although the delirium may be subtle, the mortality and morbidity remain significant. Clues that the patient is delirious include reports from caregivers of a change in coping with a waxing and waning course, in which patients seem their old selves at times, while at other times seem overwhelmed by their pain. The lack of a physiological explanation for the increased pain can also be an indicator of the need for further investigation. A delirium diagnosis must prompt a careful evaluation, not only because of the morbidity and mortality of delirium itself, but also because other conditions are sometimes more difficult to evaluate when delirium is present.

The patient with chronic pain typically takes multiple medications and often at high doses. The risk of intoxication is obvious given that opioid analgesics and benzodiazepines are frequently part of their regimen (usually prescribed for the management of insomnia, pain, anxiety, and muscle spasms). Delirium in these patients is usually more subtle than the classic presentation and often results from the toxicity of multiple interacting medications. Serum levels of any of the various medications may reach supratherapeutic or even toxic levels. Cumulative or synergistic effects also occur in which the entirety of the pharmacologic regimen is more toxic than that of any individual medication.

In these more subtle forms of delirium (particularly if it has been present for some time), the patient may develop tolerance to some of the more obvious signs of the condition. Therefore, they may not appear obviously intoxicated or markedly sedated with a decreased level of consciousness. The usual pattern of waxing and waning symptoms may be missed because the delirium has been gradually increasing or even present for long periods of time creating the illusion that no acute change has occurred.

As a result, the clinician in the ED must look for other evidence of delirium. For example, the patient may complain of a relatively acute increase in their pain or a generalization of their pain beyond its usual distribution. The patient's level of distress is markedly increased and their ability to cope with a chronic condition appears to have failed or deteriorated despite their pain having been present for years. Formal testing will demonstrate that attention and concentration are impaired. For example, the patient will not be able to perform cognitive tasks such as Serial 7 calculations or Verbal Trails B without significant errors or delays.

An initial screening step to identify problems of attention associated with delirium is to ask the patient to recite the days of the week backwards or the months of the year backwards. Another screening step would be to have the patient draw a clock face and indicate a specific time. A more structured screening test would be to administer the Confusion Assessment Method for Delirium (see Table 15.1). Understanding that an underlying delirium is present and may be responsible for the patient's presentation to the ED is critical to forming the most appropriate management plan. Also, it is important to distinguish between attention problems related to delirium and cognitive difficulty related to dementia (discussed below).

The hallmarks of delirium – a waxing and waning mental state, global dysfunction that does not follow the gradual decline seen in dementia, and alterations in the level of consciousness with hyperalert or stuporous states – can usually be appreciated with careful history and examination, but on occasion may require more patience and vigilance than is usually accommodated in a busy ED. Patients often benefit from an admission to more fully evaluate the degree of impairment and the cause.

Table 15.1. The first three criteria PLUS the fourth OR the fifth criterion must be present to confirm a diagnosis of delirium

Criteria	Evidence
1. Acute change in mental status, **AND**	Observation by a family member, caregiver, or primary care physician
2. Symptoms that fluctuate over minutes or hours, **AND**	Observation by nursing staff or other caregiver
3. Inattention	Patient history Poor digit recall, inability to recite months of year backwards
PLUS	
4. Altered level of consciousness, **OR**	Hyperalertness, drowsiness, stupor, or coma
5. Disorganized thinking	Rambling or incoherent speech

Source: Inouye S, van Dyck CH, Alessi CA, Balkin S, Siegal AP, Horwitz RI. Clarifying confusion: the confusion assessment method. A new method for detection of delirium. *Ann Int Med* 1990;**113**:941–948.

Dementia

Dementia usually refers to a gradual decline in cognitive function, but often presents to the ED when the patient becomes too difficult to manage or becomes unable to function. Most patients presenting to the ED with complications or advancement of dementia already have the diagnosis established. Early presentations of dementia are readily confused with other organic states such as delirium, described above.

Dementia needs a careful evaluation and this is particularly true with HIV patients. There is a specific dementia associated with advancing HIV disease, called HIV-associated dementia or AIDS dementia, usually seen in patients with advanced disease with T-cell (CD4-cell) counts less than 200 or a nadir of less then 200. It is characterized by affecting predominantly subcortical rather than cortical brain function, distinguishing it from Alzheimer's disease. The characteristics of subcortical dementia include apathy, mood changes, motor dysfunction, as well as memory problems. Screening tests for cortical dementia such as Alzheimer's disease (for example the Folstein mini-mental state exam) are less sensitive than those specifically directed at subcortical dementia (such as the grooved pegboard, the Trail Making B test (see Appendix at the end of this chapter), and the Modified HIV Dementia Scale). Screening tests are not diagnostic, but the presence of subcortical dysfunction in a patient with low CD-4 cells (below 200) or longstanding HIV infection raise a high index of suspicion of HIV dementia. A patient with cognitive dysfunction and suspected HIV dementia may need admission to arrange adequate supervision to make certain that they can accept or adhere to treatment. The primary treatment is highly active antiretroviral therapy (HAART), but patients with HIV dementia are often poorly able to take medications as prescribed, leading to treatment failure and even viral resistance.

Making a diagnosis of subcortical dementia is often difficult in any circumstance. In most emergency cases, co-existent medical illness also requires attention and may actually be the main reason for presenting to the ED. The prudent emergency provider should take note that the patient's ability to manage their medical illness may be significantly compromised by the onset of subcortical dementia, thereby limiting the post-ED options for

Table 15.2. Characteristics of cortical and subcortical dementia

Characteristic or function	Cortical, eg., dementia in Alzheimer's disease or Pick disease	Subcortical, eg., dementia in Huntington's disease, Parkinson's disease, or HIV infection
Alertness	Normal	"Slowed up"
Attentions	Normal early	Impaired
Language	Aphasia early	No aphasia
Episodic memory	Amnesia	Forgetfulness
Visuospatial skills	Impaired	Impaired
Calculation	Involved early	Preserve until late
Personality	Unconcerned or disinhibited if frontal type, otherwise preserved	Apathetic, inert
Mood	Euthymic	Depressed
Speech	Normal articulation	Dysarthric
Movement disorders	Absent	Common
Pathology	Primary damage to neocortex and hippocampus	Primary damage to deep gray matter structures, including the thalamus, basal ganglia, brainstem nuclei, and frontal lobe projections

Data from:
Gray KF, Cummings JL.. Dementia. In Wise MG, Rundell JR (Eds.), *The American Psychiatric Publishing Textbook of Consultation-Liaison Psychiatry*. Washington, DC: American Psychiatric Publishing Inc, 2002.
Butler C, Zeman AZJ. Neurologic syndromes which can be mistaken for psychiatric conditions. *J Neurol Neurosurg Psychiatry* 2005;**76**:i31–i38.
Lavretsky H, Chui HC. Vascular dementia. In Agronin ME, Maletta GJ (Eds.), *Principles and Practice of Geriatric Psychiatry*. Philadelphia, PA: Lippincott Williams & Wilkins, 2006.

care. Identifying or even suspecting that subcortical dementia is present can help to reinforce admission decisions (see Table 15.2).

Although lower T-cell counts are associated with AIDS dementia, cognitive impairment in HIV-infected patients can be caused by other factors. These include a variety of opportunistic infections and neoplasms, or can be the result of head trauma. In some cases, the cognitive impairment may be a reflection of baseline mental subnormality.

Elderly patients are at increased risk for both chronic pain and for dementia. While this scenario mimics the one described above in the section on delirium, some important distinctions are worth noting. First, a history of progressive cognitive decline is usually present, with manifestations such as problems remembering instructions or alternately the patient may have new history of non-compliance. This non-compliance can take a variety of forms such as taking medications inconsistently or being distracted by pain or other aspects of the experience of living with chronic pain. Upon closer scrutiny, the clinician will discover that the patient is really unable to comply with treatment. The patient who seems to be having trouble because they won't follow the medical recommendations may be someone who can't follow the treatment plan. Second, the patient with chronic pain and dementia will show evidence of deteriorating coping skills. While it is important to make sure that the underlying chronic pain condition has not worsened, the patient with dementia may slowly lose those adaptive strategies that have allowed them to function with chronic pain. Over time, the patient is less able to accommodate, accept, or adjust to their pain. Then, the final common pathway of increasing distress and decreasing function occurs. As a result, the examination of the patient should include more tests of cognitive and neurological performance such as short-term recall of three named objects or drawing of complex figures to help determine current cognitive function.

Depression

Depression is a common complication of chronic medical conditions. It is particularly common in those conditions associated with chronic inflammation, CNS injury, or tumors that elaborate cytokines. Chronic CNS inflammation has been implicated in the depression seen in HIV, hepatitis C, multiple sclerosis, and autoimmune diseases. The increased risk for depression seen in HIV is probably related to both the increased likelihood of risk behaviors in those with pre-existing depression, as well as the CNS damage caused by the HIV virus. In prevalence studies and surveys, rates of major depression in patients with HIV are much higher (our estimate was fourfold) than the base rate in the community.[2]

The diagnosis of depression is discussed elsewhere, but it is a commonly missed diagnosis in patients with comorbid medical conditions. Both clinicians and patients assume that the symptoms of depression experienced by HIV patients are related to the stresses that they experience related to the illness and the stigma of their diagnosis. It is true that patients experience depressive feelings related to living with HIV, but they also experience elevated rates of major depression. For the purposes of our discussion, we use the term demoralization for the understandable sadness and psychological response associated with medical illness (the DSM uses the term adjustment disorder) and we use the term major depression for the syndromal disease state comprised of anhedonia, low mood, decreased vital sense, decreased self-attitude, and excessive self-criticism that responds to medication. This latter state is often associated with "neurovegetative features" such as disrupted sleep, early morning awakening, poor appetite, weight change, and diurnal variation in mood.

The reason to emphasize recognition of this condition in the ED is that patients with depression often are increased emergency service utilizers and can go years without an appropriate diagnosis of depression. The patient assumes (as their primary clinician might also assume) that their depressive symptoms are caused by the burdens and stigma of their HIV diagnosis. Moreover, depressed patients are less likely to obtain good primary or preventive care and instead present with a series of crisis-related ED visits.

Depression complicates the presentation and treatment of patients with chronic pain in the ED. They often present with an inability to function or an inability to tolerate increasing levels of pain. It can be harder to discern whether the patient with a complaint of depression is sad and distressed as a result of their disease state and pain (demoralization), or whether the pain is being exacerbated by major depression. Because this distinction is difficult to make in the ED, the search for a co-existing major depression in the ED is often obscured by the requests for either opiate pain medications or more medical investigation of the cause of the pain. Many patients continue to experience persistent pain unless their major depression is diagnosed and managed. The goal in the acute care setting is to recognize the possibility of a concomitant major depression and institute an appropriate treatment plan.

Physical symptoms are common in patients suffering from major depression. Approximately 60% of patients with depression report pain symptoms at diagnosis. A depressive disorder increases the risk of developing chronic musculoskeletal pain, headache, and chest pain up to 13 years later.[3] In patients with early inflammatory arthritis, baseline symptoms of depression predicted future pain better than initial ratings of pain and disease activity.[4] The reverse is also true. Chronic pain from a long-term medical condition doubles the incidence of depression. One-third to over half of patients presenting to chronic pain clinics have a current major depression.[5] Studies of depression in medically ill populations find greater sensitivity and reliability with inclusive models of depression diagnosis in contrast to models that attempt to identify the cause of each symptom. Depression in patients with chronic pain is associated with greater pain intensity, more pain persistence, and greater interference from pain including more pain behaviors observed by others. Depression is a better predictor of disability than pain intensity and duration. The decrease in self-efficacy experienced by patients with chronic pain is highly associated with depressive symptoms.[6] Lastly, pain is more likely to be an independent risk factor for suicide in patients with head or multiple types of pain.[7]

The management of depression in the ED is discussed elsewhere, but in chronically medically ill patients and patients with chronic pain, it is often a driving factor for repeated ED visits and prolonged lengths of stay. These patients are frustrating, and the usual opiate pain treatments only amplify their problems. It is usually beyond the scope of the ED to begin treatment with antidepressants, but it is possible to develop a treatment plan that includes next-day or urgent referral to an outpatient clinic that can appriopriately diagnose and manage depression in complex patients.. A relationship with a psychiatric and substance use clinic that can accept walk-in patents the next day can allow the ED to help patients better engage in appropriate treatment.

Depression with comorbid pain is more resistant to treatment.[8] Pain often subsides with improvement in depressive symptoms. In patients over age 60 with arthritis, antidepressants and/or problem-solving oriented psychotherapy not only reduced depressive symptoms but also improved pain, functional status, and quality of life.[9] In addition to having greater efficacy for the treatment of neuropathic pain, serotonin-norepinephrine reuptake inhibitors (SNRIs) and tricyclic antidepressants (TCAs) are associated with effective resolution of symptoms of major depressive disorder.[10]

Anxiety

Patients with chronic pain syndromes have increased rates of anxiety symptoms and concurrent anxiety disorders such as generalized anxiety disorder, panic disorder, agoraphobia, and posttraumatic stress disorder.[11] Almost 50% of patients with chronic pain report anxiety symptoms and up to 30% of patients have an anxiety disorder. One prospective study of 1007 young adults found a baseline history of migraine was significantly associated with an increased risk (OR=12.8) of panic disorder.[12] In patients with non-cardiac chest pain, the presence of panic disorder significantly worsened health-related quality of life.[13] Anxiety symptoms and disorders are associated with high levels of somatic preoccupation and physical symptoms. Almost two thirds of patients with panic disorder report at least one current pain symptom. Pain is related to higher levels of anxiety symptoms, panic frequency, and cognitive features of anxiety. Anxiety and depression increase pain intensity in rheumatoid arthritis independent of disease activity. Pain severity, pain-related disability, and health-related quality of life are significantly worse in patients with chronic musculoskeletal pain and comorbid anxiety or depression.[8]

The patient with chronic pain may present to the ED with complaints of severe generalized anxiety or attacks of panic that they will attribute to anticipation of increased pain. The patient will often describe a vicious cycle of easily exacerbated pain and uncontrolled anxiety that further limits their ability to engage in productive activities and worsens their physical deactivation. The patient often presumes that the answer lies in more aggressive analgesia to lessen pain and abort the cause of anxiety. Alternately they take ever-increasing doses of benzodiazepines or muscle relaxants to increase their function despite the presence of pain. Neither strategy usually results in improvement and the patient continues to deteriorate, which prompts them to seek more medication and the cycle continues.

Posttraumatic stress disorder (PTSD) is increasingly presented as a comorbid condition with significant consequences for patients with medical illnesses, especially chronic pain disorders.[14] Over half of fibromyalgia patients reported clinically relevant PTSD-like symptoms that were significantly associated with greater levels of pain, emotional distress, interference, and disability. PTSD symptoms and other psychological factors were the strongest predictors of the development of chronic pain in people who suffered severe accidents three years earlier.[15]

In the ED, patients will complain of being overwhelmed with their illness or will report in some way that they suffer from flashbacks or nightmares about some aspect of their chronic pain such as the inciting trauma or situations associated with exacerbations of pain. As in many of these presentations, the patient will seek analgesics to decrease pain or benzodiazepines to suppress their anxiety so that they can return home. While it is true that some beneficial effect can be attained, it will be short lived and will not address the underlying disorder. The more significant problem is that the patient's medication-seeking behavior will be reinforced and will become that much more difficult to extinguish if the medications are given. Therefore, the better approach is to engage the patient in a productive dialogue about learning how to tolerate their symptoms and begin addressing the provocations of their symptoms so that they can begin a process of adaptive coping. Patients with personality problems and addictions frequently present with a complaint of PTSD, and will need careful evaluation to make certain that they get appropriate treatment (see discussion below).

Personality disorders

Patients with personality problems are often the most problematic in acute care settings. These patients are notable for the emotional response they provoke in the clinicians caring for them. Their goal in the ED is frequently unclear, as they often present with an ever-changing list of complaints wishes, and demands. As described by Sydenham in the seventeenth century, "All is caprice. They love without measure those whom they will soon hate without reason. Now they will do this, now that; ever receding from their purpose."[16] They often come with complaints of suicidal feelings, unexplained medical symptoms, and chronic pain. They exhaust resources with manipulative, demanding, and sometimes coercive behaviors, and they are less likely to be satisfied and more likely to file complaints than other patient populations. They are often given pejorative labels, and many physicians come to fear and avoid them because the interactions are so unsatisfying for both the patient and the clinician.

Personality disorders are found at increased prevalence in several medical conditions. Personality disorders also increase the risk for HIV infection, as well as other conditions associated with impulsivity. A disturbing trend in the HIV epidemic has been the persistence of modifiable risk factors among persons who are HIV infected. The fact that knowledge of HIV and its transmission is insufficient to deter these individuals from engaging in HIV risk behaviors suggests that certain personality characteristics enhance the tendency to engage in such behaviors.

Personality is a complex amalgamation of learned behavior, natural tendency, and executive choice. The natural tendencies that underlie personality have been termed "temperament." The traits of temperament have been described as being adaptive for certain environments and maladaptive for others. While they are overall seen as "neutral," they make people "vulnerable" in specific environments. One measurable element of temperament has been termed the introversion-extraversion axis. Extraversion is that property of temperament that increases the salience of feelings, events occurring in the present time, and rewards. The opposite trait, introversion, increases the salience of function, the future, and consequences. Because of what is salient to them, extraverts are more likely to engage in behavior that places them at risk for HIV infection and are more likely to engage in high-risk sexual behaviors. They are less likely to plan ahead and carry condoms and more likely to have unprotected vaginal or anal sex. They are more fixated on the reward of sex and remarkably inattentive to the sexually transmitted diseases (STDs) they acquire when they do not use a condom. Extraverts are also less likely to accept the diminution of pleasure associated with the use of condoms or, once aroused, to interrupt the "heat of the moment" to use condoms. Similarly, extraverts are more vulnerable to alcohol and drug abuse. They are drawn to alcohol and drugs as a quick route to pleasure. They are more likely to experiment with different kinds of drugs and to use greater quantities. Extraverts are also more likely to experiment with injection of drugs and develop into regular users. Introverted personalities appear to be relatively less likely to engage in risk behaviors, and therefore are less represented in HIV populations.

Personality disorder can be described as occurring when the prevailing style of personality, including underlying temperament and learned behavior, becomes maladaptive. Prevalence rates of personality disorders among HIV-infected patients (19%–36%) and individuals at risk for HIV (15%-20%)[17] are high and significantly exceed rates found in the general population (10%). The most common personality disorders among HIV-infected patients are antisocial and borderline types.[18] Antisocial personality disorder is the most common and is a risk factor for HIV infection.[19] Individuals with personality disorder, particularly antisocial personality disorder, have high rates of substance abuse and are more likely to inject drugs and share needles compared with those without an Axis II (personality disorder) diagnosis. Approximately half of drug abusers may meet criteria for a diagnosis of antisocial personality disorder. Individuals with antisocial personality disorder are also more likely to have a greater number of lifetime sexual partners, engage in unprotected anal sex, and contract STDs compared with individuals without antisocial personality disorder.[20]

Although introverts develop chronic pain, extraverted patients are more likely to develop disordering chronic pain syndromes and more likely to develop addictive behaviors related to prescribed medications. They are more easily conditioned by the positively reinforcing effects of narcotics, disability payments, and attention, than are introverts. They often develop what Izzy Pilowski referred to as "abnormal illness behaviors," which are behaviors attached to illness that can persist when the illness is no longer present. These behaviors persist particularly when they are positively reinforced, such as with narcotics, benzodiazepines, and attention. These patients are directed at comfort over function and easily see themselves as victims, a position that is less conducive to rehabilitation. The prevalence of personality disorders ranges from 31–81% in chronic pain patients and is greater than in the general population or in populations with either medical or psychiatric illnesses.[21,22] We discuss a behavioral approach to the management of patients with personality difficulty and manipulative behavior below.

Substance abuse and chronic pain

Substance abuse plays a major role in the dissemination of HIV, both via contaminated needles and impaired judgment. High-risk sexual behaviors are associated with using intoxicating drugs and multiple partners. Adherence to antiviral medications is adversely affected by drug addiction, alcohol use, and prescribed narcotic overuse. Patients presenting to the ED with HIV frequently come for addiction-related problems. This is further complicated by the high frequency of chronic pain in HIV infected patients. As many as 30–50% of HIV patients suffer from neuropathy related to HIV or caused by antiretroviral therapy. These patients may have a history of addiction that precedes the development of chronic pain, but are often iatrogenically addicted to prescribed opiate pain medication.

The prevalence of substance dependence or addiction in patients with chronic pain is difficult to ascertain due to the difficulty of defining overuse in patients with chronic pain. The core criteria for a substance use disorder in patients with chronic pain include the loss of control in the use of the medication, excessive preoccupation with the medication despite adequate analgesia, and adverse consequences associated with its use. The Researched Abuse, Diversion and Addiction-Related Surveillance System (RADARS) reported that prescription opioid abuse is widely prevalent.[23] However, reliance on medications that provide pain relief can result in a number of stereotyped patient behaviors that overlap with those seen in addictions. These behaviors have been termed pseudoaddiction, that is, addiction-like behavior that results from therapeutic dependence on opiates in the setting of inadequate pain control.

Patients often display their concern about medications with several patterns of non-adherence to, or misuse of, prescribed medications.[24] One common pattern, the taking of more medication than prescribed, was associated with patients' increased concerns about addiction, tolerance, withdrawal, and excessive scrutiny by others of their medication use, as well as a greater perceived need for medication.

During the first five years after the onset of a chronic pain problem, patients are at increased risk for developing new drug use problems and disorders. The risk is highest among those with a history of drug use disorder or psychiatric comorbidity. Patients with substance use disorders have increased rates of chronic pain and are also at the greatest risk for stigmatization and under-treatment. Opioid-dependent patients with chronic pain have even higher rates of drug use than those without chronic pain.[25,26] Surprisingly, 84% of patients with chronic pain who abused prescription opioids entering a drug abuse treatment facility reported that they had legitimately received a prescription from a physician for the treatment of pain.[27] However, 91% had purchased prescription opioids through illegitimate sources and 80% had altered the delivery system of the prescription drug, suggesting severe forms of addiction. Integrating care for chronic pain with innovative stepped-care models of substance abuse treatment would likely improve outcomes by tailoring the intensity of treatment to individual patients' needs.[28]

In the ED, patients with chronic pain and substance dependence disorders present with the usual symptoms but the goal may not be pain relief, rather drug effects such as euphoria or sedation. The patient may not focus on getting an adequate medical evaluation, but instead on access to narcotics. The treatment demanded by the patient will often be narrowly defined, such as IV opioids or a particular named medication. Attempts to deviate from the patient's demands will result in anger and agitation. Non-verbal pain behaviors will be inconsistent and often fade when the patient is distracted or indirectly observed by staff. Collateral information as may be gained from family members, outside clinicians, or medical records that will corroborate a pattern of aberrant medication-taking behaviors is critical.

Management of difficult patients with HIV or chronic pain in the ED

Although discussed elsewhere in this chapter, the issue of the management of chronic pain is central to the task of dealing with difficult patients in the ED. Patients with acute pain are usually relatively straightforward to manage, while those with chronic pain are far more difficult. Chronic pain is not usually the result of ongoing tissue damage, but rather the result of altered sensory and sympathetic nervous function. Patients are often given opiates at ever-increasing doses to try to combat their pain, and while some may benefit, many become increasingly intoxicated and exhibit more dysfunction as the dose increases. Unfortunately, the efforts to make pain a vital sign and to ensure that all pain is relieved have led to a massive overuse of narcotics and escalating problems of iatrogenic addiction.[29]

Non-malignant chronic pain is often not relieved with chronic opiates, and can be made worse by chronic opiate use.[30] While some patients benefit from chronic opiate administration, it is increasingly clear that many do not. Alternative methods of pain management may be more useful for patients with chronic pain.[31]

For the emergency physician, it is important to remember that pain has two components, a sensory element and an affective element. The affective element produces the distress associated with pain and often provides the drive to seek "emergency" treatment. As described above, patients with depression have an increased sensitivity to pain, particularly the affective component. Patients with significant extraversion or instability are more reactive to the distress associated with pain, and will tolerate a lower level of function in their effort to eliminate pain. They are at increased risk for addiction and medication overuse that produce recurrent cycles of craving, medication seeking, and maladaptive reinforcement.

Patients with chronic pain often are in the "difficult patient" category. Providers and the patient are often focused entirely on the goal of pain relief to the detriment of improving function. They arrive in the ED demanding escalating doses of opiates with the supposed hope of finally achieving pain relief. Usually, these patients are given comfort-directed pharmacologic interventions such as opiates, benzodiazepines, and other sedative-hypnotics. The goal becomes a rapid disposition of the patient with return home and follow-up in their usual outpatient clinic. Unfortunately, this approach does not lead to long-term positive change for the patient but reinforces a dysfunctional coping strategy and ongoing abnormal illness behavior and disability. Below, we discuss a behavioral approach to the management of chronic pain and related conditions.

A behavioral approach to difficult patients

In the early 1900s, Ivan Pavlov described the ability to change behavior in animals by association with a particular stimulus. He was able to measure salivation in dogs in response to food, but then by pairing the food with a tuning fork, he was able to elicit salivation in response to the tuning fork. This has been described as classical conditioning, and occurs passively. This type of conditioning has been observed with patients in many settings. Patients who have had several exposures to chemotherapy will often develop nausea and may even vomit upon arriving at the cancer treatment center.[32] It is possible to condition changes in immune function,[33] condition asthma attacks,[34] and to condition neutral stimuli to cause pain.[35] Classical (or Pavlovian) conditioning occurs when a patient associates a behavior with a desirable or undesirable stimulus or experience.

Operant conditioning, described later by BF Skinner, occurs when a behavior performed by the patient is reinforced with a specific consequence. This type of conditioning results in increasing or decreasing the likelihood of the associated behavior. As an example, a pigeon pecks a key and receives a food reward. This results in more frequent and faster key-pecking behavior. Skinner described "shaping," where reinforcements/consequences are used in stepwise fashion to develop increasingly complex behaviors, behaviors with multiple steps, or behaviors that require molding from the original. For example, pigeons can be "shaped" to peck a ball into a slot for food. The pigeon is first reinforced for pecking the ball. Once this behavior is established, the reward pattern is altered and given only when it pecks the ball in a specific direction. Skinner described four types of conditioning, as shown in Table 15.3. In this way, the sought behaviors are increased if the consequence of the behavior is a reward (positive reinforcement) or the removal of something noxious (negative reinforcement). The behaviors are decreased if the consequence of the behavior is the removal of the reward (extinction) or the delivery of something noxious (punishment). Removal of rewards can ultimately completely extinguish a behavior. However, the effect of punishment is not so effective as it often merely suppresses behavior that will re-emerge when the threat or experience of punishment is gone.

All of these conditioning paradigms have been described for doctor-patient interactions. A patient who throws a tantrum in your office and demands narcotics has probably been reinforced for that behavior by the previous delivery of narcotics in the same situation. Subtle reinforcement of illness behaviors such as limping, splinting, moaning, crying, and even falling can occur with patients who are vulnerable to the reinforcing effects of particular responses. Interestingly, when the subject perceives that the reinforcement schedule weakens, as may occur when providers withhold or give

Table 15.3. Four types of conditioning

Quality of the consequence	Positive (rewarding)	Negative (noxious)
Delivery of consequence	Positive reinforcement Increased behavior	Punishment Decreased behavior
Withdrawal of consequence	Extinction Decreased behavior	Negative reinforcement Increased behavior

smaller prescription amounts, the maladaptive behavior, in this case antics associated with drug seeking, actually increases. This is an important principle to understand, as when positive reinforcers are withdrawn in an attempt to extinguish a behavior, that very behavior initially intensifies.

A caveat here is that reinforcement works only when the consequence or reward being employed to shape behavior has salience to the person being shaped. Pigeons must be hungry to work for food rewards. Pigeons who have been recently fed cannot be shaped using food rewards. Patients in a given set of circumstances are more or less vulnerable to the reinforcing effects of narcotics, attention, praise, encouragement, criticism, relief from distress, and diagnostic labels. A person with a good job may be eager to return to work and perceive an excuse from work as aversive and therefore understate their discomfort, while a person who is unhappy at work may find a note excusing them a reward and overestimate their discomfort. Physicians are constantly shaping their patients. All doctor-patient interactions subtly shape behavior. What is important to understand is that the reinforcement is in the "eye of the beholder." The clinician doesn't define what is perceived as reward to noxious stimuli, or punishment. Rather, the clinician needs to understand the patient's perception of these circumstances and environment. Consider the example of a patient who is in an unpleasant marriage, has a job he detests, and essentially lives to play softball. He describes going to the ED after hurting his ankle at a softball game, where he received a "shot" of Demerol, a note for three days off from work, and directions to his wife to bring him things for a couple days in bed. His next visit to the ED a few weeks later results in similar management, and he now looks forward to his third injury. He relates that after a while he became a frequent visitor to emergency rooms and pain clinics. He ultimately lost his job, his wife, and his home. When he comes for treatment, he now looks back on his job and wife with a newfound affection as the best time in his life. In retrospect, it is clear that he had major depression, which more than likely influenced his view of his job and marriage in a negative way. His circumstances, his temperament, and his depressive disorder had made him vulnerable to the reinforcing effects of the attention and narcotics he received in the ED.

Patients are positively reinforced by opiate and sedative hypnotic medications, attention from doctors, disability payments, and by permission to express prohibited feelings. The relief of pain through the use of narcotics, relief from insomnia through sedative hypnotics, and relief from the expectations and demands at work and at home are each strong negative reinforcers. This will increase medication-seeking, doctor-seeking, and pain-related behavior. This will also shape patients to be less committed to recovery.

Fortunately, these same behavioral tools can be used to shape recovery-related and function-related behaviors. Izzy Pilowsky described illness-related behaviors in the absence of ongoing pathology, with the term "abnormal illness behavior."[36] Many of these behaviors are conditioned to occur as described above. Ignoring abnormal illness behaviors will help result in their extinction. Rewarding healthy behaviors such as rehabilitation, function, and coping will encourage them to develop. Examples of this include the use of letters, forms, attention, and personal approval as positive reinforcers of specific behavior. Patients on chronic opiate treatment for pain might be required to demonstrate 40 hours of structured activity a week to stay on opiates. Rehabilitation of chronic pain using these techniques was described by William Fordyce in 1968,[37] and the operant conditioning approach has been a standard (although sadly underrecognized) approach to chronic pain.[38,39] It is also important to recognize that patients condition their physicians as much as we condition them. In a seminal study of prescription writing behavior, Turk showed that non-verbal pain behaviors have a potent influence on the prescription writing behavior of doctors.[39]

The deliberate application of behavioral techniques to treatment of difficult patients takes much of the emotional element out of the picture. A first step is to focus on what the patient is doing, and not on what he or she is feeling. Five steps have been described as essential for successful treatment, similar to those for addictions. Prior to beginning treatment, a full evaluation for medical and psychiatric conditions must be completed. It is critical to know all aspects of the case when starting treatment with difficult patients.

Treatment begins with a role induction. This consists of describing to the patient the entire formulation of the physician impression. Include the medical and psychiatric elements in the discussion. Allow lots of time for the patient to ask questions about what each condition is, and the evidence that supports the diagnosis as well as how each condition affects them. Avoid allowing patients to derail the discussion or argue about the diagnosis. When patients attempt to argue about the diagnosis, explain things fully, and inform them that they can arrange to get a second opinion. It is important not to allow the patient to short circuit the discussion of diagnosis by leaping to treatment. The discussion of treatment begins after the patient has heard the diagnostic formulation completely. The typical approach: describe the medical problems first, then note how these are complicated by the lack of reward in major depression, subsequently explain how amplification of sensation is due to temperament and the lack of coping skills, describe how aversive experiences have made it difficult to receive appropriate treatment, and finally clarify the manner in which conditioning has systematically incapacitated the patient. Offer an optimistic discussion of treatments even though they are often contrary to the patient's requested treatments, but explain how they will result in better outcome. Stress the losses and indignities the patient has suffered from their illness and how important it is to try to recover their lives. Finish the role induction by pointing out that it is possible the diagnosis could be wrong, and that the patient will need to decide if they want to seek treatment elsewhere, or engage in the treatment prescribed. This approach is paternalistic, but also establishes the critical core of the doctor-patient relationship. Patients can fire you and go elsewhere, but they cannot prescribe their own treatment.

The next step involves detoxification if needed, and the development of a set of behavioral goals with associated rewards and consequences. Thus, the equivalent of the detoxification step in addictions treatment in which the sustaining behavioral rewards that maintain abnormal illness behavior are removed.

The initiation of medical and psychiatric treatments (equivalent to the treatment of comorbid conditions in addictions) is critical to the success of the overall treatment. This is done in concert with the initiation of behaviorally based rehabilitation. Treatment often includes an opiate taper, physical therapy, and comprehensive rehabilitation for chronic pain, chronic bowel dysfunction, or any other chronically deconditioned organ system. Finally, relapse prevention in the form of a program to prevent the recrudescence of the pathological response to the underlying illness is required. Almost all "difficult patients" will have a chronic medical problem that will continue to need attention and treatment. Without ongoing care, the pattern of behavioral reinforcement for disability and deconditioning is likely to recur.

Summary

Patients in the ED with HIV or chronic pain usually present with an underlying illness that has been made worse by psychiatric conditions that exacerbate the illness and lead to disability, but also by a system that rewards poor medical care, focuses on symptoms rather than on conditions, and directs treatment at comfort rather than function. A comprehensive diagnostic formulation that includes comorbid psychiatric conditions allows clinicians to develop treatment plans that overcome the barriers to successful medical treatment. The route to success is to focus on the patient's medical treatment and their behavior, and to pay less attention to their feelings, their emotional provocations and manipulations, and their comfort. Unfortunately, these patients require more time, are less satisfied, use more resources, and are less able to pay for their treatment. The current medical care system does not adequately reward clinicians for their care, nor does it provide an incentive for successful treatment. The growing emphasis on "customer" satisfaction, financial efficiency, and allowing patients to prescribe their own treatment has been a disservice to these patients in particular. It is tragic to watch these patients flail against those who want to help them, and exploit every weakness in the system to their own detriment.[40] Clinicians are discouraged from engaging with difficult patients by a system that can actually penalize clinicians for caring for them appropriately.[41]

Because these patients are often conditioned to engage in self-defeating behavior, they may sabotage their own care to hurt a clinician when they are angry about something, even though, as Sydenham observed, they tend to recede from their purpose.[16] It has become politically popular to see difficult patients in terms of their rights,[42] but a patient who is difficult may be suffering from impaired autonomy and is not making decisions in an autonomous fashion. There is also a growing literature discussing the characteristics of physicians who have their difficulty with patients,[43–45] suggesting a view that difficult patients are a product of clinician failure. Certainly, better skills are helpful in managing difficult patients, but mastery of treating the underlying problem is necessary to rehabilitate patients to full function. "Understanding" how the patient feels may be comforting but no more therapeutic than having the orthopedic surgeon "understand" your fracture. Ultimately, the best way to manage a difficult patient is to get them better, but many patients will need to hear the same message repeatedly before they are ready to accept the treatment plan most likely to succeed. Patient advocacy, oddly enough, sometimes involves advocating for something that the patient does not want but certainly needs.

References

1. Gallego L, Barreiro P, López-Ibor JJ. Diagnosis and clinical features of major neuropsychiatric disorders in HIV infection. *AIDS Rev.* 2011;**13**(3): 171–179.

2. Treisman G, Angelino A. Interrelation between psychiatric disorders and the prevention and treatment of HIV infection. *Clin Infect Dis.* 2007;**45**(Suppl 4): S313–S317.

3. Larson SL, Clark MR, Eaton WW. Depressive disorder as a long-term antecedent risk factor for incident back pain: a 13-year follow-up study from the Baltimore Epidemiological Catchment Area sample. *Psychol Med.* 2004;**34**(2):211–219.

4. Schieir O, Thombs BD, Hudson M, et al. Symptoms of depression predict the trajectory of pain among patients with early inflammatory arthritis: a path analysis approach to assessing change. *J Rheumatol.* 2009;**36**(2):231–239.

5. Dersh J, Polatin PB, Gatchel RJ. Chronic pain and psychopathology: research findings and theoretical considerations. *Psychosom Med.* 2002;**64**(5):773–786.

6. Rahman A, Reed E, Underwood M, Shipley ME, Omar RZ. Factors affecting self-efficacy and pain intensity in patients with chronic musculoskeletal pain seen in a specialist rheumatology pain clinic. *Rheumatology (Oxford).* 2008;**47**(12): 1803–1808.

7. Ilgen MA, Zivin K, McCammon RJ, Valenstein M. Pain and suicidal thoughts, plans and attempts in the United States. *Gen Hosp Psychiatry.* 2008;**30**(6):521–527.

8. Bair MJ, Wu J, Damush TM, Sutherland JM, Kroenke K. Association of depression and anxiety alone and in combination with chronic musculoskeletal pain in primary care patients. *Psychosom Med.* 2008;**70** (8):890–897.

9. Lin EH, Katon W, Von Korff M, et al; IMPACT Investigators. Effect of improving depression care on pain and functional outcomes among older adults with arthritis: a randomized controlled trial. *JAMA.* 2003;**290**(18): 2428–2429.

10. Rosenzweig-Lipson S, Dunlop J, Marquis KL. 5-HT2C receptor agonists as an innovative approach for psychiatric disorders. *Drug News Perspect.* 2007;**20** (9):565–571.

11. McWilliams LA, Cox BJ, Enns MW. Mood and anxiety disorders associated with chronic pain: an examination in a nationally representative sample. *Pain.* 2003;**106**(1–2):127–133.

12. Breslau N, Davis GC. Migraine, physical health and psychiatric disorder: a prospective epidemiologic study in young adults. *J Psychiatr Res.* 1993;**27** (2):211–221.

13. Dammen T, Ekeberg Ø, Arnesen H, Friis S. Health-related quality of life in non-cardiac chest pain patients with and without panic disorder. *Int J Psychiatry Med.* 2008;**38** (3):271–286.

14. Liebschutz J, Saitz R, Brower V, et al. PTSD in urban primary care: high prevalence and low physician recognition. *J Gen Intern Med.* 2007;**22**(6):719–726.

15. Jenewein J, Wittmann L, Moergeli H, Creutzig J, Schnyder U. Mutual influence of posttraumatic stress disorder symptoms and chronic pain among injured accident survivors: a longitudinal study. *J Trauma Stress.* 2009;**22**(6): 540–548.

16. Sydenham T. *The works of Thomas Sydenham MD, translated from the Latin edition of Dr. Greenhill.* London: The Sydenham Society, 1850.

17. Hansen NB, Cavanaugh CE, Vaughan EL, et al. The influence of personality disorder indication, social support, and grief on alcohol and cocaine use among HIV-positive adults coping with AIDS-related bereavement. *AIDS Behav.* 2009;**13**: 375–384.

18. Bennett WR, Joesch JM, Mazur M, et al. Characteristics of HIV-positive patients treated in a psychiatric emergency department. *Psychiatr Serv.* 2009;**60**: 398–401.

19. Weissman MM. The epidemiology of personality disorders: a 1990 update. *J Personal Disord.* 1993;**7** (suppl):44–62.

20. Ladd GT, Petry NM. Antisocial personality in treatment-seeking cocaine abusers: psychosocial functioning and HIV risk. *J Subst Abuse Treat.* 2003;**24**: 323–330.

21. Vendrig AA. The Minnesota Multiphasic Personality Inventory and chronic pain: a conceptual analysis of a long-standing but complicated relationship. *Clin Psychol Rev.* 2000;**20**:533–559.

22. Vendrig AA, Derksen JJ, de Mey HR. MMPI-2 Personality Psychopathology Five (PSY-5) and prediction of treatment outcome for patients with chronic back pain. *J Pers Assess.* 2000;**74**:423–438.

23. Cicero TJ, Inciardi JA, Surratt H. Trends in the use and abuse of branded and generic extended release oxycodone and fentanyl products in the United States. *Drug Alcohol Depend.* 2007;**91**:115–120.

24. McCracken LM, Hoskins J, Eccleston C. Concerns about medication and medication use in chronic pain. *J Pain.* 2006;7:726–734.

25. Peles E, Schreiber S, Gordon J, Adelson M. Significantly higher methadone dose for methadone maintenance treatment (MMT) patients with chronic pain. *Pain.* 2005;113:340–346.

26. Rosenblum A, Joseph H, Fong C, Kipnis S, Cleland C, Portenoy RK. Prevalence and characteristics of chronic pain among chemically dependent patients in methadone maintenance and residential treatment facilities. *JAMA.* 2003;289:2370–2378.

27. Passik SD, Kirsh KL, Donaghy KB, Portenoy RK. Pain and aberrant drug-related behaviors in medically ill patients with and without histories of substance abuse. *Clin J Pain.* 2006;22:173–181.

28. Clark MR, Stoller KB, Brooner RK. Assessment and management of chronic pain in individuals seeking treatment for opioid dependence disorder. *Can J Psychiatry.* 2008;53:496–508.

29. Devi S. USA hones in on prescription drug abuse. *Lancet* 2011;378(9790):473–474.

30. Ossipov MH, Lai J, King T, Vanderah TW, Porreca F. Underlying mechanisms of pronociceptive consequences of prolonged morphine exposure. *Biopolymers.* 2005;80 (2–3):319–324.

31. Clark MR. Psychiatric issues in chronic pain. *Curr Psychiatry Rep.* 2009;11 (3):243–245.

32. Stockhorst U, Steingrueber HJ, Enck P, Klosterhalfen S. Pavlovian conditioning of nausea and vomiting. *Auton Neurosci.* 2006;129(1–2):50–57.

33. Exton MS, von Auer AK, Buske-Kirschbaum A, Stockhorst U, Göbel U, Schedlowski M. Pavlovian conditioning of immune function: animal investigation and the challenge of human application. *Behav Brain Res.* 2000;110(1–2):129–141.

34. Bouhuys A, Justesen DR. Allergic and classically conditioned asthma in guinea pigs. *Science.* 1971;173(991):82.

35. Greeley J. Pavlovian conditioning of pain regulation: insights from pharmacological conditioning with morphine and naloxone. *Biol Psychol.* 1989;28(1):41–46.

36. Pilowsky I. Abnormal illness behaviour. *Br J Med Psychol.* 1969;42(4):347–351.

37. Fordyce WE, Fowler RS, DeLateur B. An application of behavior modification technique to a problem of chronic pain. *Behav Res Ther.* 1968;6(1):105–107.

38. Turk DC, Swanson KS, Tunks ER. Psychological approaches in the treatment of chronic pain patients – when pills, scalpels, and needles are not enough. *Can J Psychiatry.* 2008;53(4): 213–223.

39. Turk DC, Okifuji A. What factors affect physicians' decisions to prescribe opioids for chronic noncancer pain patients? *Clin J Pain.* 1997;13(4):330–336.

40. Fee C. Death of a difficult patient. *Ann Emerg Med.* 2001;37(3):3.

41. Sonnenberg A. Personal view: passing the buck and taking a free ride – a game-theoretical approach to evasive management strategies in gastroenterology. *Aliment Pharmacol Ther.* 2005;22(6):513.

42. Reeves RR, Douglas SP, Garner RT, Reynolds MD, Silvers A. The individual rights of the difficult patient. *Hastings Cent Rep.* 2007;37(2):13; discussion 13–15.

43. Krebs EE, Garrett JM, Konrad TR. The difficult doctor? Characteristics of physicians who report frustration with patients: an analysis of survey data. *BMC Health Serv Res.* 2006;6:128.

44. Batchelor J, Freeman MS. Spectrum: the clinician and the "difficult" patient. *S D J Med.* 2001;54(11):453–456.

45. Haas LJ, Leiser JP, Magill MK, Sanyer ON. Management of the difficult patient. *Am Fam Physician.* 2005;72(10):2063–2068.

Appendix

Trail Making Test (TMT) Parts A & B

Instructions:

Both parts of the Trail Making Test consist of 25 circles distributed over a sheet of paper. In Part A, the circles are numbered 1–25, and the patient should draw lines to connect the numbers in ascending order. In Part B, the circles include both numbers (1–13) and letters (A–L); as in Part A, the patient draws lines to connect the circles in an ascending pattern, but with the added task of alternating between the numbers and letters (i.e., 1-A-2-B-3-C, etc.). The patient should be instructed to connect the circles as quickly as possible, without lifting the pen or pencil from the paper. Time the patient as he or she connects the "trail." If the patient makes an error, point it out immediately and allow the patient to correct it. Errors affect the patient's score only in that the correction of errors is included in the completion time for the task. It is unnecessary to continue the test if the patient has not completed both parts after five minutes have elapsed.

Step 1:	Give the patient a copy of the Trail Making Test Part A worksheet and a pen or pencil.
Step 2:	Demonstrate the test to the patient using the sample sheet (Trail Making Part A – SAMPLE).
Step 3:	Time the patient as he or she follows the "trail" made by the numbers on the test.
Step 4:	Record the time.
Step 5:	Repeat the procedure for Trail Making Test Part B.

Scoring:

Results for both TMT A and B are reported as the number of seconds required to complete the task; therefore, higher scores reveal greater impairment.

	Average	Deficient	Rule of thumb
Trail A	29 seconds	>78 seconds	Most in 90 seconds
Trail B	75 seconds	>273 seconds	Most in 3 minutes

Sources:

- Corrigan JD, Hinkeldey MS. Relationships between parts A and B of the Trail Making Test. *J Clin Psychol.* 1987;**43**(4):402–409.
- Gaudino EA, Geisler MW, Squires NK. Construct validity in the Trail Making Test: what makes Part B harder? *J Clin Exp Neuropsychol.* 1995;**17**(4):529–535.
- Lezak MD, Howieson DB, Loring DW. *Neuropsychological Assessment.* 4th ed. New York: Oxford University Press, 2004.
- Reitan RM. Validity of the Trail Making Test as an indicator of organic brain damage. *Percept Mot Skills.* 1958;**8**:271–276.

Trail Making Test Part A

Patient's Name: _____   Date: _____

Trail Making Test Part A – *SAMPLE*

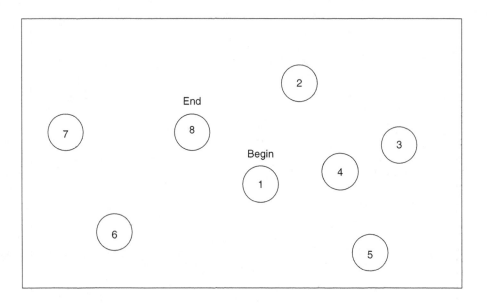

Trail Making Test Part B

Patient's Name: _____   Date: _____

Trail Making Test Part B – *SAMPLE*

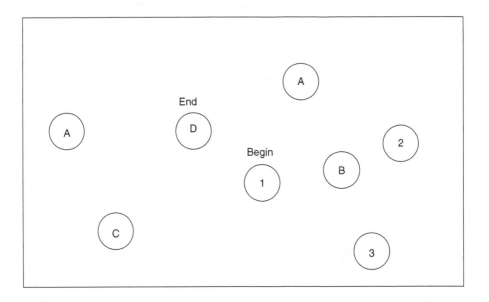

Death and dying

Catherine A. Marco and Valerie R. Lint

Introduction

Death in the emergency department (ED) occurs frequently. Approximately 249,000 patients die in EDs annually (0.2% of ED visits).[1] Emergency care of dying patients and survivors presents numerous unique challenges to emergency physicians and other front line providers. Management of end-of-life (EOL) symptoms, communication, cultural sensitivity, attention to spiritual needs, and psychosocial support for grieving survivors are essential skills for emergency physicians.

Caring for dying patients is challenging. The American College of Emergency Physicians (ACEP) acknowledged this and provided some guidance when they issued a Policy on Ethical Issues at the End-of-life, in 2008. Within that policy, the college succinctly summarized the importance of compassionate end-of-life care by stating, "Emergency physicians should respect the dying patient's needs for care, comfort, and compassion."[2] In this chapter, we review the basic issues of death and dying in the ED and provide some strategies for management.

As imminent death is identified, several issues should be considered. Attempts should be made to obtain the patient's advance directives, or gain an understanding of the patient's wishes. These can be gleaned either directly from the patient when he or she is lucid and able to comprehend the gravity of the situation, or from a surrogate who can fairly represent the patient's wishes. In their policy statement regarding EOL care in the ED (2008), the ACEP identified some key points for emergency physicians to consider when caring for a dying patient:

- Respect the dying patient's needs for care, comfort, and compassion.
- Communicate promptly and appropriately with patients and their families about EOL care choices, avoiding medical jargon.
- Elicit the patient's goals for care before initiating treatment, recognizing that EOL care includes a broad range of therapeutic and palliative options.
- Respect the wishes of dying patients including those expressed in advance directives. Assist surrogates to make EOL care choices for patients who lack decision-making capacity, based on the patient's own preferences, values, and goals.
- Encourage the presence of family and friends at the patient's bedside near the EOL, if desired by the patient.
- Protect the privacy of patients and families near the EOL.

Emergency Psychiatry, ed. Arjun Chanmugam, Patrick Triplett, and Gabor Kelen. Published by Cambridge University Press. © Cambridge University Press 2013.

- Promote liaisons with individuals and organizations in order to help patients and families honor EOL cultural and religious traditions.
- Develop skill at communicating sensitive information, including poor prognoses and the death of a loved one.
- Comply with institutional policies regarding recovery of organs for transplantation.
- Obtain informed consent from the appropriate surrogate(s) for postmortem procedures.

Providers must consider patient and family desires in dealing with EOL issues, however there are other issues that must be included in the decision-making process. Stewardship of medical resources and interventions at the EOL are also an important physician responsibility and must be balanced with the patient's condition. The wise and prudent application of rapidly advancing technologic capabilities such as therapeutic hypothermia, extracorporeal membrane oxygenation, implantable defibrillators, among others, is of increasing importance, especially as these technologies can often temporize a patient's condition, even if it is for a very short time.

An example of an intervention that can prolong life is cardiopulmonary resuscitation (CPR), which is frequently undertaken for ED patients in cardiac arrest. Because of the variable nature of prognosis in cases of cardiac arrest, the risks, benefits, and duration of resuscitative efforts should be carefully considered. In some cases, CPR can be used to successfully resuscitate a patient who may survive to have a reasonable quality of life. In other cases, patients may have reached a condition whereby the prolongation of life will result in a continuation or worsening of their pre-event state or can only prolong life for a very short period of time before death will occur. Emergency providers must carefully balance the patient's condition, the availability of resources, and the likelihood of a positive outcome all within the context of the dignity of the patient and their wishes. Individual patient treatment plans must include an unbiased analysis of the risks and benefits of proposed medical treatments and a realistic appreciation of likely outcomes. In summary, EOL decisions should be made in the context of well-established data, patient and family wishes, and professional judgment.[3]

For some resource-intense interventions, or highly scarce resources, institutional or departmental guidelines are used to help emergency providers with EOL decision-making. In other cases, legislative policy or regulatory mechanisms will dictate the conditions when patients will be eligible for specific resources. Emergency providers should familiarize themselves with these institutional, legislative, and regulatory policies, before encountering patients who require immediate decision-making. Managing dying patients is difficult, so having an understanding of the available resources and the policies regarding their utilization can help to more effectively deliver the most appropriate care.

Emergency providers should be familiar with the complex and evolving technologies that may be available for resuscitating patients. They should also be part of the process for developing institutional and legislative policy and regulatory mechanisms to address the appropriate allocation of resources at the EOL. Participation in advocacy of national, regional, or state policy can help providers gain familiarity with EOL issues. Involvement with departmental or institutional procedure and policy review as well as ongoing education about novel interventions should be augmented whenever possible to help providers become more comfortable at the bedside and to aid in the decision-making process during what must be regarded as a critical time for patients, families, and staff.

Some providers advocate withholding "futile" EOL interventions. The term "futility," although commonly used, has fallen out of favor, due to difficulties in definition and inconsistencies in interpretation. Because of the continuing controversy over the meaning of the term "futility," it may be preferable to avoid the term and to refer instead to interventions as medically "non-beneficial," "ineffectual," or "low likelihood of success." Dilemmas regarding non-beneficial interventions may arise as a result of inadequate or ineffective communication between physician, patient, and family.[4] When a difference of opinion exists, first steps toward resolution should include improved communication, education, and joint decision-making.

Many individuals and organizations agree that physicians are under no obligation to render treatments which they believe will provide little or no benefit to the patient. There have been numerous published opinions supportive of the position of providing only those treatments judged to be of likely medical benefit. The AMA Council on Ethical and Judicial Affairs states that CPR may be withheld, "when efforts to resuscitate a patient are judged by the treating physician to be futile."[5] Withholding interventions requested by the patient or family when judged of little benefit to the patient is a controversial practice.[6–8] The ACEP states in policy that, "physicians are under no ethical obligation to render treatments that they judge have no realistic likelihood of medical benefit to the patient," and that judgments should be unbiased, based on scientific evidence and societal and professional standards.[9]

There may be disagreement about the level of invasive and aggressive medical care at the EOL. In some cases, the family may desire more aggressive action than recommended by the physician. For such cases, The American Medical Association Council on Ethical and Judicial Affairs recommends a process-based approach to addressing futility.[10] Although this policy may have limited utility in the ED environment, it is reasonable to have an understanding of the recommendations, as there may arise opportunities to employ these recommendations in some fashion. The recommendations are as follows:

- Deliberation and resolution.
- Joint decision-making with physician, and patient or proxy.
- Assistance of a consultant or patient representative.
- Utilization of an institutional committee (i.e. ethics committee)

When specific interventions or therapies are withheld, for any reason, as required by professionalism and standard of care, the health care team of course should continue to provide compassionate, attentive, and situation-appropriate medical care for the patient.

Advance directives

An *Advance Directive* is a legal document to communicate individual treatment wishes, to be carried out if patients are unable to communicate their preferences. Some examples of advance directives are the *Do Not Resuscitate* (DNR) order, living will, and durable power of attorney for health care. Many states have passed legislation to recognize state-approved DNR orders and identification. A *Living Will* is a record declaring a patient's provisions for care in the specific cases of a terminal illness or permanent vegetative state. A *Durable Power Of Attorney* for health care assigns a surrogate decision-maker in the event that a patient is incapable of making medical decisions. In essence, patients may elect as their durable power of attorney any person of their choosing, although most often this falls to a spouse or other close family member.

Many individuals have strong personal preferences regarding cardiopulmonary resuscitation and EOL care. Without advance directives, providers and families often are unable to accurately state the patient's EOL wishes.[11–13] Recent research suggests that full resuscitative efforts are not universally desired by patients, and that trends toward societal consensus in hypothetical resuscitation scenarios can be identified.[14–15] Unfortunately, however, there are challenges to the widespread use of advance directives, including inaccurate public knowledge, low rates of completion, and lack of understanding of implications.[16–20] If there are no DNR/POA/LW or health care surrogates available, then it is up to the emergency providers to judge the wishes of the patient to the best of their ability and to use professional judgment to determine which interventions are most appropriate for the given circumstance.

End-of-life emergency medical care

Medical care at the EOL should focus on patient comfort, communication, psychosocial, cultural, and spiritual support. This allows such patients to shift focus from their terminal condition to optimizing the remainder of life. Palliative care, or care that is designed to improve the quality of life as opposed to prolonging survival, is often mistakenly believed appropriate only when life-prolonging care ends. However, medical care and palliative care are not always mutually exclusive. In reality, the World Health Organization's definition of palliative care, which follows, is much broader: "Palliative care is an approach that improves the quality of life of patients and their families facing problems associated with life-threatening illness, through the prevention and relief of suffering by means of early identification and impeccable assessment and treatment of pain and other problems, physical, psychosocial, and spiritual." In acute care settings there are at least three major palliative issues that can be addressed for patients receiving EOL care.

First, pain control is an integral element and an issue of high consequence for many receiving EOL care in emergency settings. Standard means to assess patients' pain such as the visual analog scale, verbal numeric scale, or adjective scale, etc., remain the mainstay for all patients. Some may be concerned that the use of pain medications such as opioid analgesics or sedative agents may hasten a patient's death. However, many ethicists agree that the principle of "double effect" is morally, legally, and ethically acceptable, if the provider's intent is to relieve suffering in an EOL care situation.[21–24]

Second, dyspnea is also common at the EOL, particularly in the elderly, who may have underlying impaired respiratory function. Dyspnea is often undertreated, and may lead to a sense of panic and anxiety.[25] Treatment options for dyspnea should first be directed at standard approaches to symptom control such as providing supplemental oxygen, non-invasive positive pressure ventilation, and specific treatments to control underlying conditions (e.g., CHF). As adjuncts, or if such measures are unsuccessful, palliative use of opioids and anxiolytics, in addition to oxygen therapy, are appropriate.[26]

Finally, depression is a common symptom near the EOL. Unfortunately, many doctors minimize or ignore symptoms of depression or anxiety as a natural reaction in the terminally ill or dying patient.[27–28] Providers in the ED can play a useful role in seeking evidence for unrecognized or undermanaged depression/anxiety. Specific instruments that may be helpful to identify depression include the Hospital Anxiety and Depression Scale, a visual analog scale, or simply asking "Are you depressed?"[29–30]

Disposition

Some patients will expire in the ED. Whenever possible providers should seek to provide an appropriate setting and provide the necessary resources for patients and family, including spiritual support, social services, privacy, and a setting for grieving. Other patients require another disposition for longer term care, such as inpatient admission, or hospice and palliative care settings. Palliative care settings offer many services to patients and their families in the EOL setting. Many communities offer hospice and palliative services at acute and chronic care facilities, in the hospital, or in the patient's home.[31] In the future, it is likely that hospice and palliative care will evolve and transfers from acute care settings such as EDs may become more common. Education of patients and families about options, and communication with admitting and primary care providers, are important responsibilities of the emergency physician. Emergency providers will be the key figures in advising patients and families during the time of the ED visit. For those patients who will leave the ED, the emphasis should be on the continuum of care and the team approach involving input from the other providers, especially those that will inherit primary responsibility for the medical care of the patient.

Family presence during resuscitative efforts

Traditionally, it was felt by most health care personnel that having family present during a resuscitation, especially that of a child, would create more angst and stress for all parties involved. This belief has been challenged over the past decade, and a new era was established regarding the concept of family presence at the bedside during resuscitation. Research articles have been published introducing the psychological benefits of family presence during resuscitation and organizations began to establish protocols on the subject. In 1994, the Emergency Nurses Association (ENA) developed an educational booklet to facilitate programs allowing family presence during resuscitation.[32] In 1995, the association followed with a position paper that was the official statement on the guidelines for family presence during invasive procedures and cardiopulmonary resuscitation. This has since been revised and updated several times.[33] The ENA continues with its strong position, recently revising its first educational program in 1995, entitled *Presenting the Option for Family Presence*.[34] And finally, the American Heart Association (AHA) followed suit with its support for family presence as taught during the Pediatric Advanced Life Support Course starting with its 2002 update as one of the evidence-based changes. In its 2005 guideline, the AHA states, "In the absence of data documenting harm and in light of data suggesting that it may be helpful, offering select family members the opportunity to be present during a resuscitation seems reasonable and desirable (assuming that the patient, if an adult, has not raised a prior objection)."[35]

Despite national recognition of the desirability of family presence through policy pronouncement and scholarly evidence of benefits, many health care providers remain very uncomfortable and unconvinced. In 2003, a 30-item survey on family presence was mailed to 1500 members of the American Association of Critical Care Nurses and 1500 members of the ENA. In the 984 surveys returned, there was no universal acceptance or guideline for family presence at the bedside despite the heightened awareness with the subject matter.[36] Only 5% of the respondents worked on units that had a written policy allowing family presence during resuscitation. Some 45% responded that their institution did not have policies related to family presence, but that their unit did allow for such practice. In contradistinction, 29% reported that family presence during resuscitation was prohibited on their unit because of an unwritten rule. Interestingly, 31% stated that a patient's family had asked whether they could be present during CPR a mean of three times during the past year. In February 2007, the American College of Critical Care Medicine published formal guidelines supporting family-centered care in critical care of adult patients.[37]

There are a number of underlying concerns associated with allowing family presence during resuscitation and invasive procedures. Some clinicians are distressed about the possibility of parental interference with patient care, although there is literature that provides evidence to the contrary.[38] Parents who have been present during procedures or resuscitations have indicated that they would choose to be present in the future if allowed,[39] but unfortunately they are not routinely asked to be present. Additionally, those clinicians who are opposed to parent presence speculate that the procedure will create a very emotional, upsetting environment, which in turn will generate anxiety with the physician and/or the child.[40] Others raise concerns of redirected attention to tasks such as responding to unnecessary questions, hindering of educational training, potential violation of patient confidentiality, and lastly, that this practice may trigger litigation by inexperienced observers who may misunderstand medical procedures and terminology.

Despite these concerns, several other position statements have been published in regards to family presence, especially related to the care of children. A consensus of recommendations regarding pediatric procedures and cardiopulmonary resuscitation was approved in concept by the American Academy of Pediatrics (AAP) and the Ambulatory Pediatrics Association (APA) in 2003 as part of a conference that included representatives from 18 national organizations.[41] The consensus recommendations specifically included the consideration of family presence as an option during pediatric procedures and cardiopulmonary resuscitation after assessing mitigating factors. If a family is not offered the option of presence, the recommendations suggest documenting the reasons why.

Despite the national recognition, family inclusion is not yet a universal process. There is some data to suggest that providers are supportive of the concept but are not well prepared for the actual process. In a study by Gold et al., the authors set out to look for support for this emerging practice among the pediatric population.[42] They randomly selected 1200 pediatric critical care and emergency medicine providers from professional association mailing lists. Of the 521 who responded, 83% reported participation in pediatric resuscitation with family members present and of those, more than half thought it was helpful for the family, and two thirds believed that parents wanted the option. Ninety-three percent would allow family presence in some situations, which were not clearly defined. It does appear that family presence during resuscitation has become a more favorable consideration but that additional research and education about the process is needed.

Acute care settings such as EDs face even more hurdles, due to the inherent fast paced, high acuity, time limited environment typical of most EDs. Other issues such as overcrowding and limited resources can further complicate the issue. All of these factors conspire to impede upon the relatively short period of time where the emergency providers can develop a relationship with the patient and/or family to explore the personal, spiritual, cultural, and religious beliefs. Despite these challenges, achieving rational implementation of family presence during invasive procedures and resuscitation is possible in the ED. If appropriate policies are well developed and implemented, and providers are given the appropriate education and training, family presence can be addressed, as well as anywhere in the hospital with the focus being on family communication.

Pediatric issues

Pediatric deaths pose specific challenges in the ED. Of the estimated 40,000 American children less than 15 years old who die each year, 20% die or are pronounced dead in outpatient sites, primarily the ED.[43] Many of these deaths are sudden and unexpected, but a substantial percentage of these cases will have a chronic component to their disease process. In the acute setting, these EOL issues are compounded by the lack of an established patient-physician relationship. However, there is an obligation to support the bereaving family while coinciding with the emotional, religious, and legal issues inevitably involved. The American Academy of Pediatrics and American College of Emergency Physicians recognized this difficulty and collaborated on a joint policy statement, *Death of a Child in the Emergency Department*. They agreed on recommendations on the principles of care after the death of a child in the emergency department.[44–45] Additionally, providing and organizing child and family centered care at the time of death is the subject of the Institute of Medicine (IOM) report *When Children Die: Improving Palliative and End-of-Life Care of Children and Their Families*.[46] In this report, the IOM describes a number of challenges to providing palliative and EOL care for children and families. Perhaps the most prevailing obstacle is the inadequate amount of research addressing this issue.

Fortunately, the number of pediatric deaths overall is low. As a result, there are very few physicians with any depth of experience with managing the bereaving process of families. Moreover, physicians lack training in palliative, EOL, and bereavement care.[47] One of the major recommendations from the IOM reports is that education be provided to health care professionals including scientific and clinical knowledge and skills, interpersonal skills and attitudes, ethical professional principles, and organizational knowledge skills.[46]

A team approach that includes nursing staff, hospital chaplain(s), and social workers is considered optimal. This team approach will not only provide an organized means for providing the necessary details to any EOL situation, but it will facilitate the necessary time for attention that may be needed to address further explanation, discussion, and effective counseling. Just as in the previous discussion regarding family presence during resuscitation, encouragement should be provided to maintain contact with their most recent deceased loved one by physical presence, whether it be a child or a spouse.[48] This may be the beginning of the healing process.

Cultural and spiritual issues

Cultural issues relating to medical care, especially at the EOL, are becoming increasingly significant as our population becomes more diverse. EOL decision-making and utilization of health care resources should be in harmony with cultural standards and the beliefs of the patient. Awareness of various cultural beliefs, attitudes, and traditions is important; however, it is equally important to avoid generalizations that all members of a culture espouse the same specific beliefs and traditions. Individual assessments and personal communications regarding cultural backgrounds and perspectives are as important as understanding individual preferences regarding medical interventions.

Communication of bad news is an area of focus that may vary among cultures. In the US, traditionally, providers are expected to fully disclose the patient's condition and prognosis. However, in some cultures, patients may be protected from full disclosure, with the belief that bad news may be excessively traumatic. Awareness of such traditions should be respected, but this should not limit honesty with patients. Frank and open discussion with the family and the patient often is the best course of action in the context of cultural sensitivity. Communication of ethical and legal obligations regarding disclosure and honesty may be important to support ongoing healthy physician-patient relationships and help to promote open discussion, especially in the acute care setting.

Spiritual beliefs and traditions play an important role at the EOL for many patients. The definition and scope of the term "spirituality" is highly variable. Attention to religious issues important to individual patients and families can help promote a meaningful EOL experience. Similarly to cultural awareness, the provision of spiritual care at the EOL should be viewed as a personalized process between health care providers, patients, and families, rather than a set of prescribed rules.[49] Individualized communication regarding religion, spiritual beliefs, prayer, or other religious observances, can be helpful in assisting the patient with meeting spiritual goals at the EOL.

Communication with survivors

Effective communication with patients and loved ones is an essential component of compassionate medical care at the EOL. An accurate understanding of the patient's goals and expectations of medical treatment can improve the physician's ability to provide the best care possible, in accordance with the patient's wishes. When communicating bad news (diagnosis, prognosis, or death), effective techniques include using eye contact, addressing patients or family members by name, using understandable layperson language, non-verbal communication to demonstrate empathy, and employing active listening techniques.[50–52]

Conclusions

Emergency physicians play important and multifaceted roles in EOL care in the ED (see Table 16.1). In addition to the provision of competent medical care, the physician must also appropriately address palliative care, symptom relief, patient education, communication, empathy, and cultural and ethical issues. Emergency providers can improve EOL skills through education as well as through familiarity with the ongoing research, advocacy issues, and the developments in palliative care. EDs may benefit providers and patients by establishing policies and procedures that support the compassionate provision of EOL care.

Table 16.1. Summary of end-of-life care in the emergency department

Provision of a dignified, comfortable, and private environment

Education of patients and families regarding disease state and prognosis

Communication with patients and families regarding treatment preferences

Encourage presence of family and friends at the bedside

Competent and compassionate medical care

Symptom relief

Cultural sensitivity

Psychosocial support

Spiritual support

References

1. Pitts SR, Niska RW, Xu J, Burt CW. National Hospital Ambulatory Medical Care Survey: 2006 emergency department summary. National health statistics reports; no 7. Hyattsville, MD: National Center for Health Statistics, 2008.

2. American College of Emergency Physicians. Ethical issues in emergency department care at the end-of-life. *Ann Emerg Med.* 2008;**52**:592.

3. Marco CA, Larkin GL, Moskop JC, Derse AR. The determination of "futility" in emergency medicine. *Ann Emerg Med.* 2000;**35**:604–612.

4. Goold SD, Williams B, Arnold RM. Conflicts regarding decisions to limit treatment: a differential diagnosis. *JAMA.* 2000;**283**:909–914.

5. AMA Council on Ethical and Judicial Affairs. Guidelines for the appropriate use of do-not-resuscitate orders. *JAMA.* 1991;**265**:1868–1871.

6. Gampel E. Does professional autonomy protect medical futility judgments? *Bioethics.* 2006;**20**:92–104.

7. Paris JJ, Reardon FE. Physician refusal of requests for futile or ineffective interventions. *Cambridge Quarterly of Healthcare Ethics.* 1992;**2**:127–134.

8. Jecker NS, Schneiderman LJ. Futility and rationing. *Am J Med.* 1992;**92**: 189–196.

9. ACEP Policy Statement. *Nonbeneficial ("futile") emergency medical interventions.* American College of Emergency Physicians, Dallas, Texas, 1998.

10. AMA, Council on Ethical and Judicial Affairs: medical futility in end-of-life care. *JAMA.* 1999;**281**:937–941

11. Wenger NS, Phillips RS, Teno JM et al. Physician understanding of patient resuscitation preferences: insights and clinical implications. *J Am Geriatr Soc.* 2000,**48**:S44–51.

12. Layde PM, Beam CA, Broste SK et al. Surrogates' predictions of seriously ill patients' resuscitation preferences. *Arch Fam Med.* 1995;**4**:518–523.

13. Beach MC, Morrison RS. The effect of do-not-resuscitate orders on physician decision-making. *J Am Geriatr Soc.* 2002;**50**:2057–2061.

14. Hamel MB, Lynn J, Teno JM et al. Age-related differences in care preferences, treatment decisions, and clinical outcomes of seriously ill hospitalized adults: lessons from SUPPORT. *J Am Geriatr Soc.* 2000;**48**: S1:76–82.

15. Marco CA, Schears RM. Societal preferences regarding cardiopulmonary resuscitation. *Am J Emerg Med.* 2002;**20**:207–211

16. Silviera M, DiPiero A, Gerrity M, Feudtner C. Patients' knowledge of options at the end-of-life: ignorance in the face of death. *JAMA.* 2000;**284**(19):2483–2488.

17. Teno J, Lynn J, Wenger N, et al. Advance directives for seriously ill hospitalized patients: effectiveness with the patient self-determination act and the SUPPORT intervention. SUPPORT Investigators. Study to Understand Prognoses and Preferences for Outcomes and Risks of Treatment. *Am Geriatr Soc.* 1997;**45** (4):508–512.

18. Taylor DM, Ugoni AM, Cameron PA, McNeil JJ. Advance directives and emergency department patients: ownership rates and perceptions of use. *Intern Med J.* 2003;**33**(12):586–592.

19. Llovera I, Ward MF, Ryan JG et al. Why don't emergency department patients have advance directives? *Acad Emerg Med.* 1999;**6**:1054–1060.

20. Tulsky JA. Beyond advance directives: importance of communication skills at the end-of-life. *JAMA.* 2005,**294**:359–365.

21. Castellano G. The criminalization of treating end-of-life patients with risky pain medication and the role of the extreme emergency situation. *Fordham Law Rev.* 2007;**76**(1):203–234.

22. Gallagher A, Wainwright P. Terminal sedation: promoting ethical nursing practice. *Nurs Stand.* 2007;**21**(34):42–46.

23. Boyle J. Medical ethics and double effect: the case of terminal sedation. *Theor Med Bioethic.* 2004;**25**(1):51–60.

24. Lo B, Rubenfeld G. Palliative sedation in dying patients: "we turn to it when everything else hasn't worked". *JAMA*. 2005;**294**(14):1810–1816.

25. Hall P, Schroder C, Weaver L. The last 48 hours of life in long-term care: a focused chart audit. *J Am Geriatr Soc*. 2002; **50**(3):501–506.

26. LeGrand SB, Khawam EA, Walsh D, Rivera NI. Opioids, respiratory function, and dyspnea. *Am J Hosp Palliat Care*. 2003; **20**(1):57–61.

27. Emanuael EJ. Depression, euthanasia, and improving end-of-life care. *J Clin Oncol*. 2005;**23**(27):6456–6458.

28. Goy E, Ganzini L. End-of-life care in geriatric psychiatry. *Clin Geriatr Med*. 2003;**19**:841–856.

29. Lees N, Lloyd-Williams M. Assessing depression in palliative care patients using the visual analog scale: a pilot study. *Eur J Cancer Care*. 1999;**8**:220–223.

30. Chochinov HM, Wilson KG, Enns M, Lander S. "Are you depressed?" Screening for depression in the terminally ill. *Am J Psychiatry*. 1997;**154**:674–676.

31. Ahern P. End-of-life – not end of story. *Mod Healthcare*. 2007;**37**(25):24.

32. Meyers TA, Eichhorn DJ, Guzzetta CE. Do families want to be present during CPR? A retrospective survey. *J Emerg Nurs*. 1998;**24**:400–405.

33. Emergency Nurses Association. Position statement: family presence at the bedside during invasive procedures and cardiopulmonary resuscitation. Revised October 2005. Dallas, TX: Emergency Nurses Association, 2005.

34. Eckle, N. (Ed.), *Presenting the Option for Family Presence*. Dallas, TX: Emergency Nurses Association; 2007.

35. American Heart Association. 2005 American Heart Association guidelines for cardiopulmonary resuscitation and emergency cardiovascular care. *Circulation*. 2005;**112**:Supp IV-1–IV-211.

36. MacLean SL, Guzzetta CE, White C, et al. Family presence during cardiopulmonary resuscitation and invasive procedures:

practices of critical care and emergency nurses. *Am J Crit Care*. 2003;**12**:246–257.

37. Davidson JE, Powers K, Hedayat KM, et al. Clinical practice guidelines for support of the family in the patient-centered intensive care unit: American College of Critical Care Medicine Task Force 2004–2005. *Crit Care Med*. 2007;**35**(2) 605–622.

38. Dingerman RS, Mitchell EA, Meyer EC, Curley MAQ. Parent presence during complex invasive procedures and cardiopulmonary resuscitation: a systematic review of the literature. *Pediatrics*. 2007;**120**(4):842–854.

39. Sacchetti A, Paston C, Carraciio C. Family presence during invasive procedures in the pediatric intensive care unit: a prospective study. *Arch Pediatr Adolesc Med*. 1999;**153**;955–958.

40. Bauchner H, Waring C, Vinci R. Parental presence during procedures in an emergency room: results from 50 observations. *Pediatrics*. 1991;**87**: 544–548.

41. Henderson DP, Knapp JF. Report of the National Consensus Conference on family presence during pediatric cardiopulmonary resuscitation and procedures. *J Emerg Nurs*. 2006;**32**:23–29.

42. Gold KJ, Gorenflo DW, Schwenk TL, Bratton SL. Physicians experience with family presence during cardiopulmonary resuscitation in children. *Pediatr Crit Care Med*. 2006;**7**(5):428–433.

43. Knapp J, Mulligan-Smith D, American Academy of Pediatrics Committee on Pediatric Emergency Medicine. Death of a child in the emergency department. *Pediatrics*. 2005;**115**(5):1432–1437.

44. American Academy of Pediatrics and American College of Emergency Physicians, Committees on Pediatric Emergency Medicine. Death of a child in the emergency department, a joint statement by the American Academy of Pediatrics and the American College of Emergency Physicians. *Ann Emerg Med*. 2002;**40**:409–410.

45. American Academy of Pediatrics and American College of Emergency

Physicians, Committee on Pediatric Emergency Medicine. Death of a child in the emergency department a joint statement by the American Academy of Pediatrics and the American College of Emergency Physicians. *Pediatrics.* 2002;**110**:839–840.

46. Institute of Medicine, Committee on Palliative and End-of-Life Care for Children and Their Families. In Field MJ, Behraman RE (Eds.), *When Children Die: Improving Palliative and End-Of-Life Care for Children and their Families.* Washington, DC: National Academy Press, 2003.

47. Greenberg LW, Oschsenschlager D, Cohen GJ, et al. Counseling parents of a child dead on arrival: a survey of emergency departments. *Am J Emerg Med.* 1993:**11**:225–229.

48. Meert KL, Thurston CS, Briller SH. The spiritual needs of parents at the time of their child's death in the pediatric intensive care unit and during bereavement: a qualitative study. *Pediatr Crit Care Med.* 2005;**6**(4):420–427.

49. Daaleman TP, Usher BM, Williams SW, et al. An exploratory study of spiritual care at the end-of-life. *Ann Fam Med.* 2008;**6**:406–411.

50. O'Mara K. Communication and conflict resolution in emergency medicine. *Emerg Med Clin North Am.* 1999;**17**:451–459.

51. Ong LM, de Haes JC, Hoos AM et al. Doctor-patient communication: a review of the literature. *Soc Sci Med.* 1995;**40**: 903–918.

52. Olsen JC, Buenese ML, Falso W. Death in the emergency department. *Ann Emerg Med.* 1998;**31**:758.

Chapter 7

The emergency management of women with psychiatric illness

Karen Schwartz

Overview

Women seek acute care and come to the emergency department (ED) for many of the same psychiatric concerns as men. However, there are several psychiatric illnesses that are more common in women than in men and, therefore, are more likely to be encountered in EDs. Some disorders apparently more common in women include: major depression, rapid cycling bipolar disorder, eating disorders, panic disorder, phobias, generalized anxiety disorder, somatization, and borderline and histrionic personality disorder. Women also have a higher rate of suicide attempts and parasuicides (suicide gestures and deliberate self-harm). In addition, there are psychiatric conditions that are accentuated or precipitated by pregnancy. It is important for the acute care physicians to be aware of these illnesses when evaluating and treating women in these types of settings.

Affective disorders

Affective or mood disorders are illnesses in which a significant change in mood is the primary feature. The most common affective disorder is **major depression**. Although the incidence of depression is approximately equal for girls and boys in childhood, depression becomes more common in females during puberty and is twice as common in women as it is in men.[1-2]

Diagnosis of depression is difficult as the range of clinical presentation is broad and there are no ancillary tests to help guide the clinician. However, there are a number of clinical conditions, including medications and drugs, that mimic or precipitate mood disorders (see Chapter 8). Thus, even if the patient's acute condition is known to parallel previous presentations, a directed medical evaluation including ancillary testing may be appropriate to rule out an organic cause. That said, the diagnosis of psychiatric based mood disorder is based on a clinical history and a mental status examination. In the case of depression, the principal features are a sad mood or anhedonia, and a lack of interest in and the inability to enjoy usual activities. One of these features must be present for at least two weeks to meet diagnostic criteria in the DSM-IV-TR[3] in addition to five or more neurovegetative symptoms (Table 17.1).

The presence of symptoms for at least two weeks helps to distinguish a major depressive episode from an adjustment disorder often seen in response to a stressful life event, such as the death of a loved one. An adjustment disorder is usually self-limited, often responds to

Emergency Psychiatry, ed. Arjun Chanmugam, Patrick Triplett, and Gabor Kelen. Published by Cambridge University Press. © Cambridge University Press 2013.

Table 17.1. Diagnostic criteria of depression

Major symptoms (at least one)

Low mood (sadness) or anhedonia

Neurovegetative symptoms (at least five)

Sleep disturbances (insomnia or hypersomnia)

Appetite change (increased or decreased)

Fatigue or energy loss

Psychomotor change (agitation or retardation)

Feelings of guilt, worthlessness, or hopelessness

Concentration impairment

Suicidal ideation or passive death wish

Decreased sexual interest

supportive therapy, and usually does not require medication. However, in the ED, it is more important to assess the severity of symptoms than the time course of the illness.

Postpartum depression has the same clinical features as a major depressive episode, but by definition it begins after labor and delivery. According to the DSM, the onset of depression must occur within four weeks of delivery; however, other literature sources allow postpartum depression to begin up to a year after delivery. Additionally it is common for postpartum depression to actually begin during the pregnancy, especially during the third trimester. It is important to look for postpartum depression in the ED because the prevalence (10–20% of women) is fairly high.[4] It is more common in women with a history of major depression or women with a previous history of postpartum depression.[5–6] It is distinguished from the "baby blues", a self-limited, common phenomenon occurring in 80% of women a few days after birth and resolving in 1–2 weeks. Symptoms of postpartum blues include the heightening of emotion, tearfulness, mood lability, and a feeling of being overwhelmed in the first week or two after delivery.

Bipolar disorder is another affective disorder that commonly presents in the ED. Although the prevalence of bipolar disorder is equal in men and women, rapid cycling bipolar disorder (four or more mood episodes in 12 months) is more common in women.[7] Bipolar disorder comprises both depressed and manic episodes. The depressed episodes experienced are identical to those described for major depression. The manic episodes experienced are characterized by a persistently elevated, expansive, or irritable mood for at least one week. Additionally, three hyperdynamic symptoms (four, if the patient's mood is irritable rather than elevated) must be present (Table 17.2).

Often these patients overspend money, drive recklessly, and participate in promiscuous sexual behavior while experiencing a mania.

The spectrum of bipolar disorder includes several different forms of the illness. Bipolar disorder, type I, is the classic form of the illness which contains both depressed and manic episodes. Bipolar disorder, type II includes depressed and hypomanic episodes. **Hypomania** is a less severe form of mania (see Chapter 8), in which similar symptoms occur but do not cause marked impairment in social or occupational function, do not necessitate hospitalization, and psychotic features are not present. Additionally, symptoms only have to be

Table 17.2. Diagnostic criteria for mania

Major symptoms (at least one week)

Persistently elevated, expansive, or irritable mood

Additional symptoms (three or more [four or more if primary mood is irritable])

Grandiosity (inflated self esteem)

Decreased need for sleep

Increased (goal related) activity

Increased or pressured speech

Flight of ideas, or racing thoughts

Distractibility

Increased risk behaviors (including sexual indiscretion)

present for four days to qualify as hypomania. Another mood state seen in bipolar disorder is a mixed state, in which the patient experiences depressed and manic symptoms simultaneously. This is a very uncomfortable state for the patient, as she will usually feel energized or on edge but also be extremely distressed or down. This particularly dangerous mood state is attended by increased suicide risk and substance use.[8] Another form of bipolar disorder, mentioned above, is a rapid cycling type, in which mood states switch rapidly with four mood episodes occurring within 12 months.

Women with a history of bipolar disorder who are not on medication during pregnancy are at an increased risk of developing postpartum psychosis. Postpartum psychosis is a very serious mood state which presents with psychosis, confusion, and other symptoms of mania, generally in the first three months postpartum. Women usually have a severe worsening in function, disorganized behavior, and often limited insight into their illness. Although postpartum psychosis is extremely rare, occurring in only 0.05–0.1% of all deliveries, there is a 20–30% likelihood of a woman with bipolar disorder developing postpartum psychosis.[9-10] Postpartum psychosis is considered a psychiatric emergency with potentially grave outcomes for the patient and her baby if she is not treated appropriately and rapidly. The mother should be hospitalized immediately and care of the baby should be transferred to another caretaker until she is stabilized.

Anxiety disorders

Anxiety disorders are common psychiatric disorders with a mean age of onset in the late second (adolescence) or early third (young adulthood) decade of life. Many patients do not seek treatment for these disorders and often present to non-psychiatric physicians with complaints about the somatic manifestations of their anxiety disorder. With the exception of obsessive-compulsive disorder (OCD), all anxiety disorders are more commonly diagnosed in women than in men. Women are three times more likely to experience phobias, 1.5 times as likely to develop panic disorder with agoraphobia, and twice as likely to suffer from generalized anxiety disorder (GAD). The reason for these gender differences is unknown.[11]

The anxiety condition most likely to present to the ED is a panic attack, characterized by a sudden onset of intense fear, lasting several minutes. Four acute anxiety oriented or adrenergic symptoms also must be present (Table 17.3).

Table 17.3. Diagnostic criteria for panic attack

Major symptom

Sudden-onset intense fear lasting at least several minutes.

Additional symptoms (at least four)

Palpitations

Diaphoresis

Trembling

Paresthesias

Chills or hot flushes

Shortness of breath or feeling of choking

Chest pain

Nausea

Dizzy or lightheaded

Derealizaton (feelings of unreality) or depersonalization (feeling detached from oneself)

Fear of losing control or "going crazy"

Fear of dying

Panic attacks can be seen with any anxiety disorder. In panic disorder, a patient has recurrent, unexpected panic attacks that become associated with anticipatory anxiety of future attacks. This leads to a change in behavior to try to avoid future attacks. A woman with panic disorder is susceptible to abusing alcohol to try to "self-medicate" her anxiety symptoms.[12]

GAD is another common anxiety disorder. GAD is described as excessive worry for at least six months about a number of activities, such as work or school. The worrying leads to an impairment in functioning. Patients with GAD also experience restlessness, difficulty concentrating, irritability, muscle tension, sleep disturbance, and easy fatigability. It is also possible, but less likely, for a woman with OCD to present to the ED. While OCD is common, it rarely becomes so intrusive as to require ED evaluation and management. OCD is characterized by obsessions or anxiety provoking, recurrent, unwanted, intrusive thoughts or images and compulsions or repetitive behaviors that the patient feels driven to perform to decrease a feeling of tension or anxiety. A patient realizes that the fear is excessive or irrational and tries to resist it. Examples of obsessions include a fear of germs or a fear of committing a shameful act. Common compulsions are hand washing, checking, and counting.

Anxiety disorders can be exacerbated during times of hormonal change, such as during the premenstrual, pregnancy, and postpartum periods. Pregnancy and the postpartum period have been specifically associated with a 30% increase in cases of pre-existing panic disorder and OCD.[12]

Behavioral disorders

Behavioral disorders involve self-reinforcing or addictive behaviors which are goal directed and which become the prevailing concern of the patient. The most common behavioral disorders in women are the cluster of **eating disorders**: anorexia nervosa, bulimia nervosa, and binge eating disorder. Women are ten times more likely to experience anorexia or bulimia than men. Young white women, especially from middle to upper classes in Western cultures, are at the highest risk for anorexia or bulimia. However, rates of eating disorders are on the rise in men and in other racial and socioeconomic groups.[13]

Anorexia nervosa has been described as an "addiction to starvation."[14] It is characterized in the DSM by self starvation, with a refusal to maintain body weight above 85% of normal for the patient's age and height. The patient also has a psychological preoccupation with a fear of fatness. Women afflicted misinterpret their body and its shape. By definition, there is endocrine dysfunction leading to at least three consecutive months of amenorrhea. Bulimia nervosa has the same fear of obesity and body dissatisfaction as in anorexia nervosa, but the patient also engages in binge eating episodes and recurrent, inappropriate compensatory or purging behaviors in order to prevent weight gain. Compensatory behaviors include self-induced vomiting, misuse of laxatives, diuretics or enemas, fasting or excessive exercise. Purging behaviors can also occur in anorexia nervosa. Anorexia is distinguished from bulimia by the patient being underweight and amenorrheic, not by specific behaviors. Binge eating disorder has some similarity to bulimia because in both disorders the patient gorges or overindulges. However, binge eating disorder is different in that compensatory behaviors are not present. Thus, patients with binge eating disorder tend to be obese. It is not uncommon for women to slide between diagnoses over the course of a lifetime.

Eating disorders are often underdiagnosed because patients tend to hide signs and symptoms due to shame and conflicts over whether they want to give up the behaviors. The physiologic signs of an eating disorder are usually related to starvation or purging behaviors. Signs of starvation are low body weight, bradycardia, hypotension, chronic constipation, delayed gastric emptying, osteoporosis, and menstrual irregularities. Signs of purging behaviors are electrolyte abnormalities which can lead to seizures, dental problems, parotid gland hypertrophy, and gastrointestinal problems. Any woman with unexplained excessive thinness or emaciation who presents with any of the above findings should be closely screened for an eating disorder. It is especially important to consider this diagnosis in women, because eating disorders have the highest mortality rate of any psychiatric disorder. Patients with anorexia tend to die from starvation or suicide and bulimics tend to die from hypokalemia-associated arrhythmias or suicide. When screening, it is important to ask about the patient's highest and lowest weight, her dieting behaviors, and extensive questions about bingeing and purging.

The psychological effects from an eating disorder can be secondary to the eating disorder or can be seen as a separate psychiatric disorder. Studies have shown that starvation itself causes a depressed mood, low libido, and social isolation. These symptoms resolve with refeeding and a return to a normal weight.[15] Still, even when a normal weight is achieved, patients with eating disorders are at an increased risk for psychiatric comorbidities. Comorbid depression or dysthymia is seen in 50–75% of patients with anorexia and 24–88% of patients with bulimia.[16] Eating disorder patients are also at risk of anxiety disorders, substance abuse, and personality disorders.

Substance abuse is another category of behavior disorders that frequently present to the ED. The rate of substance abuse is higher in men, however, a significant number of women abuse substances as well. Among adult women, 5% have a serious alcohol problem and 6% abuse other substances.[17] The rate of abuse may be higher in women than reported. Research has shown that physicians are less likely to take a substance abuse history or detect alcohol abuse in women than in men.[18] Additionally, many standard diagnostic questionnaires rely heavily on occupational and legal issues when assessing substance abuse. These problems are often not evident in women who work in the home, leading to further underdiagnosis. Research also suggests that gender differences are narrower among younger age cohorts.[19]

Substance abuse is defined as the continued use of a substance that results in repeated adverse social consequences, such as failure to meet work, family, or school obligations, interpersonal conflicts, or legal problems. A patient is considered substance-dependent when she experiences withdrawal symptoms if the substance is discontinued. Tolerance should be considered when there is a need for increased amounts of the substance to produce the desired effects. When tolerance is suspected, the substance of abuse is taken in larger amounts and efforts to cut back its use are unsuccessful.

Although substance abuse includes the use of illicit street drugs and the misuse of prescription drugs such as narcotics, the most commonly abused substance in the United States is alcohol. Alcohol abuse may be different in women compared to men. Women who abuse alcohol are more likely to drink alone and are less likely to have a history of violence. They are more likely to be victims of physical and sexual abuse and to develop posttraumatic stress disorder.[20] Women are also more likely to have an alcoholic partner than men and are often influenced significantly by their partner. Women develop alcohol-related medical problems more quickly and with less alcohol intake than men because of lower levels of gastric alcohol dehydrogenase and a higher ratio of body fat to water volume.[21] Women experience cirrhosis, hypertension, fatty liver, gastrointestinal bleeding, cardiac problems, cognitive impairment, stroke, and malnutrition earlier than men. It is thought that a woman consuming 1.5 alcoholic drinks daily is equivalent to a man having four drinks per day.[22]

Women who abuse one substance are much more likely to abuse other substances simultaneously. Furthermore, women who abuse substances have a high rate of psychiatric comorbidity. Psychiatric disorders that often occur with alcohol abuse include mood disorders, eating disorders, and anxiety disorders. One study showed that the prevalence of depression in alcoholic women was 19% compared to 7% in non-alcoholic women.[23] Women with mood and anxiety disorders report drinking to "self-medicate" uncomfortable mood states. If relief from these symptoms occurs, it is short lived. Overall, using substances exacerbates psychiatric disorders and makes them difficult to treat. A patient often must be abstinent for several weeks before mood returns to its baseline. In addition, compared to the general population, women who abuse alcohol are much more likely to attempt suicide, particularly in an intoxicated state.

Psychotic disorders

Schizophrenia is an illness which afflicts approximately 1% of the population and is marked by positive symptoms, including delusions, hallucinations, and disorganized thought, and negative symptoms, including a flat affect and avolition. It is not uncommon for a patient with an exacerbation of schizophrenia, especially the positive symptoms, to present to the ED. These patients are frequently paranoid or appear internally preoccupied by voices in their heads. Schizophrenia is equally prevalent in men and women; however the onset of the illness differs between the two sexes. The peak age of onset in women is 25 to 35 years old, whereas the onset for men is earlier. Adolescent boys are twice as likely as girls to develop the illness, but women over 50 are seven times more likely to develop late-onset schizophrenia. Women with schizophrenia are more likely to marry and have children than men with the illness. Women also experience more mood symptoms, paranoia, and auditory hallucinations, while men experience more negative symptoms.[24]

The pregnancy rate for women with schizophrenia is increasing and is close to that of the general population. Additionally, women with schizophrenia are thought to have more unplanned pregnancies and receive less prenatal care. They are more likely to have poor nutrition and use more alcohol, tobacco, and illicit drugs than women without schizophrenia.[25] Exacerbations of schizophrenia are not uncommon during pregnancy, especially as there are data to suggest that a majority of women with psychotic illness are not linked to psychiatric services during their pregnancies.[26] Postpartum psychosis, described above, is highly linked to mood disorders, especially bipolar disorder. However, women with schizophrenia are also at risk for a psychotic episode after delivery. McNeil found that 24% of patients with schizophrenia had a postpartum relapse. Pregnancy-related psychotic symptoms for women with schizophrenia occur later than in women with mood disorders who generally become symptomatic in the first three months postpartum.[27]

Delirium

Delirium is an underrecognized and underdiagnosed clinical disorder that occurs both in men and women. It should be considered in any patient who presents to the ED with psychiatric symptoms. The hallmark symptom of delirium is a change in consciousness along with global cognitive impairment. Its onset is usually abrupt and it follows a waxing and waning course. Patients often present with disorientation, attention difficulties, behavioral disturbances, hallucinations and delusions, and sleep-wake cycle disturbances. It can be the consequence of any medical illness, however, patients with pre-existing brain damage who are taking multiple medications and are over the age of 60 are more susceptible to delirium.[28] Additionally, patients who have a history of substance abuse are more likely to become delirious. Delirium is common in the setting of benzodiazepine and alcohol withdrawal.

Victims of domestic violence (intimate partner violence)

Domestic violence is not a psychiatric disorder, but it can have an impact on mental health. Although the incidence of domestic violence is virtually impossible to measure, it is thought that approximately one in four women will experience domestic violence in her lifetime. The number of males who are victims of domestic violence is increasing, but women are still at a much higher risk.[29] Pregnant women experience domestic violence at a similar rate as non-pregnant women. Studies have found that 4% to 17% of pregnant women experience domestic violence during their pregnancy.[30]

Not all victims of domestic violence have access to health care, but most do. Victims of domestic violence commonly use health care services at a higher rate than the general population. A recent study showed that after adjusting for age, education, and other factors, victims of domestic violence had 50% higher ED visits, twice as many mental health visits, and six times the use of drug and alcohol services than those without a history of domestic violence. They also had 14% to 21% more visits to primary care and specialty care clinics. Even five years after the abuse had ceased, women with a history of domestic violence use health care services 20% more often than women with no history of domestic violence.[31]

All women, despite their presenting complaint, should be screened for abuse and domestic violence in the ED. In fact, ED screening of all women for intimate partner violence is a requirement of the The Joint Commission. Not only do these women present to the ED with physical injuries from abuse, they also experience more headaches, chronic pain, gastrointestinal and gynecologic problems, and anxiety and depression than other women.[31] It is impossible to know who is suffering from domestic violence and, therefore, all women should be screened. Although the ED can be a hectic environment with many challenges often preventing a meaningful discussion about domestic violence, there are techniques to improve communication between physicians and patients. Women are more likely to admit abuse when: the health care provider probes or asks more than one question about abuse, asks open ended questions and provides an opportunity for response, picks up on patient clues such as current social stressors, and follows up on these with specific questions.[32]

Assessment and acute management

The often hectic high-paced environment of the ED poses specific management challenges for acute psychiatric presentations. In patients who were victims of violence in the past, an aggressive approach by providers can evoke memories of the violence and worsen the patients' condition overall. Unfortunately, this often leads to even more aggressive management which in turn upsets the patient further and the cycle continues.[33]

Several actions will enhance patients' feelings of safety and help to minimize confrontational, erratic, or escalating behaviors. As with all ED patients, those with a primary psychiatric concern should be informed about their course of care as much as possible, including routine registration and other procedures before and as they occur. Coercion should be minimized. Patients should be given choices and their wishes should be implemented whenever possible. Specifically, gender preference in staff-patient interactions, especially when being searched, should be followed. Special consideration should be given to all patients with a history of trauma, as the use of physical restraints or coercion can trigger traumatic memories leading to increased agitation. Restraints and seclusion should only be used when absolutely necessary and for the minimum amount of time possible. An assessment of a patient should be done as soon as possible so more appropriate, detailed treatment can begin.[33]

Assessment

Patients with a psychiatric presentation require a comprehensive approach in the ED. Many psychiatric conditions are a manifestation of organic (medical) disease, or are accentuated/exacerbated by underlying medical conditions. Serious medical conditions are often missed in this population.[34] Accordingly, these patients require the same diligent history and physical exam as do other ED patients. It is vital that a reliable third party informant be contacted. Patients with psychiatric complaints may not be able to accurately convey symptoms or recent history. At the same time, any potential agendas of such third party informants should be appreciated. Ancillary testing is dictated by important medical conditions within the differential diagnoses. In particular, medication effect, overdose, or withdrawal are common in the psychiatric population and should be considered as potentially explaining (or failing to explain) the patient's presentation if appropriate.

Acute management

The ED is not the appropriate environment to initiate long-term treatment for psychiatric illnesses. Rather, after assessment, and having excluded organic explanations for the presentation, the major task of the ED physician is to determine appropriate disposition. While arriving at a decision is not always straightforward, the choices are relatively simple: admission to a psychiatric facility, discharge with outpatient follow-up, specialty consultation (if available), and observation. For the most part, women and men are assessed similarly for inpatient hospitalization. The decision to hospitalize by itself is not very complicated for most patients. Hospitalization is clearly indicated for women (and men) who pose a threat to self or others, or cannot function. There are certain circumstances specific to women, such as postpartum or intra-pregnancy psychiatric disorder, for which hospitalization should be strongly considered. If there is any doubt as to patient safety or ability to provide adequate outpatient management, the woman should be hospitalized.

A woman with postpartum psychosis should be hospitalized immediately. This is considered a psychiatric emergency requiring close monitoring in a hospital setting. This condition is often associated with disorganized behavior, cognitive impairment as well as poor insight into the illness. Untreated this leads to a substantial change in her functioning with devastating consequences for the patient, her newborn, and other members of the family. Suicide is the leading cause of maternal death up to a year after delivery and occurs in 2 per 1000 mothers with postpartum psychosis.[35] Although most mothers with postpartum psychosis do not display homicidal behavior, one study found that 28–35% of women hospitalized for postpartum psychosis had delusions about their infants and 9% expressed thoughts of harming the infant.[36] In addition to careful monitoring of mothers with postpartum psychosis, treatment of the illness includes the use of antipsychotic medications, mood stabilizers, and electroconvulsive therapy (ECT), depending on the patient's underlying diagnosis and treatments in the past.[37] Obviously, care for her newborn and other children should be arranged.

Postpartum depression is another serious illness that often requires hospitalization. If a woman with depression is followed by a psychiatrist during pregnancy and the postpartum period, postpartum depression may be avoided or readily treated. Aggressive medication management, frequent appointments with the psychiatrist, and dedicated family members to observe the patient may prevent a woman suffering from postpartum depression from being hospitalized. If a woman experiencing postpartum depression presents to the ED, however, she is most likely profoundly distressed and is not obtaining appropriate treatment. She will almost certainly require hospitalization for treatment with antidepressants or ECT and to protect her safety and the safety of the newborn.

Before deciding whether to hospitalize or to link a patient to outpatient care, an ED physician may be required to manage agitation in the ED. The use of medication to control agitation is similar in men and women, except when the woman is pregnant. In pregnancy, the risks and benefits for the mother and the fetus must be weighed before treating a patient for agitation. In an ideal situation, medication would not be required to control agitation in a pregnant woman. When medication is required, it is important to know that all psychiatric medications studied to date cross the placenta and are present in amniotic fluid.[38–39] Thus, limiting the amount of medication and the number of agents used for treatment is crucial. Older medications are often preferred in the treatment of pregnant women because there are more pregnancy safety data available for these medications.

Generally antipsychotics and benzodiazepines are used for agitation in the ED. Because the atypical antipsychotics (clozapine, olanzapine, quetiapine, risperidone, ziprasidone, and aripiprazole) are fairly new medications, there are limited safety data for their use during pregnancy. Typical antipsychotics, on the other hand, have been widely used for over

40 years so the safety data are much more robust. No significant teratogenic effect has been seen with chlorpromazine, haloperidol, or perphenazine and no differences in fetal viability or birth weight were seen in newborns of mothers exposed to haloperidol.[40] Therefore, a typical antipsychotic, such as haloperidol, is recommended as the first line agent for patients who require treatment for agitation in the ED. An atypical agent might be considered first line if the patient is already taking the atypical antipsychotic regularly. The rationale for this consideration is that the fetus has been exposed to the atypical antipsychotic and has not been exposed to the traditional typical antipsychotics.

The dosage of the typical antipsychotic used should be kept to a minimum in order to decrease impact on the fetus and for other possible side effects. Medications used to treat extrapyramidal side effects caused by typical antipsychotics, such as akathisia or restlessness and dystonia or muscle rigidity, include diphenhydramine, benztropine, and amantadine. Benztropine and amantadine have not been studied systematically for safety in pregnancy. Diphenhydramine was shown to increase the risk of cleft palate in one study but has not been shown to be associated with any fetal malformations in several other studies.[41-43] Thus, diphenhydramine is a reasonable option for treating or preventing side effects caused by antipsychotics in pregnant women.

Benzodiazepines, another class of medication commonly used to treat agitation in the ED, were initially thought to increase the risk of oral clefts.[44] Even though more recent studies have not shown this association,[45-46] it is important to be mindful of potential fetal development effects if benzodiazepines must be used. When benzodiazepines are used near the time of delivery, they are associated with floppy infant syndrome, which is characterized by hypothermia, lethargy, poor respiratory effort, and feeding difficulties.[47] Neonatal withdrawal syndromes can also be seen when benzodiazepines are used around the time of delivery. These syndromes are described by restlessness, hypertonia, hyperreflexia, tremulousness, apnea, diarrhea, and vomiting.[48] *Benzodiazepines should, if at all possible, be avoided in pregnancy* except when a pregnant woman has been taking them regularly. In that situation, it is dangerous to stop the benzodiazepine abruptly as the woman will most likely experience withdrawal symptoms which can be harmful to her health and the health of the fetus.

Although it is ideal to minimize psychiatric medication during pregnancy, it is important to know that active unmanaged psychiatric illness is also considered a risk to the mother and the fetus. Pregnant women with inadequately treated or untreated psychiatric illnesses have more obstetrical complications such as increased need of forceps during deliveries, fetal distress, and low birth weight.[40] Increased newborn cortisol and catecholamine levels, delayed development,[49] and increased perinatal mortality and congenital malformations have also been observed.[50]

Pregnant patients who are safe for discharge from the ED, as a pre-requisite, must be linked to long-term psychiatric care to ensure that the psychiatric illness can be properly monitored and treated.

References

1. Angola A, Worthman CW. Puberty onset of gender differences in rates of depression: developmental, epidemiologic and neuroendocrine perspective. *J Affect Disord.* 1993;**29**:145–148.

2. Seedat S, Scott KM, Angermeyer MC, et al. Cross-national associations between gender and mental disorders in the World Health Organization World Mental Health Surveys. *Arch Gen Psychiatry.* 2009; **66**(7):785.

3. American Psychiatric Association. *Diagnostic and Statistical Manual of Mental Disorders, 4th Edition, Text Revision.* Washington, DC: American Psychiatric Association, 2000.

4. Campbell SB, Cohn JF. Prevalence and correlates of postpartum depression in first-time mothers. *J Abnorm Psychol.* 1991;**100**:594–599.

5. Frank E, Kupfer DJ, Jacob M, Blumenthal SJ, Jarrett DB. Pregnancy-related affective episodes among women with recurrent depression. *Am J Psychiatry.* 1987;**144**: 288–293.

6. Cox JL, Murray D, Chapman G. A controlled study of the onset, duration and prevalence of postnatal depression. *Br J Psychiatry.* 1993;**163**:27–31.

7. Blumenthal SJ. Women's mental health: the new national focus. *Ann NY Acad Sci.* 1996;**789**:1–16.

8. Goldberg JF, McElroy SL. Bipolar mixed episodes: characteristics and comorbidities. *J Clin Psych.* 2007;**68**:e25.

9. Gitlin MJ, Pasnau, RO. Psychiatric syndromes linked to reproductive function in women: a review of current knowledge. *Am J Psychiatry.* 1989;**146**:1413–1422.

10. Kendell RE, Chalmer JC, Platz C. Epidemiology of puerperal psychoses. *British J Psych.* 1987;**150**:662–663.

11. Yonkers KA, Gurguis G. Gender differences in the prevalence and expression of anxiety disorders. In Seeman MV (Ed.), *Gender and Psychopathology.* Washington, DC: American Psychiatric Press, 1995.

12. Pigott T. Gender differences in the epidemiology and treatment of anxiety disorders. *J Clin Psychiatry.* 1999;**60**:4–15.

13. American Psychiatric Association. Practice guideline for eating disorders. *Am J Psychiatry.* 1993;**150**(2):212–228.

14. Szmuckler GI, Tantam D. Anorexia nervosa: starvation dependence. *Br J Med Psychol.* 1984;**57**:303–310.

15. Keys A, Brozek J, Henshel A, Mickelsen O, Taylor HL. *The Biology of Human Starvation.* Minneapolis, MN: University of Minnesota Press, 1950.

16. Mitchell J, Speckler SM, de Zwaan M. Comorbidity and medical complications of bulimia nervosa. *J Clin Psychiatry.* 1991; **52**(10):13–20.

17. Substance Abuse and Mental Health Services Administration, Office of Applied Studies. *The NSDUH Report: Gender Differences in Alcohol Use and Alcohol Dependence or Abuse: 2004 and 2005.* Rockville, MD: Substance Abuse and Mental Health Services Administration, 2007.

18. Moore R, Bone LR, Gellar G, et al. Prevalence, detection and treatment of alcoholism in hospitalized patients. *JAMA.* 1989;**261**:403–407.

19. Keyes KM, Grant BF, Hasin DS. Evidence for a closing gender gap in alcohol use, abuse, and dependence in the United States population. *Drug Alcohol Depend.* 2008; **93**(1–2):21–29.

20. Brienza RS, Stein MD. Alcohol use disorder in primary care: do gender-specific differences exist? *J Gen Int Med.* 2002; **17**(5):387–397.

21. Blume SB. Women and alcohol. A review. *JAMA.* 1986;**256**:1467–1470.

22. Cyr MG, Moulton AW. The physician's role in prevention, detection and treatment of alcohol abuse in women. *Psychiatr Ann.* 1993;**23**:454–462.

23. Heizer JE, Pryzbeck TR. The co-occurrence of alcoholism and other psychiatric disorders in the general population and its impact on treatment. *J Stud Alcohol.* 1988;**49**:219–224.

24. Goldstein JM. The impact of gender on understanding the epidemiology of schizophrenia. In Seeman MV (Ed.), *Gender and Psychopathology.* Washington, DC: American Psychiatric Press, 1995.

25. Howard LM. Fertility and pregnancy in women with psychotic disorders. *Eur J Obst Gyn Repro Bio.* 2005;**119**:3–10.

26. McNeil TF, Kaij L, Malmquist-Larsson A. Women with nonorganic psychosis: mental disturbance during pregnancy. *Acta Psychiatr Scand.* 1984;**70**:27–39.

27. McNeil TF. A prospective study of postpartum psychoses in a high-risk group,

1: clinical characteristics of the current postpartum episodes. *Acta Psychiat Scand.* 1986;**74**:205–216.

28. Lipowoski ZJ. *Delirium – Acute Brain Failure in Man.* 2nd ed. New York, NY: Oxford University Press, 1990.

29. Tjaden P, Thoennes N. *Extent, Nature and Consequences of Intimate Partner Violence: Findings from the National Violence Against Women Survey.* Washington, DC: National Institute of Justice and the Centers of Disease Control and Prevention, 2000.

30. Wilt S, Olson S. Prevalence of domestic violence in the United States. *JAMWA* 1996;**51**:77–82.

31. Rivara FP, Anderson ML, Fishman ML, et al. Healthcare utilization and costs for women with a history of intimate partner violence. *Am J Prev Med.* 2007;**32**:89–96.

32. Rhodes KV, Frankel RM, Levintal N, et al. "You're not a victim of domestic violence, are you?" Provider patient communication about domestic violence. *Ann Intern Med.* 2007;**147**:620–627.

33. Stefan S. *Emergency Department Treatment of the Psychiatric Patient, Policy Issues and Legal Requirements.* New York: Oxford University Press, 2006.

34. Hall R, Gardner E, Popkin M, et al. Unrecognized physical illness prompting psychiatric admission: a prospective study. *Am J Psychiatry.* 1981;**138**:629–635.

35. CEMD. *Confidential Inquiries into Maternal Deaths: Why Mothers Die, 1997–99.* London: Royal College of Obstetricians and Gynaecologists, 2001.

36. Kumar R, Marks M, Platz C, Yoshida K. Clinical survey of a psychiatric mother and baby unit: characteristics of 100 consecutive admissions. *J Affect Disord.* 1995;**33**:11.

37. Sit D, Rothschild AJ, Wisner KL. A review of postpartum psychosis. *J Womens Health.* 2006;**15**:352–368.

38. Newport DJ, Calamaras MR, DeVane CL, et al. Atypical antipsychotic administration during late pregnancy: placental passage and obstetrical outcomes. *Am J Psychiatry.* 2007;**164**:1214–1220.

39. Hostetter A, Ritchie JC, Stowe ZN. Amniotic fluid and umbilical cord blood concentrations of antidepressants in three women. *Biol Psychiatry.* 2000;**48**: 1032–1034.

40. ACOG Committee on Practice Bulletins – Obstetrics. Clinical management guidelines for obstetrician-gynecologists, use of psychiatric medications during pregnancy and lactation. *Obstet Gynecol.* 2008;**111**:1001–1020.

41. Saxen I. Cleft palate and maternal diphenhydramine intake. *Lancet.* 1974;**1**:407–408.

42. Heinonen OP, Shapiro S, Slone D. *Birth Defects and Drugs in Pregnancy.* Littleton, MA: Publishing Sciences Group, 1977.

43. Nelson MM, Forfar JO. Associations between drugs administered during pregnancy and congenital abnormalities of the fetus. *Br Med J.* 1971;**1**:523–527.

44. Aarkog D. Association between maternal intake of diazepam and oral clefts. *Lancet.* 1975;**2**:921.

45. Eros E, Czeisel AE, Rockenbauer M, et al. A population-based case-control teratologic study of nitrazepam, medazepam, tofisopam, alprazolam and clonazepam treatment during pregnancy. *Eur J Obstet, Gynecol Reprod Biol.* 2002;**101**:147–154.

46. Lin AE, Pellar AJ, Westgate MN, et al. Clonazepam use in pregnancy and the risk of malformations. *Birth Defects Res A Clin Mol Teratol.* 2004;**70**:534–536.

47. Haram K. "Floppy Infant Syndrome" and maternal diazepam. *Lancet.* 1977;**2**: 612–613.

48. Barry WS, St Clair S. Exposure to benzodiazepines in utero. *Lancet.* 1987;**1**:1436–1437.

49. Wisner KL, Zarin DA, Holmboe ES, et al. Risk of decision making for treatment of depression during pregnancy. *Am J Psychiatry.* 2000;**157**:1933–1940.

50. Schneid-Kofman N, Sheiner E, Levy A. Psychiatric illness and adverse pregnancy outcome. *Int J Gynaecol Obstet.* 2008;**101**:53–56.

The impact of culture on the acute management of psychiatric illness

Geetha Jayaram

The goal of this chapter is to emphasize the impact of culture on the meaningful life story and behavioral perspectives of patients presenting to acute care settings, such as an emergency department (ED), in crisis. Evaluating psychiatric patients is difficult, and can be time-consuming under routine circumstances. In the ED, it is complicated by over-crowding, a fast pace, lack of privacy, and poor preparation of the patient who may be brought in under duress by family members or the police. Evaluating patients can be further complicated by language and cultural differences between the patient and examining provider. The intent of this chapter is to facilitate such an examination by focusing on the cultural differences and related aspects of interviewing and examining patients.

The definition of culture includes the customary beliefs, social forms, and material traits of a racial, religious, or social group. Cultural differences play a role in assessment and treatment of patients, including the attitude and behavior of both the provider and the patient regarding illness. Notions of sickness are derived from systems of medical understanding that exist within a culture. Beyond that, epistemic systems dictate how an individual expresses suffering. In many patients, their indigenous understandings of medicine and systems of coping with illness may partially or fully persist and continue to exert an influence on behavior, despite the seemingly outward expression of complete adoption of the Western system of medicine and response to illness.

The following cases illustrate how the cultural backgrounds of patients impact how they view illness, their unique coping mechanisms, and the challenge created if such differences are not well incorporated into their management.

Case example 1

A 22 year old Indian woman was brought to the ED by her new husband and her parents-in-law for new-onset odd behavior and muteness. The resident in the ED was unacquainted with the woman's culture. He conducted a routine psychiatric interview with the in-laws and husband in the room, and asked the routine questions. He was told that the patient had spilled hot oil on herself while cooking, and arranged for treatment for second degree burns on her hands. The resident decided that there was no other acute problem, gave her the name of a clinic near her home, and discharged her from the ED.

The resident reviewed the case (among others) with the attending physician who happened to be familiar with the culture of this patient. The attending physician was distressed to discover the following: the patient was not interviewed without her in-laws

Emergency Psychiatry, ed. Arjun Chanmugam, Patrick Triplett, and Gabor Kelen. Published by Cambridge University Press. © Cambridge University Press 2013.

in the room, was not examined for other injuries, was not considered as a possible abuse victim, and was not referred to social work or the police. Also, the patient was not given the opportunity for psychiatric follow-up. The resident defended his actions by stating that the woman denied all symptoms and appeared to be in no significant distress.

The attending physician pointed out that the patient may be in the US through an "arranged marriage," which meant that she may not have known much about her husband or her in-laws before her arrival in the US. "Bride burning" incidents are common in India, particularly when conflicts arise about dowries to the groom's family. These conflicts can lead to physical and emotional abuse. The woman was isolated from her family in India and was likely without any other social support in the US. She may have had an unstable visa status, and may have had some distress trying to adjust to a new marriage in a new country. It is possible she may have been subject to emotional abuse and may have attempted suicide or engaged in self-harm by burning herself. Self burning is a common mode of suicide in the Asian subcontinent. Furthermore, many South Asians may not be particularly open to discussing personal problems with a stranger, especially a male physician. The presence of her husband and in-laws in the examining room may have intimidated the patient enough to silence her about her concerns. Finally, those who come from a rural background are often unaware of means to access psychiatric assistance and may not even know the term to use for anxiety and depression in an alien culture. An important opportunity to help the patient and avoid potential loss of life was lost because of ignorance about the patient's cultural norms.

Case example 2

A Korean-American psychiatrist well known to his colleagues was deeply depressed. He was under the care of a Caucasian physician. He was also estranged from his family. His involvement in the Korean community was not known to his care provider. The patient was sufficiently ill to engender close scrutiny by his friends. They kept in close contact with him by taking turns with checking in with him and providing personal support; but outwardly, he appeared to be doing well. His friends became more confident about his condition, as he had been noted to be laughing and smiling and appeared to be communicating well. He even continued to treat patients himself. When he did not come into work as scheduled, it was a surprise to his friends and colleagues that he was found dead in his apartment having cut his throat in a completed suicide.

The matter of shame and loss of face in one's community is an Asian concept that is critical in the evaluation of Asian patients. For some cultures, seeing a psychiatrist carries a stigma. Consequently, patients may choose to see their primary care provider for medications. Often they are undertreated. Therapy is not sought except by very Westernized, educated professionals. To see a primary care provider for a few minutes every few weeks may not be sufficient for a seriously ill patient who could be suicidal. In many cases, due to stigma, these individuals prefer talking to friends or a priest at a church or temple, instead of seeking help from a counselor, therapist, or psychiatrist. In some cases, the patients may recognize the need for professional assistance, but may consider a primary care or ED visit to be sufficient. Both primary care and emergency providers need to be vigilant that although patients such as the one above may admit to some difficulty with coping, they may not be as forthcoming as to the extent of the problem. These patients may minimize their symptoms, but if acute care providers are thorough in their evaluation, they can help the patient by creating the most appropriate treatment plan, which may include inpatient treatment as an option.

Case example 3

A young Hispanic woman whose husband was a migrant worker without permanent resident status was brought to the ED by her friends for severe abdominal pain. She did not speak English, but was extremely tearful. She reported that her husband drank daily and spent his wages on alcohol, spending excessive time in bars with his co-workers. The patient was verbally abused by him if she questioned his loyalty to her and their young son. She felt trapped in an alien culture and was hopeless, felt overwhelmed, and was constantly tearful. She feared for her young son's future.

In the ED, she was evaluated for her abdominal pain and was seen by the social worker. With the help of a bilingual translator she was given much-needed counseling. Her abdominal pain improved with minimal interventions. She was offered additional outpatient resources, both medical and psychiatric, including a clinic that provided her with a support system through the local church for Spanish-speaking people. The social worker helped her in obtaining information about housing alternatives and other resources.

Case example 4

A 50 year old African-American woman who had grown up living and working in rural North Carolina had recently moved to Baltimore to live closer to her city relatives. These family members brought her to the ED because they were concerned she had been "talking out of her head" for several days. The patient thought that her neighbors were "working roots and putting spells" on her. The belief of "working roots" has similarities to (but is not the same as) voodoo. Depending on the strength of the belief that "root working" can cause harm, it can manifest as delusions, persecutory hallucinations, anxiety, and agitation. Although the cultural belief of "working roots" may be mistaken for a delusion, in this case it was the primary misconception that the someone in the neighborhood was working the roots that was the significant delusion. The patient's relationship with her neighbors in an unfamiliar and crime-ridden environment, as well the patient's level of distress and ability to function, all needed to be fully evaluated as part of the psychiatric formulation.

Case example 5

A 23 year old black male was brought to the critical care area of a busy urban ED. He had a single gunshot to the leg, with only minor injuries noted. He was alternately yelling obscenities at the staff or crying out that he did not want to die. He refused to answer all but the simplest questions, responding with demands for food, drink, pain medications, his lawyer, and use of a telephone. Attempts to reason with him led to staff frustration. Only after speaking to him gently, reassuring him that he would be taken care of, did he begin to cry and become more reasonable with the staff.

The young man grew up in a violent, gang-ridden neighborhood. He had little parental supervision and direction. He was afraid of gang members, both his own and rival gangs. Talking to the authorities was forbidden by gang rules. Once the patient understood that the hospital staff was interested in his care and not in the gang crime details, he became less suspicious. It took time and repeated assurances before he would trust that his health care was the primary motive for the hospital staff involvement, but once he did, he became more cooperative.

Case example 6

A middle aged, single, Asian Indian woman with a PhD, who worked in a chemistry lab, was brought to the ED with a complaint of hallucinations and delusions. She had been noted to be flirtatious with her male Caucasian supervisor, and appeared to be glancing at herself in the mirror frequently, as if she was paranoid. An ED-based psychiatric assessment was requested. When interviewed by a psychiatrist who knew her language and culture, the following became apparent: the patient came from a small village in southern India. She had grown up relatively cloistered, with very little socialization with men. She had never dated. Only arranged marriages were permitted in her family. She lived with her brother in the US, who had sponsored her to obtain a work permit in the US. Her supervisor was a friendly man who often put his arm around her shoulders, encouraging her in her work. She mistook his behavior for romantic feelings towards her, which he denied on questioning. The patient had to return to her home town because the work situation became untenable. She was not delusional but she had misunderstood her supervisor's behavior.

Demographic trends

Globalization of trade, economy, and international citizenry have promoted the need for learning about and incorporating ethnic differences in treatment planning.[1] Trends in International Migration reported in the Annual Report 2010 Edition point to the fact that there is a greater diversity of immigrants in the US today.[2] One survey of the Washington DC metropolitan area published in 2009 noted that the overall immigrant population increased by 25%, with the Asian population demonstrating a 42% growth, the largest being in the Chinese and Indian groups. By the mid twenty-first century, almost half of the projected US population will be from ethnically diverse groups. The race/ethnic groups with the highest rates of increase are the Asian and Pacific Islander groups as well as the Hispanic-origin populations with annual growth rates that may exceed 2% until 2030.

More specifically, every year from now to 2050, the race/ethnic group adding the largest number of people to the population will be of Hispanic origin. In fact, after 2020, people of Hispanic origin are projected to add more people to the United States every year than would all other race/ethnic groups combined. Given the evolving demographics, it is becoming increasingly clear that the language and cultural barriers that exist have to be addressed for effective health care delivery.

Although core symptoms are the same across cultures, demographic trends are important to note because research suggests significant cultural differences in the presentation of anxiety and mood disorders.[3–5] For example, both African Americans and Hispanics are more likely to report victimization and violence in the ED assessment while victimization may be hidden by Asian women. Asian Indians may be more somatic in their illness expression.[6–10]

In order to appropriately address the needs of patients, assessments need to be completed with an awareness of cultural implications in the following three aspects of care: areas of diagnosis, medication management, and caregiver attitude and behavior.

Diagnostic issues

A diagnostic assessment consists of a thorough interview using family input and translators or other medical personnel familiar with the patient's cultural practices and language. The use of translators is not without potential problems. Family or friends should not be relied upon to provide translation. The translator must be instructed to merely translate, not interpret or judge the content of the patient's response. Family members who translate may provide translation but may also color the translation with what they believe is the diagnosis and may inadvertently mislead the treating team. Translators should be adept enough to help providers gain some familiarity of the patient's culture or pre-morbid functioning, otherwise misinterpretations can occur. For example, a psychosis may be diagnosed where none exists. Cases 4 and 6 above illustrate this point.

Distress may often be communicated in terms not generally used by the examiner, but may be typical for the patient with a specific cultural background. Acute care providers must be attuned to the fact that significant distress may be manifested differently in different cultures. For instance, panic disorder is more likely to be described in somatic terms in South Asians.[6] A critical clue is to understand how the presenting behavior is different from the patient's baseline behavior, and to thoroughly review the potential risk factors the patient may have. These include, but are not limited to, factors such as poverty, social situation, cultural beliefs, accessibility to health care, and underlying psychiatric and medical disorders.

During the evaluation, time constraints, remuneration for care rendered, and patient expectations (which can be dependent on cultural values) can impact the length of time and care provided. In addition to the expectations of the patient, family members' expectations must be managed during the interview. (In Case 1, the family's expectation was that the burns would be treated; they were not anticipating any psychiatric evaluation or social work involvement.) All of these considerations help in understanding the crisis that brought the patient to the ED, leading to a better understanding of the magnitude of the problem. If not, the care provider may be lulled into a false belief that the problem is not critical, as was seen in Case 1.

Anxiety and depression are universal, although rates of assessment vary by geographic region. Factors that place patients at risk for suicide vary across cultures.[11] In India for example, conflicts with in-laws, failure in exams, marital discord, break up of a romantic relationship, property disputes, chronic medical illnesses, and loss of a loved one may all be contributing factors. By contrast, in the United States, the following are associated with an increased risk of suicide: major depression, schizophrenia, alcoholism, recent financial or other losses, retirement, limited social support, being male and elderly, being widowed, and chronic medical or psychiatric illnesses.

Psychopharmacology/medication management

Ethnicity and culture not only play a role in the determination of a psychiatric diagnosis, but also in the differences in psychotropic drug use, metabolism, and pharmacodynamics. Not only may the response to psychotropic medications vary across different ethnic groups, but also the treatment based on the cultural background of the prescriber, as noted by Wasan et al.[12] Pi and Simpson have reported differences in drug dosing based on physician or prescriber training and culture.[13,14]

Choosing the appropriate medications to ensure compliance is dependent on patient values. The drugs that are considered acceptable, or are used in conjunction with herbal remedies, or with non-physician recommended medications given by a local healer (which are often dependent upon the prevailing culture), are dictated by norms that exist within the patient's culture. The fact that certain minority patients as noted below may be more sensitive to psychotropic drugs, are more prone to side effects, or that the side effect profile is not acceptable to some cultures, must be borne in mind. For instance, certain groups of patients, such as South Asians and elderly African Americans are less likely to use anti-depressants and more likely to suffer from side effects at lower doses for all psychotropic medications. Keh Ming Lin and Pi have both researched and presented the sensitivity of Asians to medications, with lower tolerance and greater propensity for side effects.[14,15] African Americans, particularly young males, are more prone to extra-pyramidal symptoms and dystonia. This too has been demonstrated by the same authors. Whenever possible, choices of oral or IM medications should be offered before a decision to medicate against a patient's will is made. A valuable opportunity to build rapport and promote compliance may be lost if choices are not explained or provided.

Caregiver/provider response, attitude, and behavior

In the treatment of psychiatrically ill patients in the ED, four factors must be borne in mind: (1) the danger of overlooking severe mental illness; (2) wrongly diagnosing a psychotic disorder where none exists; (3) over-treating certain ethnic groups with antipsychotic medications or under-treating them for depression; (4) failing to correctly identify the risk of suicide and taking preventive action.

Although patients' cultural background and geographic region will influence outcomes, providers must become more cognizant of the disparities found in health care, including mental health care.[16-25] For instance, many authors have noted that African Americans are more likely to be diagnosed with a psychotic disorder rather than a mood disorder.[17] They are also more likely to be given intramuscular injections in the ED, and less likely than whites to receive mental health counseling and psychotherapy, but more likely than whites to receive pharmacotherapy.[26]

As discussed earlier, sometime these disparities have a geographic basis. Medications and a focus on the diet are expected in South Asia, while psychotherapy or counseling is expected in Western countries. Women in less developed countries often have less access to treatment than men. Sartorius in 2002 pointed to barriers to treatment in underdeveloped nations, including the low value given to mental health by individuals in society, a high prevalence of mental and neurological problems, apathy toward psychosocial aspects of health and development, and chronic lack of resources. These attitudes may persist in immigrants who need psychiatric care. Attempts to obtain and provide psychiatric care may therefore be delayed until a crisis occurs. Even then, providers will have to work to overcome some of these persistent attitudes towards mental health care.

Disparities in treatment may be due to a number of factors, but this nonetheless remains an issue to be addressed. Some of these factors include differences in training, resources, and cultural attitudes of providers as well as geographic differences.[27,28] In different parts of the world, the treatment differences have been well documented. South Asian physicians in the UK are less likely to prescribe antidepressants when compared to their Western counter-parts.[29] A survey of benzodiazepine prescribing behavior and attitudes in northern Thailand revealed that a considerable proportion of general practitioners inappropriately prescribed benzodiazepines for physical illness.[30] The authors emphasized the need for improving knowledge and skills, and that somatization may be more prevalent in that local culture.

Complicating the disparity issue is that some populations are at higher risk for soma-tization. Somatic complaints may include chronic headaches, fatigue, insomnia, lethargy, palpitations, vague sensations in the head, hyperphagia, and hypersomnia. Somatization of psychological distress is common among patients in non-Western cultures. In seeking help from primary care a majority of these individuals receive inappropriate symptomatic treatment. Women from other ethnic groups may express helplessness, passive aggressive behavior, and may be reluctant to change the circumstances and environment in which they live despite counseling and interventions, unless treatment is culture-specific.[31,32]

Varieties of risk factors in relation to common mental disorders have been identified. Studies have reported that common mental disorders, such as depression and anxiety, have been strongly associated with female gender.[33] Risk factor profile, geographic differences, and cultural backgrounds of both patients and providers all conspire to add to the disparities in treatment, which if recognized, could help to improve outcomes.[34,35]

Three considerations are worthy of discussion to improve treatment for mental illness in culturally different individuals. Western pharmaceutical use may be integrated into existing cultural norms, theory, and practice congruent with the patient's belief systems, such as Ayurvedic theory (Ayurvedic medicine is a complementary and alternative medical theory that has its roots in ancient India). Second, because practitioners differ in their views of how to describe disorders to their patients, and how to treat them based on time constraints, cultural beliefs, observances, and acceptability to patients, merely recognizing and identifying treatment differences may prompt providers to consider alternative ways of both acquiring patient data and creating effective formulations. Poverty and stress create their own difficulties for acutely ill persons.[36–38] Finally, knowledge of psychiatric research in other countries or of resources to access such expertise aids in understanding cultural norms and the social context in which disease is expressed.

Suicide prevention

Essential to the evaluation in the ED is a suicide risk assessment (also see Chapter 3). Much has been written about risk factors in various geographic regions by Mann, Hawton, and others.[39,40] As noted elsewhere, the psychosocial factors that modulate risk vary among cultures. The use of alcohol and drugs, poverty, financial crises, the ending of a romantic relationship, loss of a job, spousal abuse, conflicts with in-laws, and failure in examinations must be included in the assessment of risk. Prior attempts, chronic medical illness, terminal cancer, access to guns, and knowledge of lethality of an overdose considerably increase risk. Suicidal intent is dynamic rather than static. It must be repeatedly ascertained and determined, rather than merely asked of a patient. Lethality of an attempt and knowledge of lethality must be determined. It is not sufficient to conduct a brief evaluation on a repeat visit because the patient was not suicidal some days earlier during an ED visit. Each visit must be considered a separate encounter. If the patient is discharged, take-home medications must be prescribed in non-lethal amounts until the patient is able to be seen again as an outpatient. It is prudent to err on the side of safety and admit the patient when the examining physician has insufficient data to make a prudent decision to discharge. As always, information from a family member or close friend may be helpful and must always be explored. Attempts must be made to reach others before a disposition is made.[41,42]

Planning a disposition and support services

Once the acute visit (such as an ED encounter) is over, the task of referrals and optimal care must be addressed. In performing a needs assessment, and in order to organize a service for mental health care, one needs to take into account a number of personal, cultural, geographic, and social factors that affect care delivery. Ideally, needs must be assessed through appropriately applied scientific and epidemiologic methods in any given population. In practice, such a task may not be feasible. Transportation, access to health care, dependence or restrictions due to family or cultural attitudes, the ability to negotiate the health care system, or weather conditions such as extreme temperatures may make the task of follow-up a formidable one for persons unfamiliar with the system. Inadequate resources, inadequate manpower, changing service ideology, interruption of government agencies, insurance issues, and external reporting requirements all may influence care delivery.

Among services that are rendered, one needs to identify through cultural means which segment of the population is likely to utilize services, to assimilate education, and to pass information along to others that are in need. For example, women who are case workers living in the service area may be perceived as members of the community. They would be able to freely communicate using the local language, and thus would be far more successful at disseminating information than someone who would be viewed as a stranger. Education of potential patients through local religious or other cultural organizations is another solution. Assuring continuity of care is yet another task. Such continuity requires transportation, manpower, and appropriate cultural perceptions so that outreach is not seen as an intrusion. De-stigmatizing psychiatric care and improving acceptance of appropriate screening, planning for dissemination of information through local groups such as women's groups, and dovetailing of psychiatric care into primary care are all methods of assuring continuity. Integration of such services to local celebration of holidays and generating interest and disseminating information through collaboration with local leaders serves to make a community impact.[43]

A return visit to the ED or other acute care mechanism should be encouraged for crises. Keeping options open for the patient ensures greater continuity of services. Help from local organizations that are non-medical but nevertheless provide support, education, and child care should be explored. Each local setting will likely have its own unique resources; for instance in Baltimore, the Baltimore Crisis Response Incorporated is one such agency that not only operates its own inpatient psychiatric crisis beds but also has a mobile crisis team.

Conclusions

The safe acute management of psychiatric patients consists of a thorough assessment including information from outside informants, attention to the patient's cultural norms and practices, and use of bilingual therapists or translators to fully understand the patient's distress. Critical factors, including systems of care that impact suicide risk, must be elucidated.[44] Pharmacological differences in response to medications are inherent in the physiological variations between ethnic groups and should remain a consideration. Psychosocial factors needing immediate attention vary by culture, and should be explored with the patient, and/or with the family, friends, or other members of the patient's support network. The attitude and behavior of care providers in the ED, and especially their appreciation of cultural differences, impact greatly on the outcome for safe treatment and disposition of psychiatric patients.

References

1. *SACE Final Report: Washington DeSi: South Asians in the Nation's Capital.* Washington, DC: The South Asian Community Empowerment Project, 2009.

2. Vincent G, Velkoff V. *The older population in the United States: 2010 to 2050, US Bureau of the Census, Current Population Reports, US Department of Commerce Economics and Statistics Administration.* Washington, DC: US Census Bureau, 2010.

3. Srinivasan K, Isaacs A, Thomas T, Jayaram G. Outcomes of common mental disorders in southern rural India. *Indian J Soc Psychiatry.* 2006;22:110–115.

4. Kessler RC, Aguilar-Gaxiola S, Alonzo J, et al. The global burden of mental disorders: an update from the WHO World Mental Health Surveys. *Epidemiol Psychiatry Soc.* 2009;18:23–33.

5. Green JG, Avenevoli S, Finkelman M, et al. Validation of the diagnoses of panic disorder and phobic disorders in the US National Comorbidity Survey Replication Adolescent (NCS-A) supplement. *Int J Methods Psychiatr Res.* 2011;20:105–115.

6. Bhui K, Bhugra D, Goldberg D. Causal explanations of distress and general practitioners' assessments of common mental disorder among Punjabi and English attendees. *Soc Psychiatry Psychiatr Epidemiol.* 2002;37:38–45.

7. Park L, Hinton D. Dizziness and panic in China: associated sensations of zang fu organ disequilibrium. *Cult Med Psychiatry.* 2002;26:225–257.

8. Bhui K. Culture and complex interventions: lessons for evidence, policy and practice. *Br J Psychiatry.* 2010;197:172–173.

9. Mischoulon D. Management of major depression in Hispanic patients. *Dir Psychiatry.* 2000;20:275–285.

10. Patel S, Gaw AC. Suicide among immigrants from the Indian Continent: a review. *Psychiatr Ser.* 1996;47:517–521.

11. Bhatia SC, Khan MH, Mediratta RP, Sharma A. High risk suicide factors across cultures. *Am J Social Psychiatry.* 1987;33:226–236.

12. Wasan AJ, Neufeld K, Jayaram G. Practice patterns and treatment choices among psychiatrists in New Delhi, India: a qualitative and quantitative study. *Soc Psychiatry Psychiatr Epidemiol.* 2009;44:109–119.

13. Ruiz P (Ed.), *Ethnicity and Psychopharmacology.* 1st ed. Washington, DC: American Psychiatric Publishing Incorporated, 2000.

14. Pi E, Simpson GM. Psychopharmacology: cross-cultural psychopharmacology: a current clinical perspective. *Psychiatr Serv.* 2005;56:31–33.

15. Lin KM, Poland RE, Nuccio I, et al. A longitudinal assessment of Haloperidol doses and serum concentrations in Asian and Caucasian schizophrenic patients. *Am J Psychiatry.* 1989;146:1307–1311.

16. Pavin M, Nurgozhin T, Hafner G, Yusufy F, Laing R. Prescribing practices of rural primary health care physicians in Uzbekistan. *Trop Med Int Health.* 2003;8:182–190.

17. Neighbors HW, Trierweiler SJ, Ford BC, Muroff JR. Racial differences in DSM diagnosis using a semi-structured instrument: the importance of clinical judgment in the diagnosis of African Americans. *J Health Soc Behav.* 2003;44:237–256.

18. Baker FM, Bell CC. Issues in the psychiatric treatment of African Americans. *Psychiatr Serv.* 1999;50:362–368.

19. Richardson J, Anderson T, Flaherty J, Bell C. The quality of mental health care for African Americans. *Culture, Medicine and Psychiatry.* 2003;27:487–498.

20. Bell CC, Mehta H. The misdiagnosis of black patients with manic depressive illness. *J Natl Med Assoc.* 1981;73:101–107.

21. Bhui K. The new science of cultural epidemiology to tackle ethnic health inequalities. *J Public Health (Oxf).* 2009;31:322–323.

22. Blazer DG, Hybels CF, Simonsick EM, Hanlon JT. Marked differences in antidepressant use by race in an elderly community sample 1986–1996. *Am J Psychiatry.* 2000;157:1089–1094.

23. Shankar PR, Partha P, Shenoy N. Self-medication and non-doctor prescription practices in Pokhara valley, Western Nepal: a questionnaire-based study. *BMC Family Practice.* 2002;3:1–7.

24. Lin KM, Anderson D, Poland RE. Ethnicity and psychopharmacology – bridging the gap. *Psychiatr Clin North Am.* 1995;18: 635–647.

25. Tran PV, Lawson WB, Andersen S, Shavers E. Treatment of the African American patient with novel antipsychotic agents. In Herra JM, Lawson WB, Sramek JJ (Eds.), *Cross Cultural Psychiatry.* Chichester, UK: Wiley, 1999.

26. Richardson J, Anderson T, Flaherty J, Bell C. The quality of mental health care for African Americans. *Cult Med Psychiatry.* 2003;27:487–498.

27. Moffat J, Sass B, McKenzie K, Bhui K. Improving pathways into mental health care for black and ethnic minority groups: a systematic review of the grey literature. *Int Rev Psychiatry.* 2009;21:439–449.

28. Isaac M, Chand P, Murthy P. Research, empiricism and clinical practice in low-income countries. *Int Rev Psychiatry.* 2007;19:559–571.

29. Hull SA, Aquino P, Cotter S. Explaining variation in antidepressant prescribing rates in East London: a cross sectional study. *Family Practice.* 2005;22: 37–42.

30. Srisurapanont M, Garner P, Critchley J, Wongpakaran N. Benzodiazepine prescribing behavior and attitudes: a survey among general practitioners practicing in northern Thailand. *BMC Family Practice.* 2005;6:27.

31. Linden M, Lecruiber Y, Bellantuono C, et al. The prescribing of psychotropic drugs by primary care physicians: an international collaborative study. *J Clin Psychopharmacol.* 1999;19:132–140.

32. Srinivasan K, Srinivasa Murthy R. Multiple somatic complaints in primary health care settings in tropical countries. *Tropical Doctor.* 1986;16:18–21.

33. World Health Organization. http://www.who.int/mental_health/prevention/ genderwomen/en/242.pdf. Accessed January, 2012.

34. Kishore J, Reddaiah V, Kapoor V, Gill J. Characteristics of mental morbidity in a rural primary health center of Haryana. *Indian J Psychiatry.* 1996;38: 134–137.

35. Patel V, Todd CH, Winston M, et al. The outcome of common mental disorders in Harare, Zimbabwe. *Br J Psychiatry.* 1998;172: 53–57.

36. Weich S, Lewis G. Poverty, unemployment and the common mental disorders: a population based cohort study. *BMJ.* 1998;317:115–119.

37. Mumford DB, Saeed K, Ahmad I, Mubbashar MRH. Stress and psychiatric disorder in rural Punjab. A community survey. *Br J Psychiatry.* 1997;170:473–478.

38. Mumford DB, Minhas FA, Akhtar I, Akhter S, Mubbashar MH. Stress and psychiatric disorder in urban Rawalpindi. A community survey. *Br J Psychiatry.* 2000;177:557–562.

39. Mann JJ, Apter A, Bertolote J, et al. Suicide prevention strategies: A systematic review. *JAMA.* 2005;294:2064–2074.

40. Hawton K, Harriss L. Deliberate self-harm in young people: characteristics and subsequent mortality in a 20-year cohort of patients presenting to hospital. *J Clin Psychiatry.* 2007;68:1574–1583.

41. Jayaram G, Herzog A. *Handbook on Patient Safety; SAFE MD: Practical Applications and Approaches to Safe Psychiatric Practice.* Arlington, VA: American Psychiatric Publishing, 2009.

42. Jayaram G, Sporney H, Perticone P. The utility of 15 minute checks in inpatient settings and its effectiveness. *Psychiatry.* 2010;7:46–49.

43. Jayaram G, Goud R, Srinivasan K. Overcoming cultural barriers to deliver comprehensive rural community mental health care in Southern India. *Asian Journal of Psychiatry.* (In Press) 2011.

44. Munro E. Improving safety in medicine: a systems approach. *Br J Psychiatry.* 2004;185:3–4.

Chapter 19

Understanding the psychology of difficult patients

Roshni I. Thakore

Difficult patients are encountered in acute care practices, but the impact that these patients have is different for different providers. Patients with overt psychiatric illness do not have exclusive domain over difficult behaviors. In fact many patients with difficult behavior profiles are encountered broadly in the acute care setting. For the purposes of this discussion, the "difficult patient" is defined as any patient who evokes strong emotions in the physician and other providers or with whom the physician-provider interaction is a challenge due to obstacles to a therapeutic relationship and care seemingly put in place by the patient. As Groves stated in 1978, "Emotional reactions to patients cannot simply be wished away, nor is it good medicine to pretend that they do not exist."[1] Understanding how these interactions become challenging may lead to improved patient-physician relationships and should promote favorable clinical outcomes.

Improving interactions with difficult patients is important both for providing better patient care but also for improving the job satisfaction of providers.[2] Dealing with difficult patients can be psychologically draining and greatly adds to the emotional exhaustion that contributes to provider frustration.[3] Furthermore, a study by Hinchey et al. suggested that in the difficult patient population, short-term outcomes are poor, and difficult patients report worse symptoms at two-week follow-up visits.[4] By improving the physician-patient relationship in these interactions, patients are more likely to trust the physician, which is likely to reduce physician frustration and may result in better patient compliance, with fewer self-sabotaging patient behaviors.

Characteristics and epidemiology of the difficult patient

There is scant literature regarding the epidemiology of the difficult patient in acute care settings. What literature exists is predominantly from the primary care literature. Given the partnership between emergency physicians, psychiatrists, and primary care physicians in the care of patients, the implications of these studies may also pertain to the acute care setting.

In the primary care setting, the difficult patient has been shown to be less likely to trust and less likely to be satisfied by the primary physician.[4] Such patients are also more likely to present with five or more symptom complaints simultaneously, more likely to admit to recent stress, and more likely to have a history of anxiety or depression than the comparison group of standard patients.[4]

Mas Garriga et al. studied a subset of difficult patients as identified by primary care providers. In this subgroup, they found that the 83 patients identified as "difficult"

Emergency Psychiatry, ed. Arjun Chanmugam, Patrick Triplett, and Gabor Kelen. Published by Cambridge University Press. © Cambridge University Press 2013.

represented a prevalence of 7% of the overall patient population.[5] The mean in this study was 57.8 years old with a standard deviation of 15.2 years. Of note, two thirds of the patients identified as difficult in this study were women. Strous et al. postulate that the gender difference may be secondary to two factors.[2] First, women may have atypical presentations of disease, leading in many cases to delays in diagnosis and more inaccurate diagnoses. These outcomes can lead to patient frustration and may ultimately contribute to the transformation into a difficult patient. The second speculation is that women may be more sensitive to poor communication secondary to inherent gender-based differences in communication styles.

Difficult patients have been found to be more likely to carry a diagnosis of psychiatric illness. One study found that over a third have concomitant psychiatric illness.[4] For these patients, the focus should be on treating the underlying acute psychiatric illness. The difficult behaviors will often diminish once the illness is appropriately treated. For patients whose disorders or behaviors are chronic, including personality disorders, different skill sets and approaches must be employed (see Chapter 9).

Factors associated with the difficult patient

Three main factors contribute to the making of a difficult patient: system issues, physician characteristics and response, and patient factors.[6] System factors include wait times, limited bed availability, delays due to consultants, laboratory, and radiology result times, delayed access to outside medical records, etc. For the most part, at the time of encounter, these factors are generally beyond the control of most acute care providers. Physician factors include fatigue, clinical inexperience, facility in dealing with diagnostic uncertainty, barriers to treatment, and in some situations, lack of cultural understanding. The final piece, patient factors, is the focus of the remaining discussion.

Patient factors include psychiatric illness, personality disorders, patient expectations, and certain patient behaviors. The particular patient behaviors as originally described by Groves are categorized under the following rubric: "dependent clingers," "entitled demanders," "manipulative, help-rejecting complainers," and "self-destructive deniers."[1] (Labeling patients is not endorsed by the editors of this text. The discussion presented below is a summary of an article which has some merits in trying to help provide strategies for improving understanding of potentially difficult behaviors.)

Groves' "dependent clingers," comprising about 40% of difficult patients, utilize flattery in an attempt to ingratiate themselves to physicians. They then progress to stressing the system with unreasonable and sometimes persistent demands. The dependent clinger's interactions usually pose unrealistic demands on physician and nursing time.

Groves' "entitled demanders" are challenging because they present with preconceived notions and unrealistic expectations. These patients often believe their issues must take precedence over all other priorities, which results in requests that may not be appropriate for the emergency care of a given patient.

Groves' "manipulative, help-rejecting complainers" seek to gain the trust of the physician, then proceed to reject most, if not all, of the offered interventions and assistance. This results in a particularly demoralizing effect on the treatment team.

Finally, Groves' "self-destructive denier" is, for some, the most frustrating type of patient. While there is a clear prescription for providers to improve health, such patients persist in behaviors that are harmful to their health. Examples of this include: the patient with COPD on oxygen therapy who continues to smoke, the cirrhotic patient who continues to consume alcohol, and the patient with epilepsy who is non-compliant with medications. Reasons for these maladaptive behaviors are many and the clinician should avoid emotional and judgmental response as they seek to help create the most effective management plan.

Strategy for care of the difficult patient

(1) Define the patient's agenda: What does the patient want from this health care interaction?
(2) Negotiate limits: Setting limits and boundaries to limit maladaptive behaviors and facilitate care.
(3) Find areas of commonality: Defining the common goal of both the physician and the patient can often help to develop a mutually acceptable management plan. Determining a common goal is important in facilitating an appropriate outcome.
(4) Limit bias: Biases present in many forms. Although there are many common biases in acute care settings, perhaps one that is most frequently encountered is the triage bias. A patient triaged to a lower acuity level is often allotted less time and fewer resources than a higher acuity patient. The continued assumption of a lower acuity level previously applied by other providers and nurses involved in the care of the patient is a not uncommon behavioral response, but it does set an expectation. It "frames" the patient into a certain minimal-need category. When the patient's condition requires more resources than expected, that realization can result in a natural tension.

Personal emotions and reactions should be sublimated throughout the patient visit and interactions. The difficult patient can bring out strong sentiments in a provider. Some of this is intentional on the part of the patient. Strous et al. comment on the idea of projective identification as a defense mechanism that patients use to deal with illness.[2] It is a form of regression in which the patient projects their negative feelings onto the physician in an attempt to manipulate an outcome. For example, a chronic pain patient frustrated with the management of his pain may act out towards the physician, thus inciting feelings of frustration in the physician. As noted earlier, a professional approach requires a non-judgmental response.

Groves also advocates tailoring our interactions to suit each type of difficult patient behavior.[1] Since the "dependent clinger" requests a greater portion of the resources and time from providers than available, setting boundaries is crucial in caring for this group. Similarly, coordinating care with a single primary care physician will help facilitate better management of system resources and enforce boundaries.[1]

The "entitled demanders" bring with them many expectations to the initial interaction, which are often difficult to reconcile with what is necessary and possible to facilitate their care. Reinforcing the partnership between the physician and patient is essential to ameliorate the adversarial tension that is inherently present with these patient interactions.[1]

"Manipulative, help-rejecting complainers" require a combination of limit setting and partnership as these interactions can be both resource-consuming and antagonistic.[1]

The "self-destructive deniers" are the most challenging as they are inherently resistant to accepting care. The ideal strategy for this group is continued reinforcement of the offer to participate and facilitate their care.[1]

Summary

Caring for the difficult patient can be challenging. However, better understanding this subset of the patient population will improve staff satisfaction and may also improve patient outcomes. In particular, it is important to understand that in the medical setting, the basis for the observed behaviors are multifactorial, psychological, or psychiatric-based, and not always just "character flaws." Difficult behaviors in patients should be seen as part of their symptom complex. Fortunately, there are strategies that help mitigate the overt behaviors causing disruption. Defining the patient's agenda, negotiating limits, finding common ground, limiting bias, and controlling emotions will all help to improve the physician-patient interaction in dealing with the difficult patient.

References

1. Groves JE. Taking care of the hateful patient. *N Engl J Med*. 1978;**298**: 883–887.

2. Strous RD, Ulman AM, Kotler M. The hateful patient revisited: relevance for 21st century medicine. *Eur J Intern Med*. 2006;**17**:387–393.

3. Kuhn G, Goldberg R, Compton S. Tolerance for uncertainty, burnout, and satisfaction with the career of emergency medicine. *Ann Emerg Med*. 2009;**54**: 106–113.

4. Hinchey SA, Jackson JL. A cohort study assessing difficult patient encounters in a walk-in primary care clinic, predictors and outcomes. *J Gen Intern Med*. 2011;**26**(6): 588–594.

5. Mas Garriga X, Cruz Doménech JM, Fañanás Lanau N, Allué Buil A, Zamora Casas I, Viñas Vidal R. Difficult patients in primary care: qualitative and quantitative study. *Aten Primaria*. 2003;**31**(4): 214–219.

6. Haas LJ, Leiser JP, Magill MK, Sanyer ON. Management of the difficult patient. *Am Fam Physician*. 2005;**72**:2063–2068.

Appendix: Dose recommendations for psychiatric medications commonly seen in the ED setting

These medications are not recommended for routine initiation of long-term therapy in acute care settings

Antidepressants			
Selective serotonin reuptake inhibitors			
Drug	**Initial oral dosing**		**Side effects**
	Panic disorder	**Depression**	
Fluoxetine	10 mg daily	20 mg daily	Nausea, insomnia, somnolence, tremor, prolonged QT interval
Sertraline	25 mg daily	50 mg daily	GI upset, headache, reduced libido, sexual dysfunction
Citalopram	20–30 mg daily	20 mg daily	Diaphoresis, GI upset, fatigue, dizziness
Escitalopram	10 mg daily (anxiety)	10 mg daily	GI upset, headache, sexual dysfunction, dizziness, somnolence, insomnia
Paroxetine	10 mg daily	20 mg daily	GI upset, headache, blurred vision, sexual dysfunction
Serotonin/norepinephrine reuptake inhibitors			
Venlafaxine	37.5 mg daily	75 mg daily	Hypertension, weight loss, headache
Desvenlafaxine		50 mg daily	Hypertension, hyperlipidemia, diaphoresis
Duloxetine	30 mg daily (anxiety)	20 mg BID	GI upset, hepatotoxicity
Cyclic antidepressants			
Drug	**Initial oral dosing (depression)**		**Side effects**
Amitriptyline	75 mg/day (in 1–3 divided doses)		Weight gain, constipation, dysrhythmia, agranulocytosis

Emergency Psychiatry, ed. Arjun Chanmugam, Patrick Triplett, and Gabor Kelen. Published by Cambridge University Press. © Cambridge University Press 2013.

(cont.)

Antidepressants

Doxepin	25–75 mg/day (in 1–3 divided doses)	Hypotension, somnolence, nephrotoxicity, blood dyscrasias
Nortriptyline	75–100 mg/day (in 1–4 divided doses)	SIADH, dysrhythmia, bone marrow suppression, seizure, hepatic failure

Atypical antidepressants

Drug	Initial oral dosing (depression)	Side effects
Trazodone	150 mg/day (in divided doses)	Hypotension, abnormal dreams, somnolence, blurred vision
Buproprion HCl (IR)	100 mg BID	Hypertension, dysrhythmia, insomnia
Mirtazapine	15 mg daily	Increased appetite, weight gain, somnolence
Buspirone	5 mg TID (depression/anxiety)	Confusion, nausea, dizziness, headache, nervousness

Typical antipsychotics

Drug	Acute psychosis Dosing	Maintenance dosing	Side effects/monitoring
Fluphenazine HCl	2.5–10 mg PO/IM daily divided 6–8 hours	1–5 mg PO daily	• DO NOT use decanoate formulation – not indicated for acute management
Haloperidol lactate	**Initial**: 0.5–5 mg PO/2–5 mg IM **Repeat**: 0.5–5 mg PO/2–5 mg IM Q1 HR PRN continued symptoms **Max:** PO 100 mg/day **Max**: IM dependent on response/tolerability	0.5–5 mg PO TID	• Can cause QT prolongation/ Torsades de pointes • Can cause hypotension • DO NOT use decanoate formulation – not indicated for acute management

Atypical antipsychotics

Drug	Acute psychosis dosing	Maintenance dosing	Side effects/monitoring
Aripiprazole	**Initial**: 5.25–15 mg IM **Repeat**: 5.25–15 mg IM Q2 HR PRN for continued symptoms **Max:** 30 mg PO/IM/day	10–30 mg PO daily	• Can cause weight gain, hypotension, and somnolence • Can have extrapyramidal side effects
Olanzapine	**Initial**: 2.5–10 mg IM **Repeat**: 2.5–10 mg Q2–4 HR PRN for continued symptoms **Max:** 30 mg IM/day	10–15 mg PO daily **Max**: 20 mg PO/day	• Can cause hyperlipidemia and weight gain • Can cause hypotension

(cont.)

Antidepressants			
Quetiapine	**Initial:** 25 mg PO BID Titrate to 400 mg/day as tolerated **Max:** 800 mg PO/day	300–800 mg PO BID (IR)	• Can cause orthostatic hypotension and hyperlipidemia • Can precipitate pancreatitis and diabetic ketoacidosis • Can cause extrapyramidal symptoms and neuroleptic malignant syndrome
Risperidone	2 mg PO/day (1–2 divided doses)	2–8 mg PO/day (1–2 divided doses)	• Long acting IM formulation available but provides no acute control • Doses >8 mg/day have not been shown to be more efficacious • Can cause tachycardia, peripheral edema, and GI upset • Can cause extrapyramidal symptoms and neuroleptic malignant syndrome
Ziprasidone mesylate	10 mg IM q2hours 20 mg IM q4hours **Max:** 40 mg IM/day	40–80 mg PO BID Max: 80 mg PO BID	• Convert from IM to oral therapy as soon as possible • Can cause headache, hypotension, and hyperglycemia • Can cause QT prolongation and Torsades de pointes
Mood stabilizers			
Lithium carbonate	300–600 mg PO TID	900–1200 mg PO daily	• Desired serum concentration = 1–1.5 mEq/L for acute mania vs 0.6–1.2 mEq/L for maintenance • Reduced dosing required with renal impairment • Signs of toxicity include ECG changes, seizures, electrolyte disturbances (Na+), muscle cramping, diarrhea, tinnitus, and ataxia • Dose can be adjusted to maintain therapeutic serum concentrations
Lamotrigine	**Initial:** 25 mg/day Titrate doses by 25 mg every 1–2 weeks as tolerated	200 mg PO daily as monotherapy **OR** 400 mg PO daily when combined	• ***NOTE:*** dose titration differs when patient is being treated with concomitant CYP enzyme-inducers such as valproic acid (Divalproex) • Increased seizure risk with abrupt discontinuation

(cont.)

Antidepressants

		with CYP enzyme inducers	• Can cause serious skin reactions such as TEN and Stevens-Johnsons syndrome
Divalproex	**Initial:** 750 mg/day in divided doses **Max:** 60 mg/kg/day	Doses vary based on patient weight **Target trough level** 50–125 mcg/mL	Black Box Warning for hepatotoxicity; monitor LFTs • Risk of drug toxicity with trough levels > 125 mcg/mL • Headache and gastrointestinal symptoms are common with initial therapy • Thrombocytopenia is associated with higher doses • Known teratogen; pregnancy category D

Micromedex® Healthcare Series [Internet database]. Greenwood Village, Colo: Thomson Reuters (Healthcare) Inc. 2011. http://www.micromedex.com Updated periodically
Clinical Pharmacology [database online]. Tampa, FL: Gold Standard, Inc. 2011. http://www.clinicalpharmacology.com Updated periodically
Matthew Hinton, PharmD
Melinda J Ortmann, PharmD, BCPS

Index

Note: The following abbreviations have been used: AN for anorexia nervosa; ASD for acute stress disorder; ED for emergency department; GAD for generalized anxiety disorder; OCD for obsessive-compulsive disorder; PTSD for posttraumatic stress disorder; PWIDD for people with intellectual and developmental disabilities.